JAMES RAMSDEN is a food writer and broadcaster.
He has written about food and cookery for the
Guardian, *The Times*, the *FT*, *delicious*, *Sainsbury's*
Magazine, *London Evening Standard* and many others,
and presents the Lad that Lunches on BBC Radio 1.
His supper club, the Secret Larder, is one of the most
popular in London and was described by one journalist
as "harder to get into than the Ivy". He is also the
author of *Do-Ahead Dinners*.

LOVE YOUR LUNCHBOX

JAMES RAMSDEN

101 recipes to liven up lunchtime

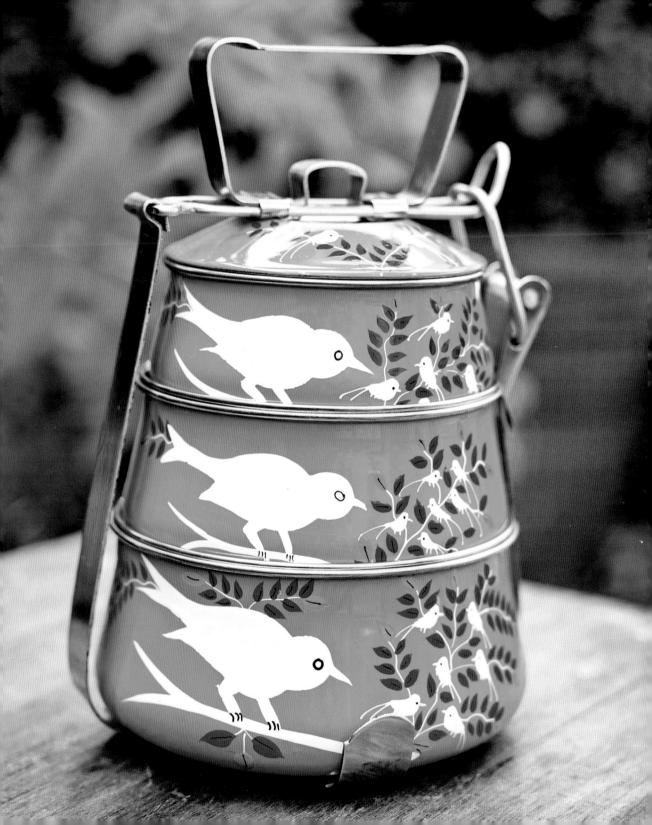

LOVE YOUR LUNCHBOX

JAMES RAMSDEN

PAVILION

101 recipes to liven up lunchtime

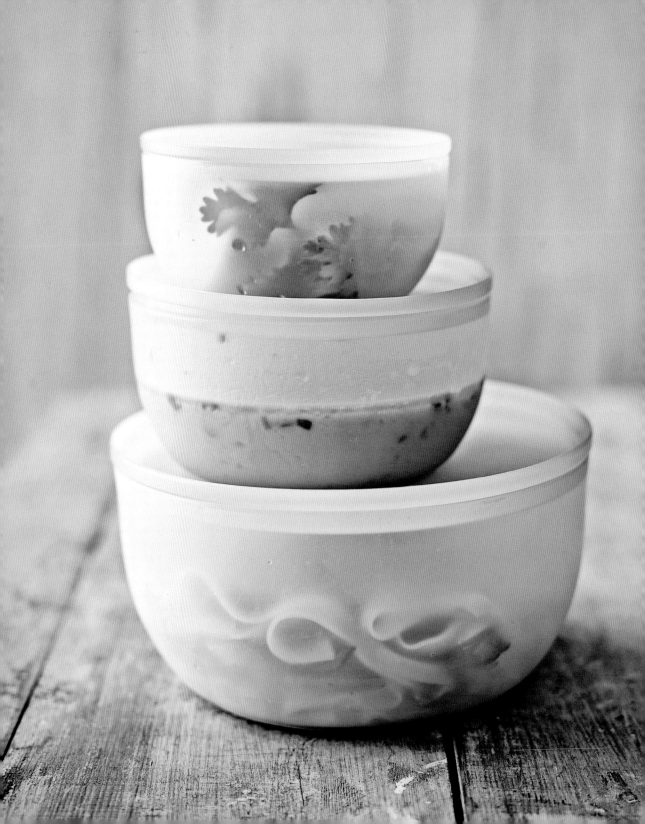

CONTENTS

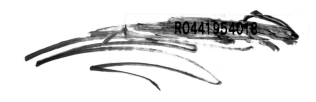

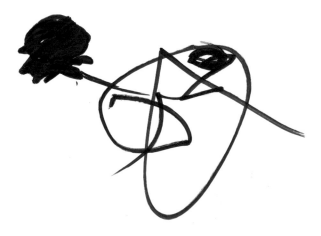

INTRODUCTION

For many children of my generation, the lunchbox was a treasured possession. My Thomas the Tank Engine one was so cool that my five-year-old self practically paraded down the street to school; its contents, whatever they were, however similar to yesterday's pickings, offered fresh promise, new excitements, and something to look forward to at midday. Would it be a cheese and pickle sandwich or a ham and lettuce bap? Would there be a chocolate biscuit or a fruit roll-up? Capri Sun or Um Bongo? Golden Delicious (thumbs up) or Granny Smith (thumbs down)? The intrigue!

With this book I want to re-inject that sense of potential, that sense of anticipation, that frisson of a well-whetted appetite to the often-too-ordinary midweek lunch. But for grown-ups. Why should kids get all the fun while the grown-ups eat the same lunch in front of their computers each day? Why not follow the Japanese and dive head first into a steaming bowl of slippery noodles, or the New Yorkers with their pastrami and rye bread, or our Mediterranean cousins with their fresh salads and nourishing grains? These lunches are resourceful, creative and practical. But in every case, it is flavour that comes first, with convenience a happy corollary and not the other way round.

Of course, moveable lunches needn't be restricted to the office – many of the dishes here will be just as happy on a beach, up a mountain, by a river, or in the park. Wherever you find yourself unwrapping your lunch, I want it to have all the delight of a Christmas stocking, and none of the disappointment. We don't want the same sandwich every day any more than we want the same pair of socks every Christmas.

Love Your Lunchbox is a book for anyone who wants better socks. Or, rather, lunch. For anyone for whom lunch is something to enjoy rather than endure, to linger over rather than bolt down, to make yourself rather than make yourself walk to the shops in the rain for. If that sounds like you, then you're in the right place.

This book is about the spirit of the lunchbox, rather than the vessel itself. A trend for vintage lunchboxes would be a happy thing (there's no shortage online), though a Tupperware and a carrier bag will do the trick. As mother always told me, it's what's on the inside that counts.

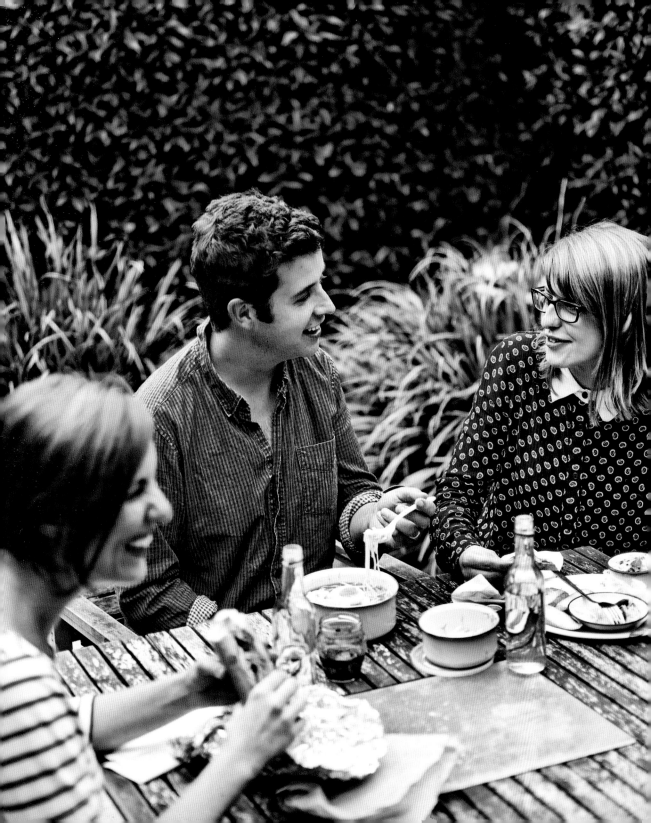

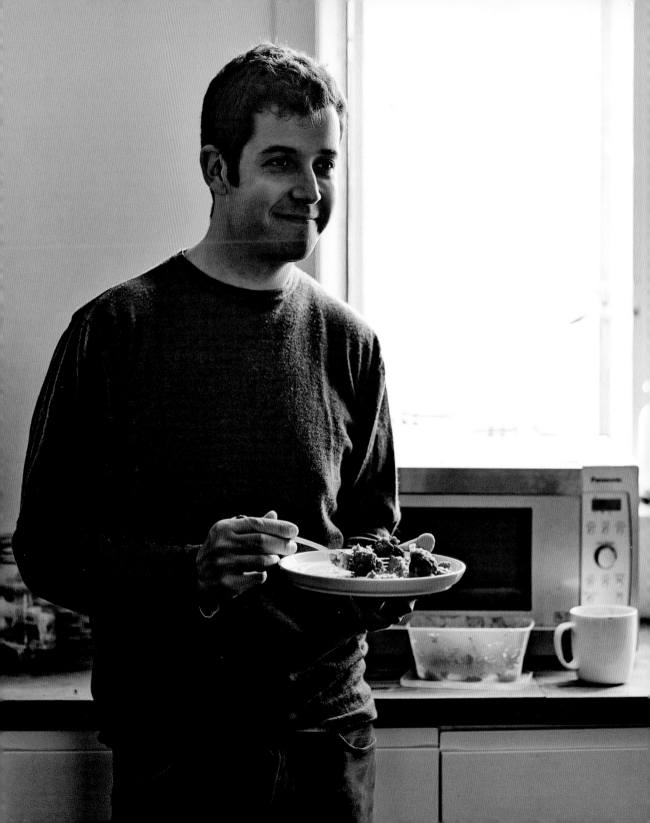

COOKING

These recipes are written to be prepared and cooked in advance and eaten later that day, or the following couple of days. Some of them are doable in a matter of minutes on the morning you plan to eat them, others may require a bit of time the evening before. This isn't necessarily a book for every day. Instead, it's for those evenings when you find you have a slice of time to prepare a lunch or two, or a Sunday afternoon to put a few bits in the freezer.

REHEATING AND EATING

Although these dishes are intended to be made in advance, clearly there is nothing stopping you devouring the thing on the spot. It would, however, get a little repetitive of me to say 'eat now or chill for later' on each recipe, so you can assume this is the case with all the recipes unless otherwise stated.

You will generally need a toaster, a microwave, or a kettle to finish those recipes that can't be eaten cold.

ON MICROWAVING

Ignore the baseless claims about microwaves 'nuking' nutrients and embrace their incredibly efficient means of heating up, and indeed cooking, food. Generally dishes should be covered with clingfilm to reheat, if only to minimize spattering, with a few holes poked in the clingfilm. Avoid putting any metal, including foil, in the microwave.

SERVINGS

Most of the recipes in this book serve two, meaning you can either lovingly prepare lunch for yourself and your other half, or lovingly prepare lunch for yourself for the next two days, or lovingly prepare yourself a single lunch of quite unnecessarily large proportions.

COST

Each recipe aims for a cost of less than £5 a head (often considerably less). At the time of writing, the average cost of lunch for an office worker is reported to be £7.81, so less than a fiver seems about right for a homemade lunch that leaves you with a few quid for a Coca Cola/Snickers fix.

A caveat: I don't know what's in your fridge or cupboard. There will be recipes in this book that cost you a little more to shop for, but that's because you may need to buy, say, rice vinegar, or a spice of which you'll use only a tablespoon. In all these cases, I've done my best to make sure such items are not perishable, and can be used and reused. Those that aren't can be frozen.

ONE LAST THOUGHT...

There has been some debate recently about the relative merits or otherwise of eating lunch at your desk, with a health minister labelling the practice 'disgusting'. I say it's entirely up to you where you strap on the nosebag, though perhaps be aware that some colleagues might object to a particularly pungent curry distracting them from crucial research on the *Daily Mail* website.

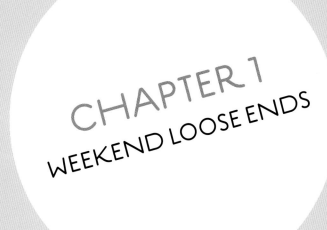

CHAPTER 1
WEEKEND LOOSE ENDS

This chapter presupposes that you will cook certain things over the weekend.
And when I say weekend, I mostly mean Sunday lunch. Your weekend may follow
many paths. There might be a bowl of pasta on Friday night, curry on Saturday,
a breakfast somewhere along the way, perhaps involving muffins and croissants
and bacon. An entire day might be lost to pints and pork scratchings,
or to prams and tantrums and takeaway pizza.

But Sundays, on the whole, are more predictable. Sundays are for a roast.
Pork belly or roast chicken or a rib of beef. There will be roast potatoes, which I've
yet to fashion into anything decent the following day, and so are absent from this
chapter, though roast root vegetables (p.12) are always very fine and very adaptable.

And, after all, Sunday is the plum day for preparing a couple of lunches
for the week ahead.

ROAST VEGETABLES WITH LENTILS, CHILLI AND FETA

The temptation with leftover roast vegetables – by which I mean any or all of: beetroot, celeriac, butternut squash, parsnip, red onion (always), garlic (ditto), swede, turnip, and so on – is to boil them briefly with stock and blend them into a soup. It's a temptation worth submitting to every now and then, creating a rich and deeply flavoured soup. But for something a little lighter and more textural, this salady number is a winner.

If you fancy making it from scratch, veg and all, then cut root veg into 2.5cm/1in cubes, toss with olive oil, salt, pepper and unpeeled garlic cloves, and roast at 200°C/400°F/Gas mark 6 for 45 minutes to 1 hour.

Prep time: 10 minutes
Cooking time: 20 minutes
Freezable? No

85g/3oz/scant ½ cup green lentils
400g/14oz roasted vegetables
a good handful of rocket (arugula)
85g/3oz feta cheese, lightly crumbled
salt and pepper
For the dressing
1 red chilli, deseeded and finely chopped
a good squeeze of lemon
4 tbsp olive oil
a handful of parsley, finely chopped

AT HOME
Rinse the lentils under running water, then cook according to packet instructions. Drain and rinse under cold water to prevent overcooking. Shake until dry.

Toss together the roasted vegetables, lentils, rocket and feta. Season with salt and plenty of pepper, and store in the fridge for up to 2 days.

To make the dressing, mix together the chilli, lemon juice, oil and parsley. Season with salt and pepper. Taste and adjust with more lemon, olive oil or salt as necessary. Store in a small pot in the fridge.

IN EACH LUNCHBOX
Portion of roast vegetable and lentil salad; portion of dressing.

TO FINISH
Dress before serving.

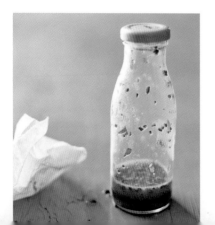

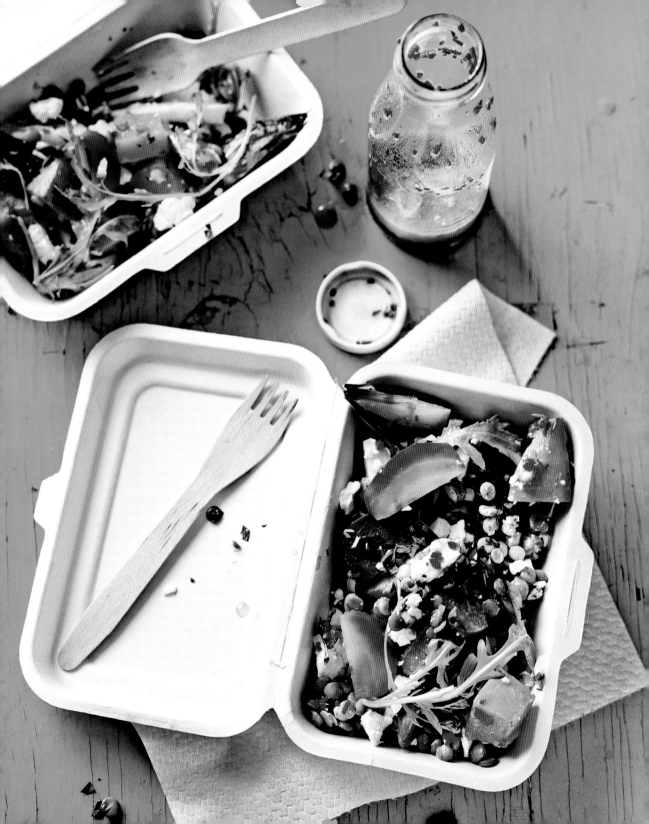

CAESAR SALAD

I was as disappointed, as no doubt you will be, to discover that this salad was not invented by the great warrior, dictator and leader of the Roman Empire Julius Caesar, but an Italian–American chap called Caesar Cardini. This excellent salad pales somewhat when you realize it wasn't concocted between invasions of Britain and bloody encounters with Gauls. But no matter. It's still a superb dish and dead easy to chuck together.

This is something of a base recipe. By all means gussy it up with whatever bits and pieces you fancy – bacon, tomatoes, squirrel...

Prep time: 15 minutes
Cooking time: 5 minutes
Freezable? No

2 tsp olive oil
a sprig of rosemary
a few small chunks of bread
crisp lettuce leaves, such as romaine, cos
    or little gem
150g/5½oz roast chicken, shredded
10 anchovy fillets (optional)
For the dressing
1 egg yolk
1 tsp Dijon mustard
100ml/3½fl oz/scant ½ cup olive oil
1 small garlic clove, peeled and crushed to a paste
15g/½oz grated Parmesan cheese
juice of ½ lemon
a few shakes of Tabasco sauce
salt and pepper

AT HOME

Heat the oil and rosemary in a frying pan over a medium heat, add the bread and fry, tossing occasionally, until golden and crisp. Drain the croutons on kitchen paper, discarding the rosemary.

Wash and dry the salad leaves if necessary, then assemble with the chicken, croutons, and the anchovies, if using. Cover and store in the fridge for up to 24 hours.

To make the dressing, whisk together the egg yolk and mustard, then very slowly add the oil, whisking continuously to emulsify. Add the garlic, Parmesan, lemon juice and Tabasco, and season with salt and pepper. Store in a jar in the fridge.

IN EACH LUNCHBOX

Portion of salad; portion of dressing.

TO FINISH

Dress the salad and eat.

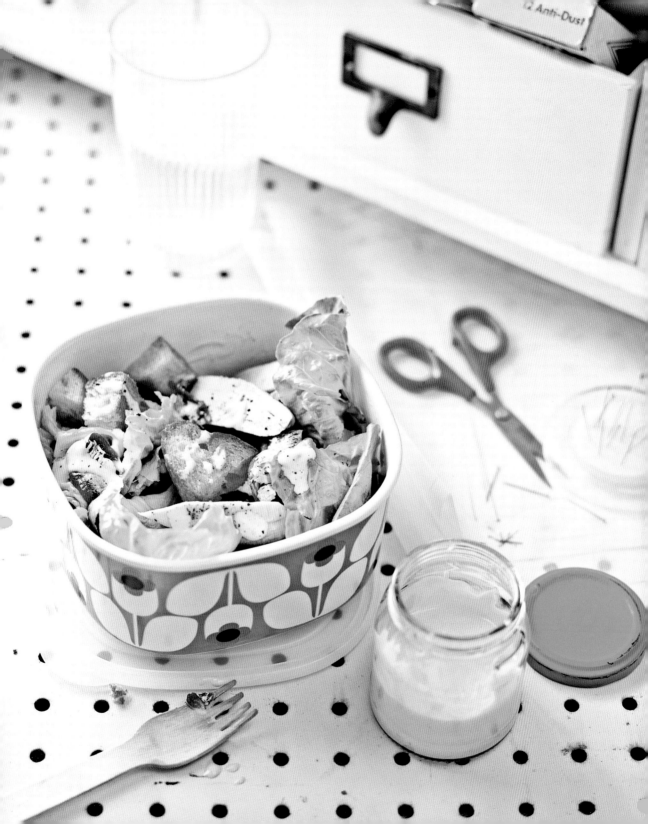

RICE AND PEAS

Also known as *risi e bisi*. For many people, Sunday lunch isn't Sunday lunch without peas. They provide comfort and nourishment and nostalgia – the hangover's enemy, the hangover sufferer's friend. I always make too much. Here's what to do with the leftovers. (And obviously it's not too onerous to cook some peas specially for this.)

Prep time: 25 minutes
Cooking time. 25 minutes
Freezable? Yes

olive oil
1 small onion or shallot, peeled and finely chopped
salt and pepper
750ml/1¼ pints/3 cups chicken or vegetable stock
125g/4½oz/generous ½ cup risotto rice
about 200g/7oz/1½ cups cooked peas
20g/¾oz Parmesan cheese, grated
a few dots of butter, to finish

AT HOME

Heat a splash of oil over a low heat and add the onion. Season with salt and pepper, and cook for 10 minutes, stirring occasionally, until soft. Meanwhile, warm the stock in another pan.

Add the rice to the onion and stir over a medium heat for a minute or two. After this, you can cook the rice in risotto fashion, stirring continuously and adding stock a ladle at a time. But if you prefer, add a third of the stock, stir, and leave to simmer for 6 minutes. Go and do something else. Perhaps stir every now and then. Add another third, simmer for another 6 minutes. Add the remaining stock and the peas. Simmer for 3 minutes, stir in the cheese, and take off the heat. It should be wetter than a risotto.

Leave to cool. Store in the fridge for up to 2 days.

IN EACH LUNCHBOX

Portion of *risi e bisi* (in a microwaveable container); a few dots of butter.

TO FINISH

Put a few dots of butter on the rice. Reheat in a microwave on medium for 4–5 minutes, stirring halfway through.

Beef and potato pasty

Ne'er was there a morsel so fraught with controversy. Devon or Cornwall? Side crimp or top crimp? Swede or no swede? These are all very important questions, but as long as the thing tastes good, I couldn't give a stuff.

Now, I'm all in favour of making your own pastry, but in this case – by which I mean the case of making your lunch – it may be a little too much to ask.

Prep time: 20 minutes
Cooking time: 30–40 minutes, plus chilling
Freezable? Yes

300g/10^1/$_2$oz shortcrust pastry

20g/^{3}/$_4$oz/1^1/$_2$ tbsp butter

1 onion, peeled and chopped

salt and pepper

1 tsp chopped thyme

2 tbsp chopped parsley

125–150g/4^1/$_2$–5^1/$_2$oz leftover beef, chopped

100g/3^1/$_2$oz cooked potato, cubed

100g/3^1/$_2$oz cooked swede (optional: use potato instead if preferred), cubed

1 egg, beaten

AT HOME

Preheat the oven to 180°C/350°F/Gas mark 4. Divide the pastry in two and roll out to about 5mm/^{1}/$_4$in thick, then cut out two rounds, each about 20cm/8in in diameter. Chill.

Melt the butter in a saucepan over a medium-low heat and add the onion. Season with salt and pepper, and cook until soft, stirring occasionally. Add the herbs, beef, potato and swede, if using. Give it a good mix. Taste for seasoning and leave to cool.

Top each pastry with the filling and fold over. Crimp to seal, then brush with the beaten egg. Prick a couple of times to let the air out, then bake for 20–25 minutes, until golden brown. Cool, cover and store in the fridge for up to 2 days.

IN EACH LUNCHBOX

A pasty.

TO FINISH

Reheat (if you wish) in an oven at 180°C/350°F/Gas mark 4 for 10 minutes. A microwave will heat it, but will also make it a little soggy.

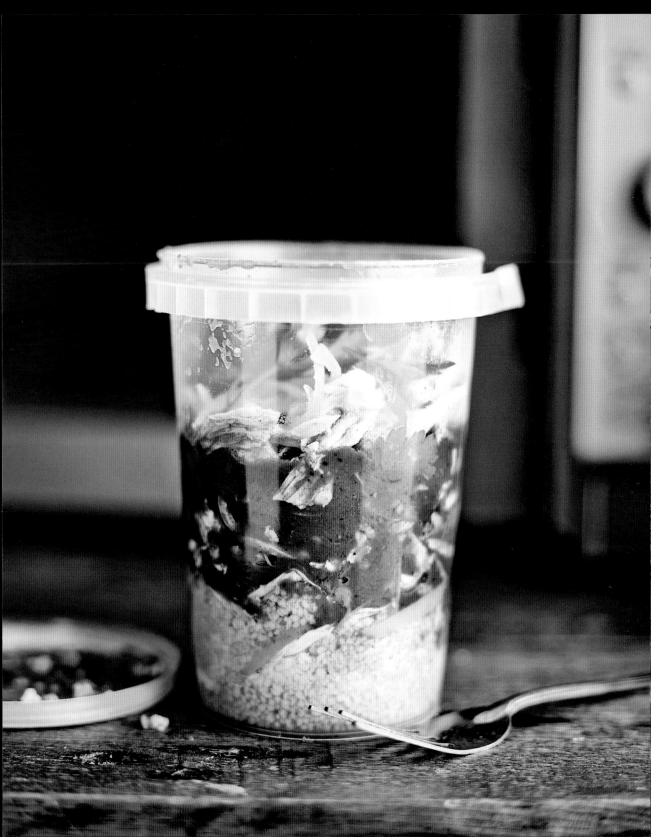

North African–style
chicken broth

SERVES 2

In truth, you could do this with any leftover meat. Lamb or beef will benefit from a longer, gentler cooking time. *Ras-el-hanout* is a North African spice blend that you can find in the spice section of most supermarkets these days.

Prep time: 15 minutes
Cooking time: 20 minutes
Freezable? Yes

olive oil
1 small onion, peeled and finely chopped
1 garlic clove, peeled and finely chopped
salt and pepper
2 tsp *ras-el-hanout*
1/2 tsp chilli flakes
400g/14oz canned chopped tomatoes
400ml/14fl oz/1 2/3 cups chicken stock
a pinch of sugar
50g/1 3/4oz/5 tbsp couscous
70–100g/2 1/2–3 1/2oz cooked chicken, shredded
2 preserved lemons, flesh discarded, peel roughly
        chopped (optional)

AT HOME

Heat a splash of oil in a saucepan over a low heat and add the onion and garlic. Season with salt and pepper, cover and cook for 10 minutes, stirring occasionally, until soft.

Turn up the heat to medium and add the spices. Stir briefly, then add the tomatoes, stock, and a pinch of sugar. Simmer for 7–10 minutes.

Meanwhile, boil a kettle and cook the couscous according to packet instructions.

Stir the cooked couscous and shredded chicken through the soup. If using, add the chopped lemon. Cool, cover, and store in the fridge for up to 2 days.

IN EACH LUNCHBOX

A portion of broth (in a microwaveable container).

TO FINISH

Microwave on medium for 4 minutes, or gently reheat in a saucepan.

CHICKEN AND PEARL BARLEY BROTH

SERVES 2

Leftover chicken can be a misused creature. Chicken risotto, for example, is often a chalky, pale, bland affair, while chicken pasta is just all kinds of wrong (is it the texture?). Some sort of brothy experience is, I reckon, best, and rather gentler on the belly than, say, a chicken sandwich, which always requires at least a litre of mayonnaise to make it not stick to the roof of your mouth like clingfilm. This is a good'un, or try the North African chicken soup on p.19.

Prep time: 15 minutes
Cooking time: 1 hour
Freezable? No

olive oil
1 small onion, peeled and finely chopped
1 celery stalk, finely chopped
1 small carrot, peeled and finely chopped
salt and pepper
50g/1¾oz/¼ cup pearl barley, rinsed
800ml/1½ pints/3⅓ cups chicken stock
a good handful of cooked chicken, shredded
a handful of finely chopped parsley
zest of ½ lemon

AT HOME

Heat a splash of olive oil in a saucepan over a low heat and add the onion, celery and carrot. Season with salt and pepper, cover, and cook for about 10 minutes, until soft.

Add the barley and stir briefly, then add the stock and bring to a boil. Simmer very gently for 45 minutes. If you need to add a splash more stock or water, go ahead.

Stir in the chicken, parsley and lemon zest. Taste for seasoning, then cool. Chill for up to 2 days.

IN EACH LUNCHBOX

A portion of broth (in a microwaveable container).

TO FINISH

Reheat in a microwave on medium for 4–5 minutes, stirring halfway through, or gently reheat in a saucepan.

LAMB PILAF

A pilaf is all about gentle spicing and comforting grains – nothing overpowering or too bullish. There's a certain amount of fear around cooling and reheating rice (have you ever met anyone who got ill from rice? Me neither), but as long as you get it in the fridge relatively sharpish after cooking, it's fine.

   You can save time by using a generic spice mix, garam masala or whatever, but if you have a spare few minutes (and that's really all it takes), then it's worth going for whole spices.

Prep time: 20 minutes
Cooking time: 25 minutes
Freezable? No

vegetable oil
1 small onion, peeled and finely chopped
salt and pepper
1 garlic clove, peeled and finely chopped
1 tsp ground cumin
2 tsp ground coriander
1 star anise
1 clove
1 cinnamon stick
about 150g/5^{1}/$_{2}$oz leftover lamb, quite
       finely chopped
125g/4^{1}/$_{2}$oz/scant ^{3}/$_{4}$ cup basmati rice, rinsed
       in a sieve under cold running water for
       a minute or so
250ml/9fl oz/1 cup chicken stock
To serve
plain yogurt
a small handful of coriander (cilantro)
a handful of flaked almonds (optional)

AT HOME

Heat a splash of oil in a saucepan over a medium heat. Add the onion, season with salt and pepper, and cook for 7 minutes, stirring occasionally, until beginning to brown, then add the garlic and spices. Stir briefly to coat the onion in spices, then add the lamb and cook until it has taken on some colour.

   Add the rice and stock, and bring to a boil. Set the heat to very low, and cover the pan. Cook for 12 minutes without lifting the lid. After 12 minutes, remove from the heat and leave for 5 minutes, keeping the lid on.

   Take off the lid and leave to stand for 2 minutes. Fluff up with a fork, cool, and store in the fridge for up to 2 days.

IN EACH LUNCHBOX

A portion of pilaf (in a microwaveable container); a little yogurt; a few coriander leaves; flaked almonds (optional).

TO FINISH

Microwave on medium for 4 minutes. Serve with yogurt, coriander and almonds.

BURRITO

The most crucial thing to remember with this behemoth is that the meat is slow-cooked. This isn't much cop with a rare slice of sirloin, which will in all likelihood come out in a single piece, leaving you with a hollow, vegetarian burrito and a piece of pink flesh hanging out of your mouth. But slow-cooked beef shin, or brisket, or shortribs, or leftover pork shoulder, all melting and wibbly, will be what is known as 'the business'.

Prep time: 15 minutes

Cooking time: 6 minutes

Freezable? No

For the beans

150g/5½oz canned black-eyed beans

vegetable oil

1 small garlic clove, peeled and crushed

½ tsp smoked paprika

salt and pepper

juice of ½ lime

For the guacamole

1 avocado

2 tbsp finely chopped red onion

2 tsp finely chopped red chilli

juice of ½ lime

a small handful of chopped coriander (cilantro)

For the rest

2 large wheat tortillas

200g/7oz slow-cooked beef or pork

a good handful of shredded lettuce

chilli sauce (I like Cholula brand)

2 tbsp sour cream

AT HOME

Gently boil the beans for 5 minutes, then drain. In the same pan, heat a little oil over a medium heat and add the garlic and paprika. Cook for 30 seconds, stirring continuously, then add the beans. Season with salt, pepper and a squeeze of lime, then mash roughly. Set aside to cool.

To make the guacamole, mash the avocado with the onion, chilli, lime juice and coriander. Season with salt.

Briefly warm each tortilla in a hot frying pan (this makes it easier to wrap), then lay on a sheet of foil. Spread the guacamole over the tortilla, then spread over the mashed beans. Lay the meat down the middle of the tortilla, and top with lettuce, a few sploshes of chilli sauce, and a spoonful of sour cream. Carefully roll up, then wrap tightly in the foil.

IN EACH LUNCHBOX

A burrito.

TO FINISH

You can eat the burrito cold — or at least at room temperature — though it's also good hot. Warm in the oven at 150°C/300°F/Gas mark 2 for 10 minutes. The foil causes problems with microwaves... ka-boom.

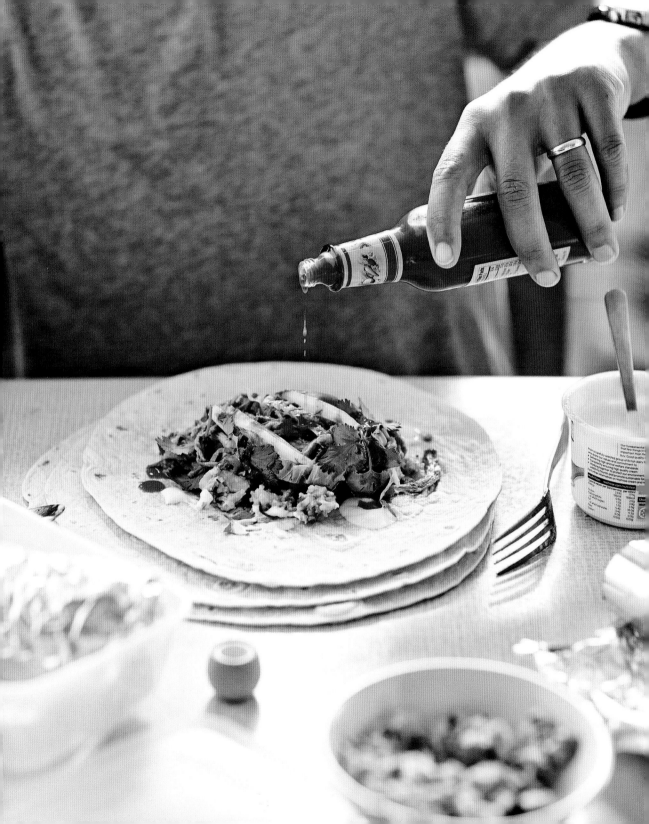

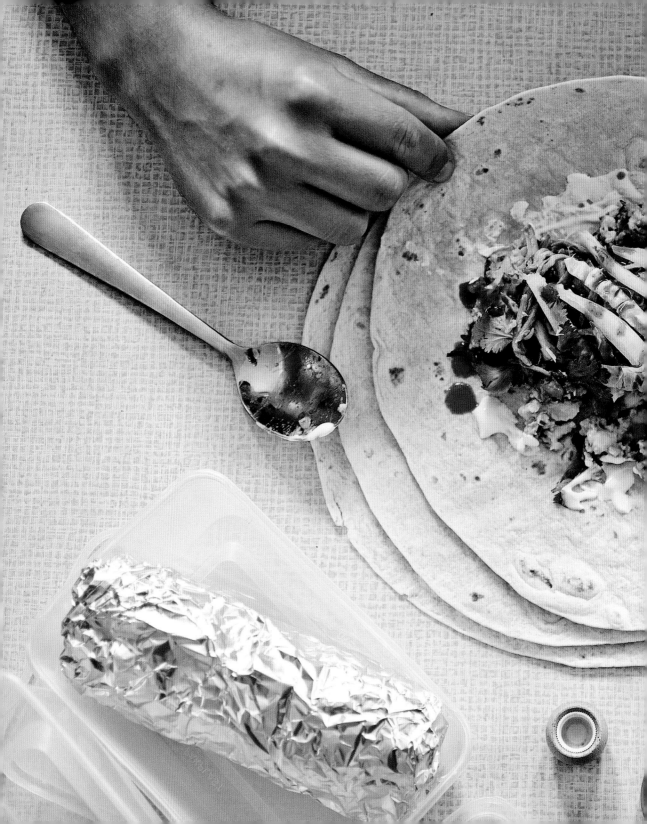

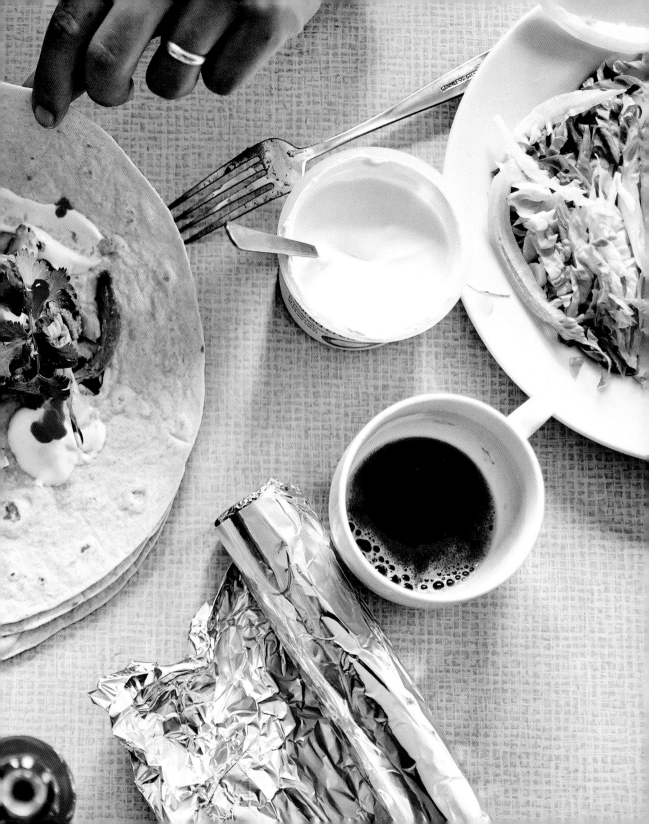

RILLETTES

Amazing how easily a joint of pork turns out to be insurmountable. What seems like an appropriate – even modest – piece of pork belly so often turns out to defeat everyone, its heady combination of rich fat and sweet meat being somewhat more filling than you'd accounted for. But no matter! Here is a quite splendid thing to do with the leftovers.

Prep time: 5 minutes
Cooking time: 45 minutes
Freezable? Yes

250–300g/9–10¹⁄₂oz leftover fatty pork
    (belly or shoulder)
2 tbsp pork fat, dripping or oil
1 tbsp brandy (optional)
a sprig of thyme
a bay leaf
a few peppercorns
a pinch of salt
To serve
toast or crusty baguette
cornichons (baby pickled gherkins)
    or pickled shallots (p.190)

AT HOME

Roughly chop the meat. Heat the fat in a saucepan over a low heat. Add the meat, brandy, herbs and pepper, and season with a pinch of salt. Cover and cook gently for 45 minutes, stirring occasionally. Don't let it colour too much, if at all.

When the meat is über-soft and tender, take it off the heat and remove the herbs and peppercorns. Tear it to shreds with a couple of forks or pulse in a blender. Press into a ramekin or bowl and cover with the liquid left in the pan. Cover and chill for up to a week.

IN EACH LUNCHBOX

A pot of rillettes; crusty bread; cornichons or pickled shallots.

TO FINISH

Take out of the fridge perhaps an hour before eating. Make some toast or tear up a good crusty baguette. Eat with cornichons or pickled shallots.

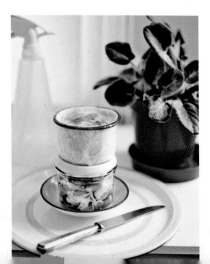

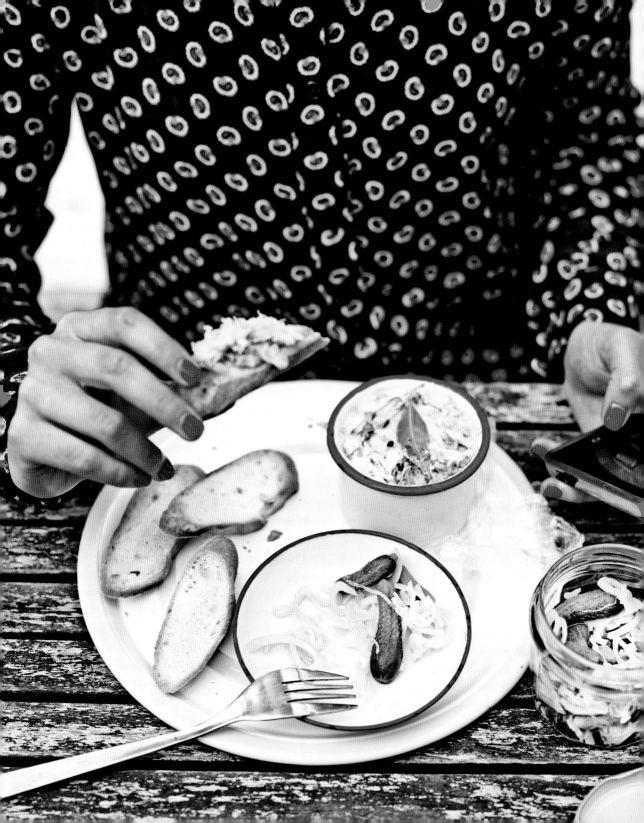

SPICED LAMB BUNS

These are quite nifty for a picnic or a long walk, particularly if made smaller, though as a big bun with a surprise filling they're deeply moreish. The recipe makes more than two people will manage at lunch, but the buns freeze very well, or alternatively will make you very popular in your office.

Prep time: 30 minutes, plus rising time
Cooking time: 40 minutes
Freezable? Yes

500g/1lb 2oz/4 cups strong white bread flour,
      plus extra for dusting
7g/¼oz/about 1 tsp fast-action dried yeast
250ml/9fl oz/1 cup warm water
4 tbsp olive oil
3 tbsp plain yogurt
1 tsp salt
For the filling
1 onion, peeled and finely chopped
olive oil
1 garlic clove, peeled and finely chopped
1 tsp ground cumin
2 tsp ground coriander
1 tsp chilli flakes
salt and pepper
400g/14oz leftover lamb, chicken or beef, chopped

AT HOME

Tip the flour into a bowl and make a well in the centre. Pour in the yeast, water, oil, yogurt and salt. Mix the wet ingredients together then, using your hand like a claw, bring in the flour, adding a little warm water or olive oil if necessary. When it has all come together, turn it onto a lightly floured surface.

Knead for about 7 minutes, until smooth and elastic. Cover with a tea towel and leave to rise in a warm place for 30 minutes.

To make the filling, cook the onion in a little oil until golden and soft, then add the garlic and spices and season with salt and pepper. Stir for a minute or so, then mix through the chopped meat.

Divide the dough into 4 large or 8 small balls. Roll out each ball on a lightly floured surface to a round about 8mm/⅜in thick. Put a good handful of the filling in the centre. Fold the outsides into the middle and pinch to seal. Place, seam-side down, on a lightly floured baking sheet. Repeat for the remaining dough, then cover with a tea towel and leave to rise in a warm place for another 30 minutes.

Preheat the oven to 220°C/425°F/Gas mark 7. Brush the tops of the buns with a little olive oil, then put in the oven. Turn the heat down to 190°C/375°F/ Gas mark 5 and bake for 25–30 minutes. Cool on a wire rack.

IN EACH LUNCHBOX

A lamb bun or two.

TO FINISH

Serve cold, or reheat in a microwave on medium for 3 minutes, or in an oven at 150°C/300°F/ Gas mark 2 for 10 minutes.

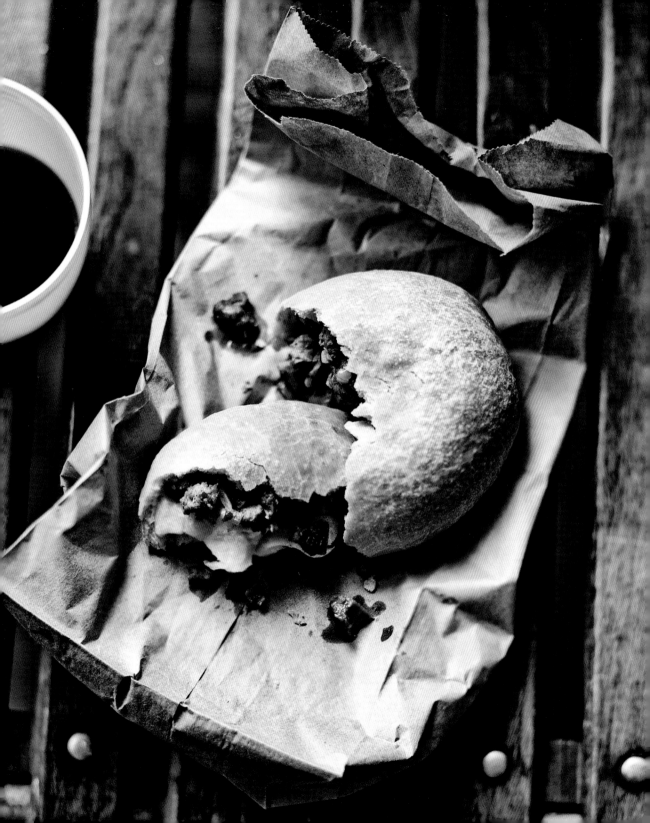

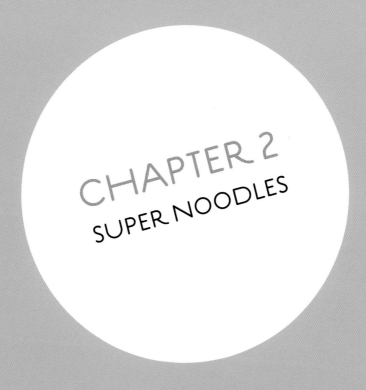

CHAPTER 2
SUPER NOODLES

A big bowl of slippery noodles is one of the finest and most comforting lunches there is, and we've seen some great strides in this country since the not-long-ago days of sachets and ominously flavoured concoctions (bacon noodles?). All the companies making these largely tasteless, synthetic and sachet-enhanced noodles are onto one thing, however, even if they don't necessarily get it right. You can inject a lot of flavour into a simple noodle and broth dish with a relatively small amount of cajolement.

Most of the recipes in this chapter come with a 'ShotPot', a little pot of concentrated flavours that you can bring to work safely, instead of having a precarious Tupperware-full of soup sloshing around on the bus. Then all you need to do is boil a kettle and pour the water over your noodles along with the ShotPot.

These recipes were tested with dried noodles, but fresh are nice, should you prefer (double the weight of noodles if using fresh).

Vietnamese beef noodle soup

My wife Rosie and I spent our honeymoon in Vietnam, an extraordinary country with some of the best food I've had anywhere. That said, it was with a degree of caution that we approached one particular lunch, at a tiny stall on a crowded backstreet in Hanoi, around which flies buzzed and on whose neighbouring stalls the viscera of countless animals hummed in the heat. It turned out to be the finest bowl of *pho*, Vietnamese noodle soup, that we had all holiday. This is my stab at that ubiquitous dish.

Prep time: 15–20 minutes

Cooking time: 30 minutes

Freezable? No

For the ShotPot

400ml/14fl oz/1²/₃ cups chicken or beef stock

2 tbsp Thai fish sauce

1 star anise

1 clove

¹/₂ tsp ground cinnamon

a few slices of fresh ginger

1 garlic clove, squashed with the flat of a knife

1 shallot, peeled and sliced

1 red chilli, deseeded and sliced

2 tsp sugar

For the rest

2 bundles (100–150g/3¹/₂–5¹/₂oz) of
    rice vermicelli noodles

200g/7oz beef rump steak

salt and pepper

vegetable oil

a handful of bean sprouts

a good handful of coriander (cilantro) leaves

lime wedges

a few Thai basil leaves (optional)

1 bird's-eye chilli, finely sliced (optional)

AT HOME

Put all the ShotPot ingredients in a saucepan and bring to a boil. Simmer over a medium-low heat until reduced to 150–200ml/5–7fl oz/about ³/₄ cup. Leave to cool. Discard the bits, and store in two jars in the fridge for up to 5 days.

Cook the noodles as per packet instructions, then run under cold water until cool. Set aside.

Season the steak on both sides, and rub with oil. Heat a heavy pan, add the steak, and cook for 2–3 minutes on each side. Set aside until cool.

Slice the meat (adding any juices to the ShotPot) and divide between two heatproof containers with the noodles and bean sprouts. Cover and store in the fridge for up to 2 days.

IN EACH LUNCHBOX

A portion of noodles, steak and bean sprouts (in a heatproof vessel); a ShotPot; fresh coriander; lime wedges; Thai basil and sliced chilli (optional).

TO FINISH

Tip the ShotPot over the noodles, then pour over 400–500ml/about 16fl oz/2 cups boiling water. Stir, then leave to stand for 1 minute. Garnish with coriander, lime, and Thai basil and chilli if using.

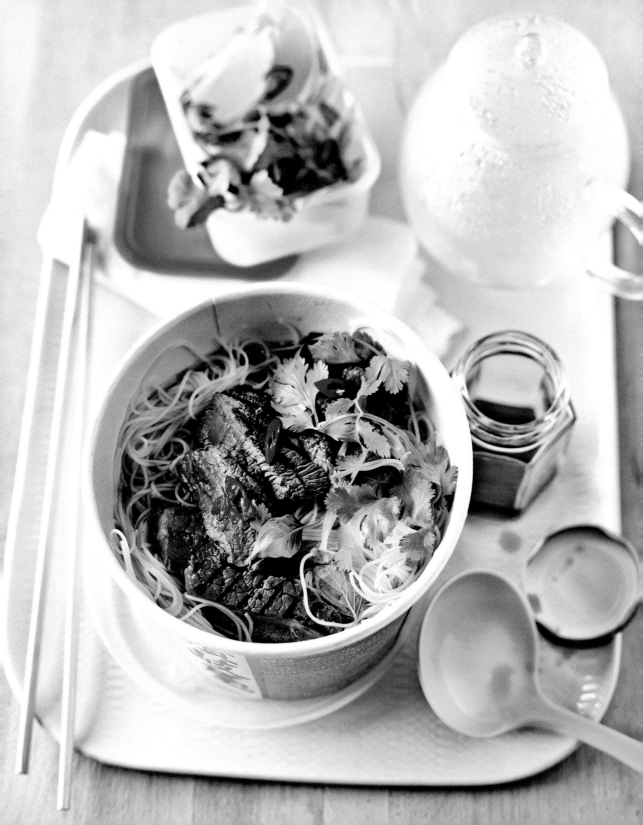

Udon noodles with miso and sesame

These big, fat noodles are pure, slippery comfort, and this recipe couldn't be more straightforward. You should be able to find miso paste at your nearest large supermarket, or order it online. The same goes for udon noodles.

Prep time: 10 minutes

Cooking time: 25 minutes

Freezable? No

For the ShotPot

400ml/14fl oz/1²/₃ cups vegetable or
        chicken stock

2 tbsp miso paste

2 tbsp soy sauce

1 tsp sesame oil

1 tsp chilli flakes

For the rest

2 bundles (100–175g/3¹/₂–6 oz) of udon noodles

4 spring onions (scallions), finely sliced

a handful of coriander (cilantro) leaves

1 tsp sesame seeds

AT HOME

Put all the ShotPot ingredients in a saucepan and bring to a boil, stirring to dissolve the miso. Simmer over a medium heat until reduced to 150–200ml/5–7fl oz/about ³/₄ cup. Leave to cool. Divide between two jars and store in the fridge for up to a week.

Cook the noodles as per packet instructions, then run under cold water until cool. Store in the fridge for up to 2 days.

IN EACH LUNCHBOX

A portion of noodles (in a heatproof vessel); a ShotPot; sliced spring onions, fresh coriander, sesame seeds.

TO FINISH

Tip the ShotPot over the noodles, then pour over 200ml/7fl oz/generous ³/₄ cup boiling water. Stir and leave to stand for 1 minute. Garnish with the spring onions, coriander and sesame seeds.

COLD SOBA NOODLES WITH RADISH AND GINGER

A light, fresh, gluten-free (as long as the soba noodles are 100% buckwheat) noodle dish.

Prep time: 10 minutes
Cooking time: 5 minutes
Freezable? No

2 bundles (100–150g/3½–5½oz) of soba noodles
1 tsp sesame oil
1 tbsp rice vinegar
2 tbsp soy sauce
100g/3½oz radishes, cut into matchsticks or grated
4 spring onions (scallions), finely chopped
2 tbsp grated fresh ginger
a few coriander (cilantro) leaves

AT HOME

Cook the noodles as per packet instructions, then rinse under running water until cold. Toss through the sesame oil, rice vinegar, soy sauce, radishes, spring onions and ginger. Garnish with coriander leaves and store in the fridge for up to 2 days.

IN EACH LUNCHBOX

A portion of soba noodle salad.

TO FINISH

Eat.

THAI CHICKEN NOODLE SOUP

There's something about Thai food – the nostril-clearing, punchy flavours combined with rich, coconutty broths and curries – that makes it irresistible. I find thigh meat far preferable, in this soup, to breast, but if you want to speed things up a bit, then just poach sliced chicken breast for 5 minutes. You could also use leftover roast chicken.

Prep time: 15 minutes
Cooking time: 1 hour
Freezable? No

For the ShotPot
vegetable oil
1 shallot, peeled and finely chopped
1 garlic clove, peeled and crushed
1 bird's-eye chilli, finely sliced
1/2 stalk of lemongrass, finely chopped
2 tsp grated fresh ginger
2 tbsp finely chopped coriander (cilantro) stalks
400ml/14fl oz/1 2/3 cups chicken stock
150ml/5fl oz/2/3 cup coconut cream
1 tbsp Thai fish sauce
zest of 1 lime
2 boneless chicken thighs

For the rest
100g/3 1/2oz flat rice noodles
50g/1 3/4oz mangetout (snow peas), roughly torn
a good handful of coriander (cilantro) leaves
2 lime wedges

AT HOME

Heat a little oil in a saucepan over a medium heat and cook the shallot, garlic, chilli, lemongrass, ginger and coriander stalks for 1 minute, stirring. Add the stock, coconut cream, fish sauce and lime zest, and bring to a gentle boil. Now add the chicken and simmer quietly for 30 minutes.

Remove the chicken. Continue to simmer the stock until reduced to about 200ml/7fl oz/generous 3/4 cup. Divide between two jars, cool and store in the fridge for up to 2 days.

Shred the cooled chicken. Cook the noodles according to packet instructions, then run under cold water until cool. Divide between two heatproof vessels, along with the mangetout and shredded chicken. Cover and chill for up to 2 days.

IN EACH LUNCHBOX

A portion of noodles, mangetout and chicken (in a heatproof vessel); a ShotPot; fresh coriander and a lime wedge.

TO FINISH

Tip the ShotPot over the noodles, then pour over 300ml/10fl oz/1 1/4 cups boiling water. Stir and leave to stand for 1 minute. Garnish with coriander and a squeeze of lime.

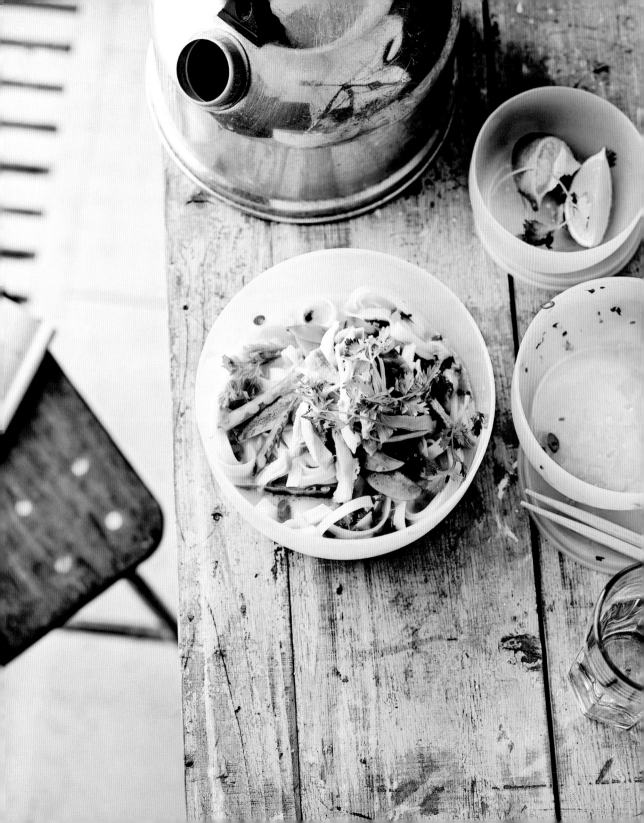

PRAWN NOODLE SALAD

Pad Thai, that backpackers' favourite, is the inspiration here, though this version is served cold. No ShotPot this time – just lots of crunch and spice and herbs and citrus.

Prep time: 15 minutes
Cooking time: 5 minutes
Freezable? No

100g/3½oz flat rice noodles
150g/5½oz cooked prawns (shrimp)
1 carrot, peeled and sliced into matchsticks
a good handful of bean sprouts
a good handful of sugar snap peas
a handful of peanuts, roughly chopped
a handful of coriander (cilantro) leaves

For the dressing
1 shallot, peeled and finely sliced
1 red chilli, deseeded and finely sliced
1 tbsp Thai fish sauce
juice of ½ lime
1 tbsp groundnut (peanut) oil
1 tsp palm or caster (superfine) sugar

AT HOME

Cook the noodles as per packet instructions, then run under cold water until cool. Divide between two Tupperwares or other lunchtime vessels along with the prawns, carrot, bean sprouts, sugar snaps, peanuts and coriander. Store in the fridge for up to 2 days.

To make the dressing, put all the ingredients in a bowl and whisk together. Store in a jar for up to 2 days.

IN EACH LUNCHBOX

A portion of salad; a portion of dressing.

TO FINISH

Dress, stir, devour.

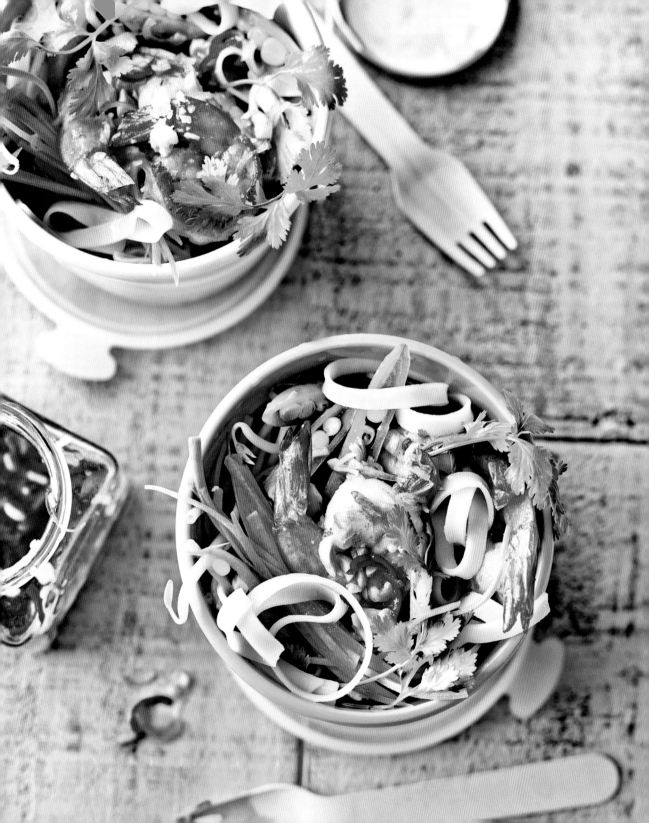

EGG NOODLES WITH TOFU, CHILLI AND LEMONGRASS

I find it rather a shame that tofu is so maligned, so misinterpreted as the pinko-vegetarian's meat substitute of choice. I and many other enthusiastic carnivores enjoy tofu for its mellow silkiness, for its unobtrusive yet very present personality, and for its pure versatility.

This is a relatively cool dish, temperature-wise, though somewhat more fiery in spice.

Prep time: 10 minutes
Cooking time: 30 minutes
Freezable? No

For the ShotPot
400ml/14fl oz/1²/₃ cups chicken stock
1 shallot, peeled and roughly chopped
1 garlic clove, squashed with the flat of a knife
¹/₂ stalk of lemongrass, finely chopped
1 red chilli, sliced
2 tbsp soy sauce

For the rest
2–4 nests (100–150g/3¹/₂–5¹/₂oz) of egg noodles
150g/5¹/₂oz silken tofu, cubed (available in
      most supermarkets)
1 red chilli, deseeded and finely sliced
2 spring onions (scallions), thinly sliced
a few coriander (cilantro) leaves

AT HOME

Put all the ShotPot ingredients in a saucepan and bring to a gentle simmer. Simmer over a medium-low heat until reduced to 150–200ml/5–7fl oz/ about ³/₄ cup. Leave to cool, strain through a sieve, then store in two jars in the fridge for up to 5 days.

Cook the noodles as per packet instructions, then run under cold water until cool. Divide between two heatproof containers along with the tofu, chilli and spring onions, and store in the fridge for up to 2 days.

IN EACH LUNCHBOX

A portion of noodles with tofu, chilli and spring onions (in a heatproof vessel); a ShotPot; fresh coriander leaves.

TO FINISH

Mix about 100ml/3¹/₂fl oz/scant ¹/₂ cup boiling water with the ShotPot, then pour this over the noodles. Stir and leave to stand for 1 minute. Garnish with coriander and serve.

HOT AND SOUR
PRAWN NOODLE SOUP

As with several of the dishes in this chapter, the protein you choose here is relatively interchangeable – you could replace the prawns with leftover chicken, beef, or even cubes of tofu.

Prep time: 12 minutes
Cooking time: 30 minutes
Freezable? No

For the ShotPot
400ml/14fl oz/1²/₃ cups chicken or
    vegetable stock
1 shallot, peeled and finely sliced
1 garlic clove, peeled and sliced
1 small thumb of fresh ginger, grated
¹/₂–1 bird's-eye chilli, finely sliced
¹/₂ stalk of lemongrass, tough outer layer removed,
    finely chopped
zest of ¹/₂ lime
1 tbsp Thai fish sauce
For the broth
100g/3¹/₂oz flat rice noodles
150g/5¹/₂oz cooked prawns (shrimp)
50g/1³/₄oz mangetout (snow peas)
To finish
a handful of bean sprouts
lime wedges
coriander (cilantro) leaves

AT HOME
Put all the ShotPot ingredients in a saucepan and bring to a boil. Simmer for 20–30 minutes, until reduced to about 200ml/7fl oz/generous ³/₄ cup. Leave to cool. Store in two jars in the fridge for up to 5 days.

    Cook the noodles as per packet instructions, then run under cold water until cool. Divide between two heatproof vessels with the prawns and mangetout, cover and store in the fridge for up to 2 days.

IN EACH LUNCHBOX
A portion of noodles, prawns and mangetout (in a heatproof vessel); a ShotPot; bean sprouts, lime wedges and fresh coriander.

TO FINISH
Pour the ShotPot over the noodles, prawns and mangetout, then add about 300ml/10fl oz/1¹/₄ cups boiling water. Stir and leave to stand for 1–2 minutes. Garnish with bean sprouts, lime and coriander.

HANOI KITCHEN'S BUN BO

This recipe comes courtesy of my friend Nigel, who runs a cracking street food stall called Hanoi Kitchen. It's one of my favourite things in the world to eat. Hopefully my version comes close to the perfection of Nigel's. Don't be put off by the long list of ingredients. This is very straightforward.

Prep time: 25 minutes
Cooking time: 30 minutes
Freezable? No

For the ShotPot

400ml/14fl oz/1 ²/₃ cups beef stock

1 tsp salt

2 tsp caster (superfine) sugar

2 tbsp rice vinegar

2 tbsp Thai fish sauce

juice of 1 lime

1 garlic clove, peeled and thinly sliced

¹/₂–1 Thai/bird's-eye chilli, finely sliced

¹/₂ stalk of lemongrass, finely chopped

For the pickled carrot

1 carrot, peeled into strips

200ml/7fl oz/generous ³/₄ cup water

3 tbsp rice vinegar

2 tbsp sugar

1 tsp salt

For the rest

200g/7oz rump steak, trimmed of excess fat

vegetable oil

100–150g/3¹/₂– 5¹/₂ oz rice vermicelli noodles

1 little gem lettuce, sliced

a handful of bean sprouts

a handful of coriander (cilantro) leaves

a handful of Thai basil leaves (or mint)

1 shallot, finely sliced

2 tbsp crushed roasted peanuts

AT HOME

Put all the ShotPot ingredients in a saucepan and bring to a boil, stirring to dissolve the sugar. Simmer over a medium–low heat for about 20 minutes, until reduced to 150–200ml/5–7fl oz/about ³/₄ cup. Cool. Store in two jars in the fridge for up to 5 days.

To pickle the carrot: mix the water, vinegar, sugar and salt until all is dissolved, then pour over the carrot strips. Set aside for at least 20 minutes.

Season the steak with salt and pepper, and rub with oil. Heat a heavy pan and cook the steak for 2–3 minutes on each side. Rest on a plate until cold, then slice. Add any juices to the ShotPot.

Cook the noodles as per packet instructions, then run under cold water until cool. Take the carrots out of their pickling juice and put in heatproof containers with the noodles, lettuce and beef. Store in the fridge for up to 2 days.

IN EACH LUNCHBOX

A portion of noodles, beef and lettuce (in a heatproof vessel); a ShotPot; bean sprouts, coriander, Thai basil, shallot and peanuts.

TO FINISH

Add the ShotPot to the noodles, then pour over about 250ml/9fl oz/1 cup boiling water. Stir and leave to stand for 1 minute. Finish with the bean sprouts, coriander, basil, shallot and peanuts.

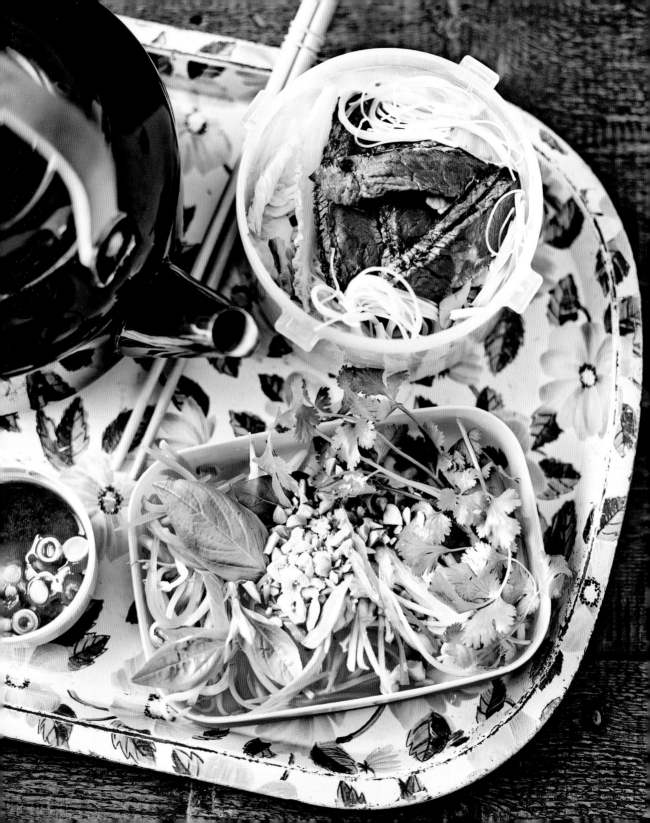

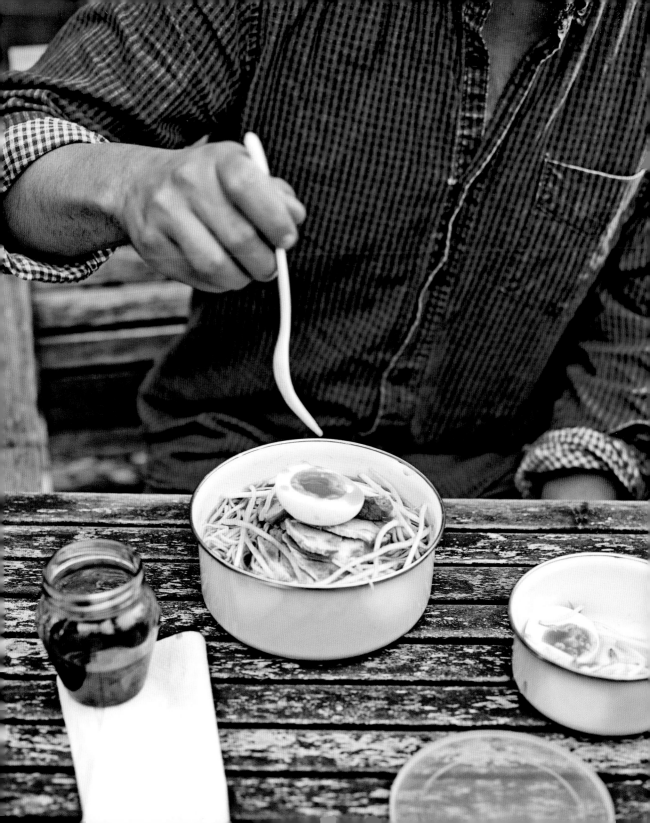

WHEAT NOODLES WITH PORK BELLY

There's quite a lot of scope for bulking this up if you fancy – sliced hearts of palm are always popular, a little finely chopped raw leek, pickled garlic... it's based on the increasingly popular Japanese ramen, which is at its best when the stock comes from a ferociously reduced pork bone broth. Pie in the sky for a midweek lunch, perhaps, but should you find yourself in possession of a pork bone, then you know what to do. (And if you don't know what to do, there are instructions for making stock on p.198.)

Prep time: 15 minutes

Cooking time: 1¹/₂–2 hours

Freezable? The pork belly is

For the ShotPot

1 litre/1³/₄ pints/4 cups ham stock

2 tbsp soy sauce

2 tbsp miso paste

1 tsp sesame oil

1 tbsp grated fresh ginger

1 tsp chilli flakes

1 garlic clove, peeled and crushed

300g/10¹/₂oz piece of skinless pork belly

For the rest

2 eggs

2 nests (100–150g/3¹/₂– 5¹/₂ oz) of wheat noodles

a handful of bean sprouts

chilli oil (shop–bought or p.188) (optional)

AT HOME

Put all the ShotPot ingredients except for the pork belly in a large saucepan and bring to a boil. Add the pork, cover, and simmer gently for 1 hour, until the meat is soft. Remove the pork and continue to simmer, uncovered, until reduced to 150–200ml/5–7fl oz/about ³/₄ cup. Divide between two jars and store in the fridge for up to 3 days.

Boil the eggs for 5 minutes, then transfer to a bowl of iced water until cool. Peel and store in a covered container in the fridge for up to 2 days.

Cook the noodles as per packet instructions, then run under cold water until cool. Slice the pork thinly and store in the fridge with the noodles for up to 2 days.

IN EACH LUNCHBOX

A portion of noodles and pork (in a heatproof vessel); a ShotPot; an egg; bean sprouts, chilli oil (optional).

TO FINISH

Pour the ShotPot over the noodles, then add 300–400ml/12fl oz/1¹/₂ cups boiling water. Stir and leave to stand for 1 minute. Garnish with bean sprouts, an egg, and a drizzle of chilli oil if you like.

Chicken noodle salad

This is based on a bang bang salad, so called because you beat the hell out of the chicken before cooking it, and then add enough chilli that the stuff explodes in your mouth. But that's entirely up to you.

Prep time: 20 minutes

Cooking time: 40 minutes

Freezable? No

For the ShotPot

1 tsp sunflower or groundnut (peanut) oil

1 shallot, peeled and roughly chopped

1 garlic clove, peeled and roughly chopped

1 Thai chilli, finely sliced

2 chicken breasts

1 tbsp rice vinegar

juice of $1/2$ lime

1 tsp salt

500ml/18fl oz/2 cups chicken stock

2 tbsp peanut butter

For the rest

2 bundles (100–150g/$3^1/2$– $5^1/2$ oz) of
    rice vermicelli noodles

1 little gem lettuce, sliced

1 carrot, peeled and cut into matchsticks

a good handful of bean sprouts

a good handful of coriander (cilantro)

a few cashew nuts

lime wedges

AT HOME

Heat the oil in a saucepan over a low heat, add the shallot, garlic and chilli, and cook gently. Meanwhile, halve the chicken breasts horizontally and put the pieces between sheets of clingfilm. Beat with a rolling pin or your fists until flattened.

Add the vinegar, lime juice, salt and stock to the pan and bring to a boil. Lower in the chicken and poach over a medium–low heat for 8–10 minutes. Remove the chicken and leave to cool. Simmer the cooking liquor for another 15 minutes, until reduced to 150–200ml/5–7fl oz/about $3/4$ cup. Stir in the peanut butter and leave to cool. Store in two jars in the fridge for up to 5 days.

Cook the noodles as per packet instructions, then run under cold water until cool. Put in your lunchboxes with the lettuce, carrot and bean sprouts. Shred the cooled chicken and chuck this in too. Cover and store in the fridge for up to 2 days.

IN EACH LUNCHBOX

A portion of noodles, chicken and vegetables; a ShotPot; fresh coriander, cashew nuts, lime wedges.

TO FINISH

Tip the ShotPot over the noodle salad and give it a good stir. Garnish with coriander, cashew nuts and lime wedges.

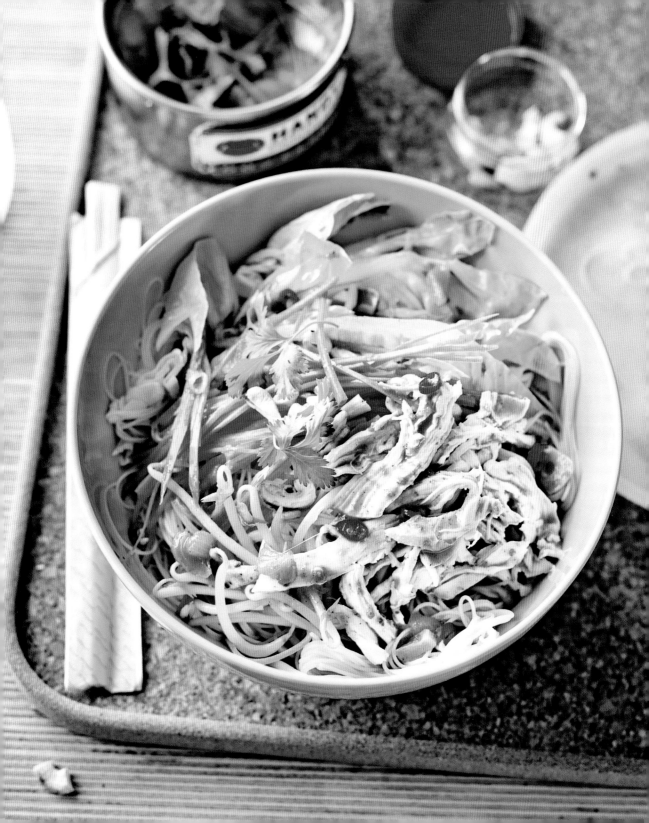

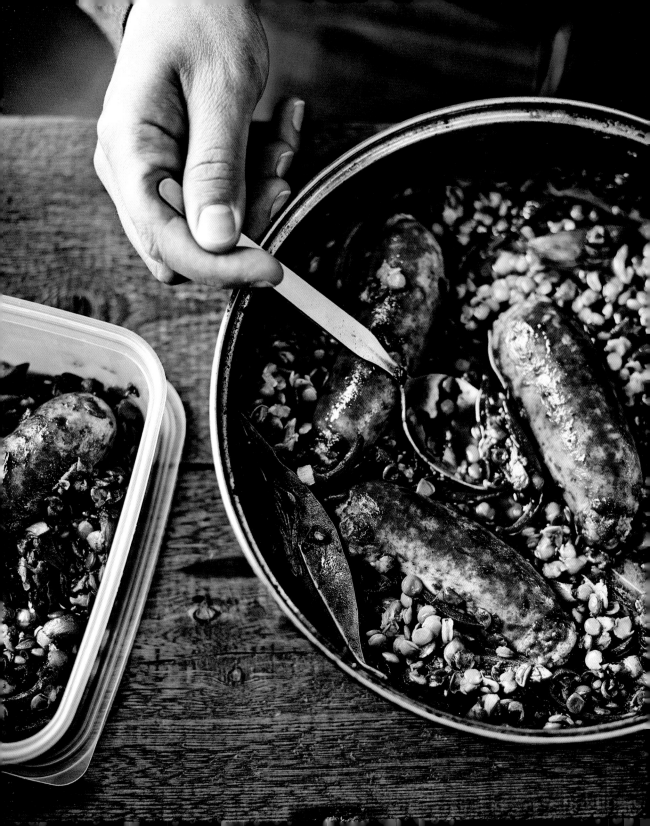

Aubergine tagine with bulgur wheat pilaf

You could get a bit more involved with this pilaf, cooking a vast amount of onion down for a long time and adding all sorts of spices, fruits and herbs. The result is delicious and worth the effort, if the timing's right, but if it's 9pm on a Monday evening you're not going to be in the mood for that, so this is a pared-down version.

Cooking time: 25 minutes

Prep time: 40 minutes

Freezable? Yes

For the tagine

olive oil

1/2 onion, peeled and finely chopped

1 garlic clove, peeled and sliced

1 tsp *ras-el-hanout* (spice blend available in most supermarkets)

salt and pepper

1 aubergine (eggplant), cut into 2.5cm/1in dice

200g/7oz chopped tomatoes (canned are fine)

For the bulgur pilaf

1/2 onion, peeled and thinly sliced

1 tsp ground cumin

2 tsp ground coriander

1/2 tsp ground cinnamon

100g/3½oz bulgur wheat

200ml/7fl oz/generous ¾ cup chicken or vegetable stock

2 tbsp raisins

2 tbsp flaked almonds or 1 tbsp pine nuts (optional)

To serve

plain yogurt

a small handful of fresh coriander (cilantro)

AT HOME

For the tagine, heat a splash of oil in a saucepan and gently cook the onion and garlic until soft. Add the *ras-el-hanout* along with a good pinch of salt and a twist of pepper, and cook over a medium heat for 1 minute, stirring continuously. Add the aubergine and tomatoes, and about 150ml/5fl oz/²/₃ cup water, stir to combine, then cover and cook for 15 minutes, until the aubergine is soft. Leave to cool. Cover and store in the fridge for up to 5 days.

For the pilaf, heat a splash of oil in a saucepan over a medium heat and cook the onion until soft and lightly browned. Stir in the spices and cook for a further minute, then add the bulgur wheat and stock. Bring to a boil, cover, and cook over the lowest heat for 15 minutes. Keeping the lid on, remove from the heat and leave to stand for 5 minutes. Stir through the raisins and almonds, if using. Cool, then cover and store in the fridge for up to 5 days.

IN EACH LUNCHBOX

A portion of aubergine tagine (in a microwaveable vessel); a portion of pilaf; yogurt and coriander.

TO FINISH

Microwave the aubergine on medium for 4 minutes, stirring halfway through. Serve with the pilaf.

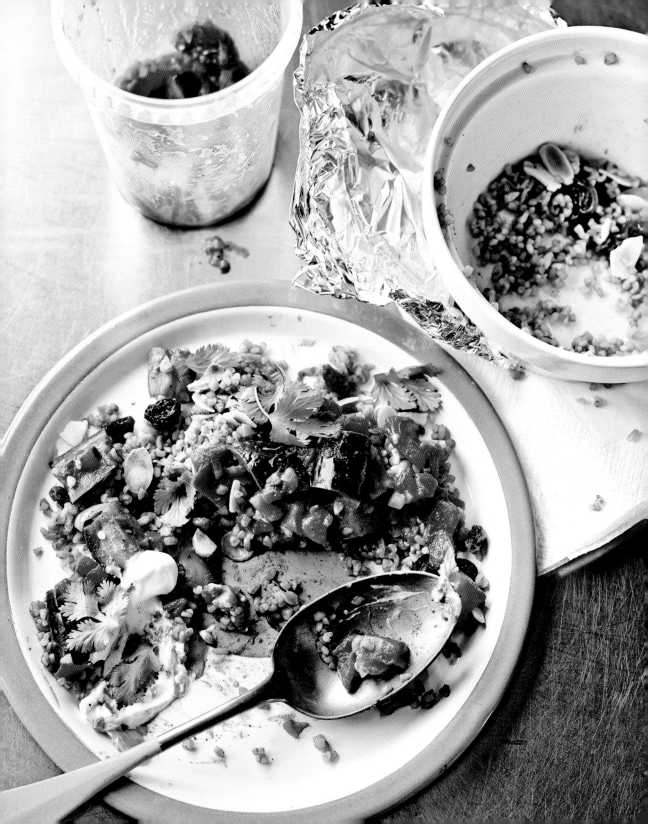

A LIGHT SMOKED MACKEREL BROTH

So-called 'comfort' food is usually associated with one or all of the following: carbohydrates, cheese, butter. Shepherd's pie, macaroni cheese, mashed potato — these are what we equate with cosseting our bellies. But it doesn't have to be so. For one thing, the season in which we need comfort is also that period when a lot of people are trying to shift the Christmas poundage. This is a light and indeed comforting broth that's low on stodge but high on gastro-hugs.

Prep time: 10 minutes

Cooking time: 20 minutes

Freezable? Yes

For the ShotPot

1 shallot, peeled and thinly sliced

1 garlic clove, peeled and thinly sliced

1/2 tsp Sichuan pepper, crushed

1 red chilli, finely sliced (deseeded if you prefer)

1 star anise

2 tbsp soy sauce

1 tbsp rice vinegar or white wine vinegar

300ml/10fl oz/1 1/4 cups chicken or vegetable stock, or 1 tbsp dashi powder with 300ml/10fl oz/ 1 1/4 cups water

For the rest

2 smoked mackerel fillets

a handful of coriander (cilantro)

2 spring onions (scallions), finely sliced

AT HOME

Put all the ShotPot ingredients in a saucepan and gently bring to a boil. Simmer for 15–20 minutes, until reduced by half. Cool and divide between two jars, discarding the star anise. Store in the fridge for up to 3 days.

IN EACH LUNCHBOX

A ShotPot; a smoked mackerel fillet; coriander and spring onions.

TO FINISH

Break a smoked mackerel fillet up into a bowl. Add the ShotPot. Boil a kettle and pour 400ml/14fl oz/ 1 2/3 cups boiling water over the mackerel. Garnish with coriander leaves and spring onions.

Bigos

Hunter's stew, or *bigos,* is a Polish dish that requires sauerkraut, but don't let that put you off. It's a useful, acidic foil to the rich sausage and various other offcuts that traditionally find their way into the stew. Leftover sauerkraut keeps well in the fridge and can be used in the sandwich on p.129.

Prep time: 15 minutes

Cooking time: 1 hour 10 minutes

Freezable? Yes

15g/¹/₂oz/1 tbsp butter

1 onion, peeled and finely sliced

salt and pepper

200g/7oz sauerkraut, drained and rinsed briefly

100g/3¹/₂oz white cabbage, finely sliced

100g/3¹/₂oz canned chopped tomatoes

100g/3¹/₂oz smoked sausage

  (*kielbasa* or *kabanos* varieties are good and
  available in Polish delis), chopped

150g/5¹/₂oz skinless pork belly, cubed

300ml/10fl oz/1¹/₄ cups beef stock

AT HOME

Melt the butter in a saucepan over a low heat, add the onion, season with salt and pepper, cover, and cook gently for 10 minutes, until soft.

Add the remaining ingredients, stir, and bring to a boil. Cover and simmer gently for 1 hour. Leave to cool and store in the fridge for up to 3 days.

IN EACH LUNCHBOX

A portion of the *bigos* (in a microwaveable vessel).

TO FINISH

Reheat in a microwave on medium for 4–5 minutes.

Pea and coriander soup

This has been a favourite since my time at Darina Allen's Ballymaloe Cookery School, upon whose recipe this one is based.

Prep time: 15 minutes
Cooking time: 15 minutes
Freezable? Yes

2 tbsp olive oil
1 small onion, peeled and finely chopped
1 small garlic clove, peeled and sliced
$^1/_2$ green chilli, deseeded and finely chopped
salt and pepper
500ml/18fl oz/2 cups chicken or vegetable stock
300g/10$^1/_2$oz/2 cups frozen peas
15g/$^1/_2$oz coriander (cilantro) leaves
plain yogurt, to serve

AT HOME
Heat the oil in a saucepan over a lowish heat and add the onion, garlic and chilli. Season with salt and pepper, cover and cook for 10 minutes, until soft. Add the stock and bring to a boil. Add the peas and simmer for 3 minutes. Stir through the coriander leaves, then blend until smooth. Leave to cool, then store in the fridge for up to 3 days.

IN EACH LUNCHBOX
A portion of pea and coriander soup (in a microwaveable vessel); yogurt.

TO FINISH
Reheat the soup in a microwave on medium for 4 minutes, stirring halfway through. Give it a good stir and serve with a dollop of yogurt.

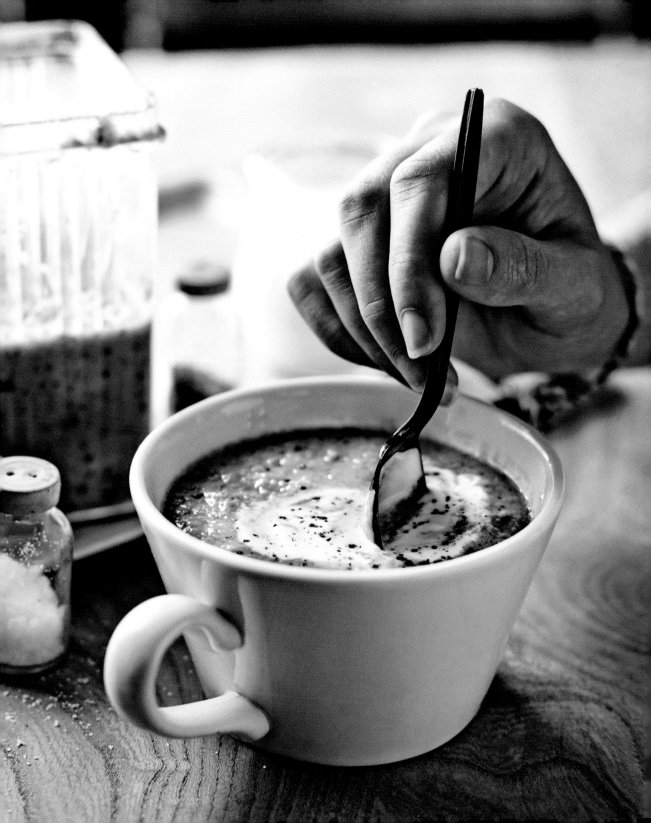

CHORIZO AND POTATOES

I love the russet hue of this dish, the soft potato on crisp, piquant chorizo, and above all its simplicity.

Prep time: 15 minutes

Cooking time: 35 minutes

Freezable? No

olive oil

125g/4½oz chorizo, chopped into big chunks

1 onion, peeled and roughly chopped

1 garlic clove, peeled and thinly sliced

1 tsp smoked paprika (sweet or hot, as you prefer)

salt and pepper

1 large floury potato (200–250g/7–9oz), cut into
  fat cubes

a sprig of thyme

a small handful of flat-leaf parsley,
  roughly chopped

AT HOME

Heat a little oil in a saucepan and fry the chorizo until crisp. Remove with a slotted spoon. Add the onion, garlic and paprika, and season with salt and pepper. Cook over a medium heat for 7–10 minutes, stirring regularly, until soft.

Add the potato, thyme, chorizo and 300ml/10fl oz/1¼ cups water. Gently simmer for 20 minutes, stirring occasionally, until the potato is tender. Cool and store in the fridge for up to 5 days.

IN EACH LUNCHBOX

A portion of chorizo and potato stew (in a microwaveable vessel); chopped parsley.

TO FINISH

Reheat in a microwave on medium for 4–5 minutes. Scatter with parsley and serve.

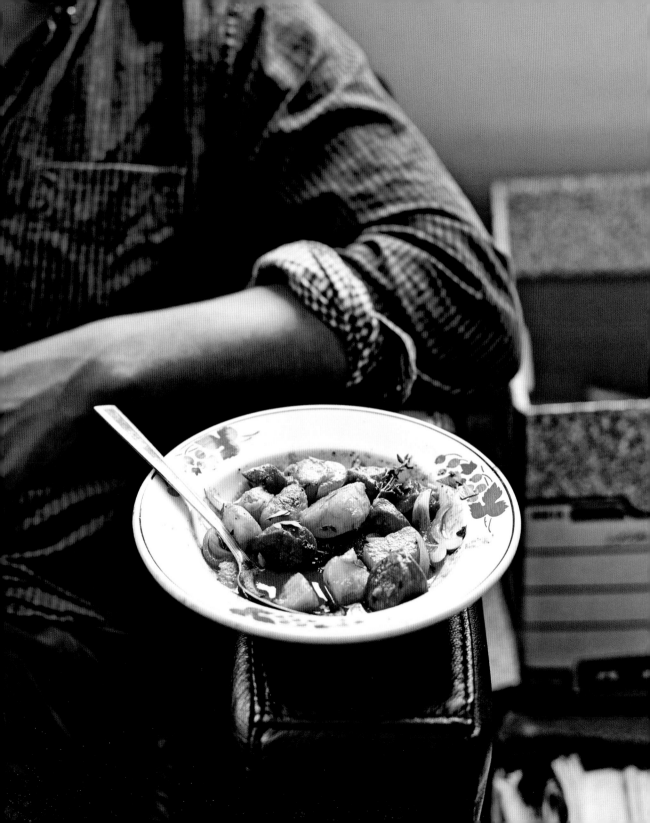

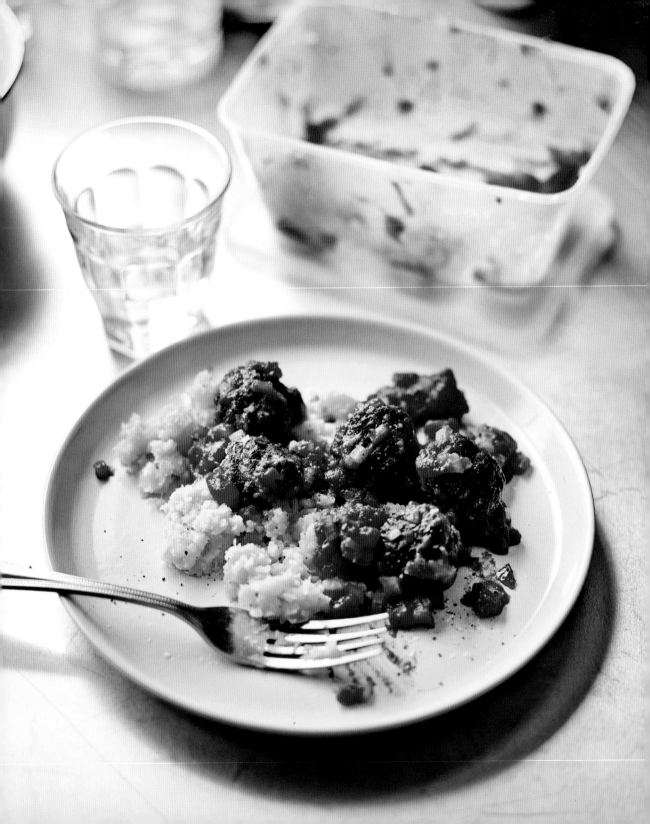

Mashed Swede with Meatballs

The poor swede is desperately under-appreciated, and I can't for the life of me work out why. Is it something to do with school food? Associations with rationing? Its deliciously pungent but undeniably unsexy aroma? Who knows? With butter and pepper, it's one of the greatest root vegetables you can pull from the earth.

Prep time: 25 minutes

Cooking time: 30 minutes

Freezable? Yes

For the meatballs

125g/4¹/₂oz fresh minced (ground) pork

125g/4¹/₂oz fresh minced (ground) beef

¹/₂ tsp chilli flakes

1 tsp fennel seeds, crushed

a small handful of parsley, finely chopped

salt and pepper

olive oil

1 small onion, peeled and very finely chopped

1 garlic clove, peeled and finely chopped

200g/7oz canned chopped tomatoes

For the mashed swede

1 small swede, peeled and cut into 2.5cm/1in dice

25–50g/1–1³/₄oz/2–4 tbsp butter

AT HOME

Mix the pork, beef, chilli, fennel and parsley, and season with salt and pepper. Form into about 10 meatballs. Heat a little oil in a sauté or frying pan and brown the meatballs all over. Remove to a plate.

Add the onions to the same pan, with another drop of oil if necessary. Season with salt and pepper, and cook gently until soft. Add the garlic and tomatoes, along with a splash of water, and bring to a gentle simmer. Return the meatballs to the pan and simmer for 10–12 minutes, until firm. Leave to cool.

Meanwhile, gently boil the swede in salted water until tender. Drain and shake off any excess liquid. Mash with the butter and plenty of pepper. Divide between two microwave-friendly containers and top with the meatballs. Cover and store in the fridge.

IN EACH LUNCHBOX

Portion of meatballs and mashed swede (in a microwaveable vessel).

TO FINISH

Reheat in a microwave on medium for 5 minutes.

KALE AND BORLOTTI
BEAN MINESTRONE

This is a somewhat slovenly dish, ideal for using up odds and ends from the fridge. If you can't find kale, or indeed borlotti, substitute savoy cabbage and butter beans or cannellini beans respectively.

Prep time: 15 minutes

Cooking time: 30 minutes

Freezable? Yes

2 tbsp olive oil

1 small onion, peeled and thinly sliced

1 garlic clove, peeled and thinly sliced

1 carrot, peeled and diced

1 celery stalk, finely chopped

a sprig of thyme

salt and pepper

100g/3½oz kale, roughly chopped

1 x 400g/14oz can borlotti beans, drained

400g/14oz canned chopped tomatoes

250ml/9fl oz/1 cup chicken stock

grated Parmesan cheese, to serve

AT HOME

Heat the oil in a saucepan over a low heat and add the onion, garlic, carrot, celery and thyme. Season with salt and pepper, cover and cook for 15–20 minutes, until good and soft.
Add the kale, beans, tomatoes and stock. Bring to a boil and simmer gently for 8 minutes. Taste for seasoning and add a pinch more salt if necessary. Leave to cool, then store in the fridge for up to 3 days.

IN EACH LUNCHBOX

A portion of minestrone (in a microwaveable vessel); Parmesan cheese.

TO FINISH

Reheat in a microwave on medium for 3–4 minutes. Scatter with Parmesan and eat.

CAULIFLOWER CHEESE

I had a brief spell of thinking I'd discovered something really quite important after making the decision to crumble Doritos over cauliflower cheese. So cheesy! So crunchy! Quite unnecessary, it turned out. Cauliflower cheese doesn't need such interference. Breadcrumbs, certainly; anchovies, ditto, though only in the right context, such as with roast lamb; mustard comes with similar caveats, or so I wrote before consulting my wife Rosie, who said mustard was crucial. Her word is final. Ultimately it's something of a blank canvas – add bells, and indeed whistles, at your discretion.

Prep time: 25 minutes

Cooking time: 30 minutes

Freezable? Yes

350ml/12fl oz/1½ cups full-fat (whole) milk

a bay leaf

a sprig of thyme

1 garlic clove, peeled and lightly squished

350g/12oz cauliflower florets

15g/½oz/1 tbsp butter, plus extra for greasing

15g/½oz/2 tbsp plain (all-purpose) flour

75g/2¾oz mature Cheddar, grated

1 tbsp English mustard

a pinch of cayenne pepper

a handful of fresh (or dried) breadcrumbs

salt and pepper

AT HOME

Preheat the oven to 180°C/350°F/Gas mark 4. Warm the milk in a small pan with the bay leaf, thyme and garlic, until just short of a boil. Set aside to infuse for 10 minutes, then discard the herbs and garlic.

Meanwhile, bring a pan of salted water to a boil and add the cauliflower. Simmer for 2 minutes, drain, and run under a cold tap until cool.

In the same pan, melt the butter and add the flour. Stir until smooth, then slowly pour in the hot milk, stirring all the while, until you have a thick, smooth white sauce. Add the cheese, a handful at a time, and stir until melted, finally stirring in the mustard and a pinch of cayenne. Season with salt and pepper.

Butter a baking dish and tip in the cooled cauliflower. Pour over the cheese sauce. Top with breadcrumbs. Bake for 25–30 minutes, until golden. Leave to cool. Store in the fridge for up to 3 days.

IN EACH LUNCHBOX

A portion of cauliflower cheese (in a microwaveable vessel).

TO FINISH

Reheat in a microwave on medium for 4–5 minutes, or in an oven at 180°C/350°F/ Gas mark 4 for 10 minutes.

BRAISED SQUID WITH BEANS AND PARSLEY

There's an old adage about squid that says something along the lines of '30 seconds or 30 minutes – everything in between is rubber'. As with a lot of 'tough cuts', this is largely true. Hot and fast or low and slow. This method is the latter, with pieces of squid gently poaching in red wine for an hour or so. It really needs very little human intervention.

Serve with crusty bread or couscous.

Prep time: 15 minutes

Cooking time: 1 hour

Freezable? Yes

olive oil

50g/1¾oz smoked lardons or chopped chorizo

1 onion, peeled and finely chopped

2 garlic cloves, peeled and finely chopped

1 dried red chilli

a sliver of orange peel

salt and pepper

300g/10½oz squid tubes, cleaned and cut into chunks

150ml/5fl oz/⅔ cup red wine

400g/14oz canned chopped tomatoes

200g/7oz canned butter beans (lima beans)

½ tsp sugar

a handful of parsley, finely chopped

crusty bread or couscous, to serve

AT HOME

Heat a little oil in a saucepan, add the lardons and fry until crisp. Add the onion, garlic, chilli and orange peel. Season with salt and pepper, cover, and cook over a low heat for 10 minutes.

Add the squid and red wine. Bring to a boil and simmer for 2 minutes, then add the tomatoes, beans and sugar. Simmer gently, uncovered, for 45 minutes, stirring occasionally, until the squid is soft. Taste for seasoning, cool, and store in the fridge for up to a day.

IN EACH LUNCHBOX

A portion of braised squid (in a microwaveable vessel); chopped parsley; crusty bread or couscous.

TO FINISH

Reheat in a microwave on medium for 4–5 minutes. Garnish with parsley and eat.

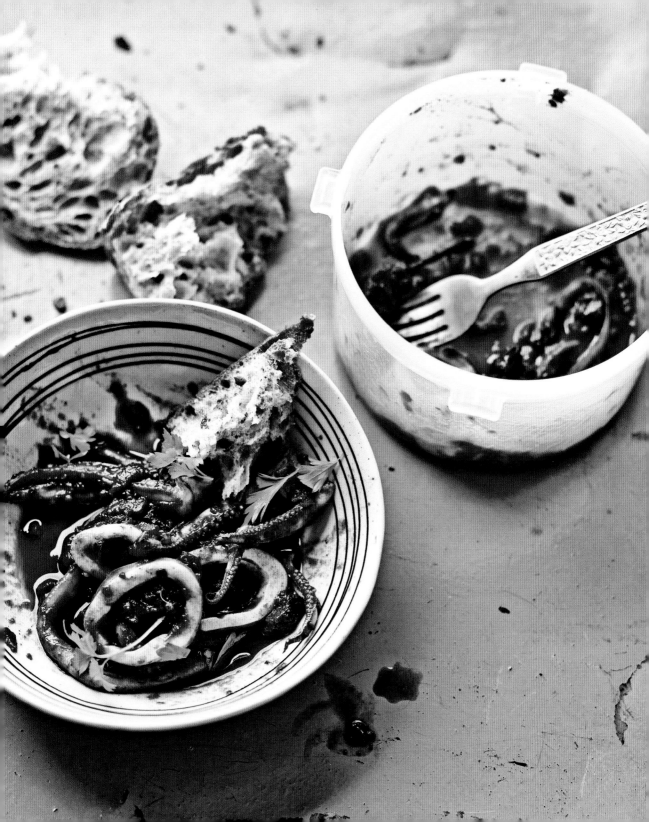

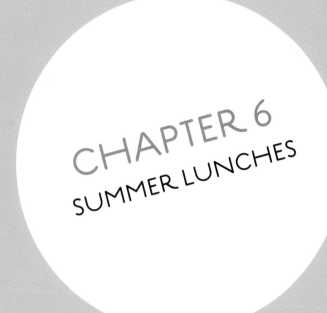

CHAPTER 6
SUMMER LUNCHES

The writing of this book was concluded during that frighteningly hot month in July 2013 (to those with foreign editions, it does indeed happen occasionally in the UK), and having spent a few days testing recipes for the previous chapter, I must admit that coming to these was something of a relief. Even with all the kitchen windows open, it was still like cooking in a Cuban casino.

The chilled soups and vibrant salads were more welcome than you can imagine, and in turn gave me the opportunity to imagine you, in your office, face inches from a fan, in desperate need of something light and cooling. With any luck, these recipes will be just the thing, though they needn't be restricted to just the hottest days. Some are wholesome, virtuous dishes for any time of year.

ONION AND ANCHOVY PIZZA

If making your own bread seems like too much of a faff, then you could use pitta bread here, or even a shop-bought pizza base. But say it's Sunday and you're planning Monday's lunch, then it's a fairly gentle afternoon recipe. Once you've got the base sussed, feel free to muck around with the toppings. I'm sure you don't need me to tell you what's good on a pizza.

Prep time: 20 minutes, plus rising time

Cooking time: 40 minutes

Freezable? Yes

For the dough

150g/5½oz/1¼ cups plain (all-purpose) flour

1 tsp fast-action dried yeast

a pinch of salt

75ml/2½fl oz/5 tbsp warm water

1 tbsp olive oil

For the topping

olive oil

2 large onions, peeled and thinly sliced

salt and pepper

12 anchovies

a handful of pitted black olives, sliced

To serve

a handful of rocket (arugula) leaves

balsamic vinegar

AT HOME

To make the dough: mix the flour, yeast and salt, then add the water and oil. Mix to form a dough. Knead for 5 minutes, until smooth and elastic. Cover with a tea towel and leave for 45 minutes.

Meanwhile, make the topping: heat a good glug of oil in a large pan and add the onions. Season with salt and pepper, and cook over a medium-low heat for 20–30 minutes, stirring occasionally, until soft and golden.

Preheat the oven to as high as it will go. Divide the dough in two and roll out to form rough circles, about 3mm/⅛in thick (the thickness of a pound coin). Transfer to a large, lightly floured baking sheet. Top with the onions, anchovies and olives, and bake for 5–10 minutes, until crisp and golden. Leave to cool, cover, and store in the fridge for up to 2 days.

IN EACH LUNCHBOX

A pizza, rocket leaves, balsamic vinegar.

TO FINISH

I'd eat this cold quite happily, though if you prefer, warm in an oven at 180°C/350°F/Gas mark 4 for 5 minutes. I tried reheating this in a microwave and it's perfectly fine, but somewhat floppy. Serve with salad leaves and a few drops of vinegar.

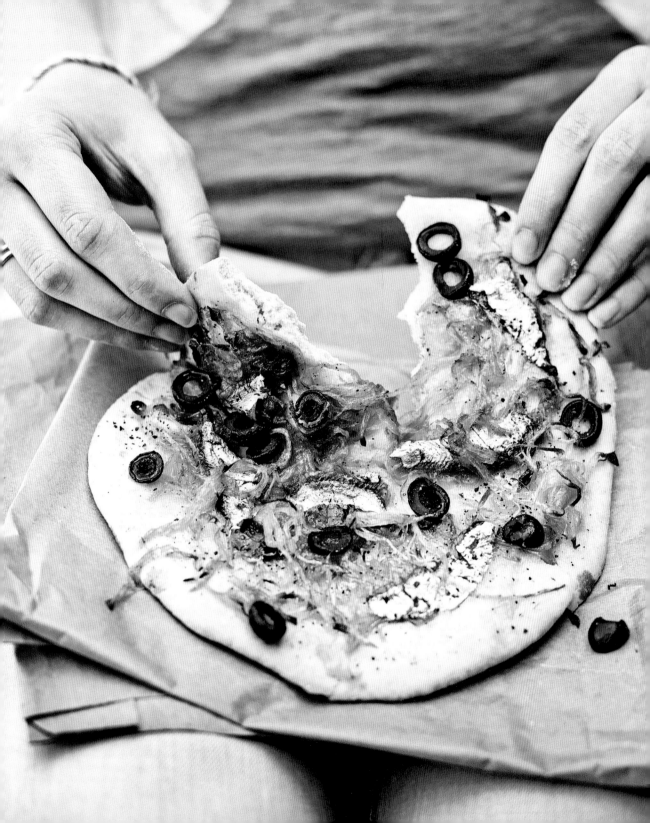

ORZO WITH CRISPY CABBAGE AND LEMON AND PINE NUTS

Amazing how easy it is to borrow a recipe without realizing it.

'I'm not entirely sure where this recipe came from', I began this introduction. 'Possibly just some strange and hungry backwater of my mind. Orzo is a kind of pasta that looks like fat grains of rice. If you can't find it, use macaroni instead...'.

After cooking it one evening, however, my wife Rosie pointed out that there is a recipe in her own book, *The Recipe Wheel*, that is nigh-on identical, save for the fact that she uses macaroni instead. So there you go. It's still here because, well, it's rather nice. But thanks to Ro for the idea.

Prep time: 5 minutes

Cooking time: 10 minutes

Freezable? No

200g/7oz orzo

salt and pepper

4 tbsp olive oil

1 garlic clove, peeled and thinly sliced

200g/7oz savoy cabbage, very finely sliced

zest and juice of ½ lemon

1 tbsp pine nuts

grated Parmesan cheese, to serve

AT HOME

Bring a pan of salted water to a boil and cook the orzo according to packet instructions. Drain and run under a cold tap until cool.

Meanwhile, heat the oil in a large frying pan or saucepan over a medium–high heat, and briefly fry the garlic. Add the cabbage and season with salt and pepper. Cook for 5–7 minutes, stirring frequently, until the cabbage is cooked and crisp here and there. Stir in the lemon zest and juice and set aside.

In a dry frying pan, toast the pine nuts over a medium–high heat, taking care not to burn. Stir these and the cabbage through the pasta. Leave to cool and store in the fridge for up to 3 days.

IN EACH LUNCHBOX

A portion of orzo salad; grated Parmesan.

TO FINISH

Serve with a little grated Parmesan.

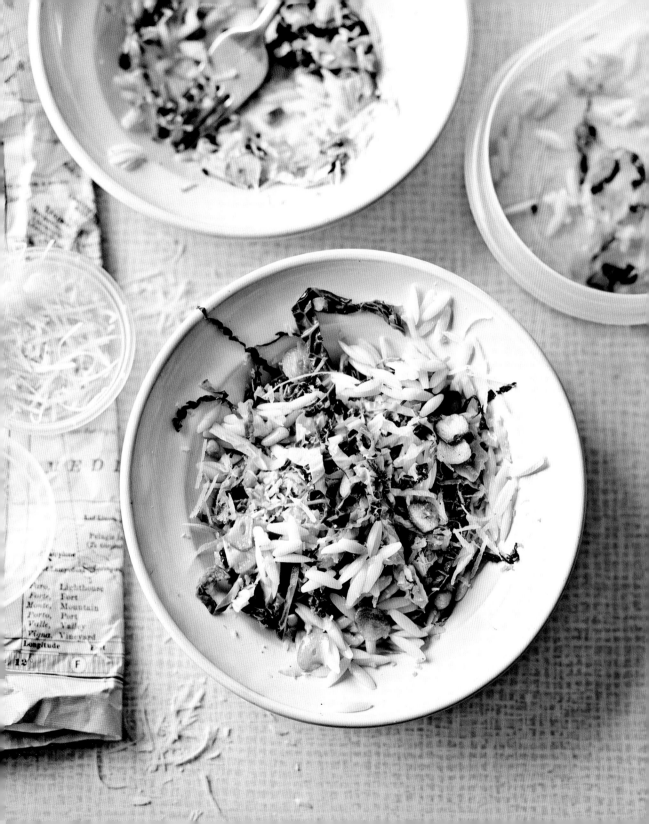

A RAW SALAD OF ROOTS AND TOASTED NUTS

I once briefly – in the name of research – endured a raw vegan diet. A slightly barmy friend had assured me it would give me energy, clear skin, enormous brain power, and no beer belly. I can tell you, after two weeks all it gave me was a sense of despair and a very short temper. It did, however, leave me with a new appreciation of the beauty of raw roots, and particularly beetroot, in my view the star of the show here.

Prep time: 20 minutes

Cooking time: 2 minutes

Freezable? No

1 tsp cumin seeds, lightly crushed

1 tsp coriander seeds, lightly crushed

1 tbsp sesame seeds

1 tbsp pumpkin seeds

2–3 tbsp chopped hazelnuts

2–3 tbsp chopped pistachios

1 beetroot, peeled and grated

1 large carrot, peeled and grated

1 fennel bulb, finely sliced

a good handful (about 20g/³⁄₄oz) of parsley leaves

salt and pepper

For the dressing

juice of 1 lemon

3 tbsp olive oil

AT HOME

Put a dry frying pan over a medium–high heat and add the spices, seeds and nuts. Toast, shaking the pan occasionally, until fragrant. Take care not to burn but equally don't be too ginger – you want a bit of colour.

Put the beetroot, carrot and fennel in a bowl, scatter over the chopped parsley and toasted nuts and spices, and season with a little salt and pepper. Store in the fridge for up to 2 days.

For the dressing, shake together the lemon juice and olive oil in a jar, along with salt and pepper.

IN EACH LUNCHBOX

A portion of salad; a portion of dressing.

TO FINISH

Toss the dressing through the salad and eat.

CHILLED ROAST TOMATO AND BREAD SOUP WITH A SOFT BOILED EGG

This is an ever-so-slightly bastardized version of the Andalusian *salmorejo*, a cousin of gazpacho that uses only tomato and is blended instead of left rough and ready. I've cooked the onion and garlic so as to take the edge off – without this the soup tends to, er, linger – but you needn't bother.

Prep time: 10 minutes

Cooking time: 15 minutes

Freezable? Yes

5 tbsp olive oil

1 garlic clove, peeled and very thinly sliced

1/2 onion, roughly chopped

salt and pepper

50g/1¾oz stale-ish bread, cut into small chunks

2 eggs

500g/1lb 2oz tomatoes, roughly chopped

1 tbsp red wine vinegar

AT HOME

Heat a little of the oil in a small pan and add the garlic and onion. Season with salt and pepper, then cook over a low heat for 10 minutes, until softened, then set aside to cool for a couple of minutes.

Meanwhile, toss the remaining oil with the bread and leave to stand. Boil the eggs for 5 minutes, then cool in a bowl of iced water. Once cold, peel and set aside.

Put the tomatoes in a blender along with the onions and garlic, bread and vinegar, and blend until smooth. Taste for seasoning. Chill in the fridge for up to 2 days.

IN EACH LUNCHBOX

A portion of tomato soup; an egg.

TO FINISH

Carefully cut the egg in half and place on top of the soup.

RED CAMARGUE RICE WITH
MINT AND ALMONDS

This hardy, nutty rice is grown in the south of France and is a new favourite of mine. Come to that, it's pretty new to most people, having only been grown for 50 or so years. It's a little more expensive than your average rice, but worth the cheddar, in my opinion. Some recommend you cook it like risotto, but here the whole thing's a little more straightforward.

This recipe was inspired by one knocked out by Yotam Ottolenghi. What isn't, these days?

Prep time: 15 minutes

Cooking time: 35 minutes

150g/5½oz/generous ¾ cup red Camargue rice
    (I like the stuff mixed with wild rice)

5 tbsp olive oil

1 onion, peeled and finely chopped

salt and pepper

50g/1¾oz flaked almonds, toasted

50g/1¾oz dried apricots, finely chopped

a good handful of fresh mint

a good handful of rocket (arugula),
    roughly chopped

juice of 1 lemon

AT HOME

Cook the rice according to packet instructions, then rinse under a cold tap until cool.

Meanwhile, heat a splash of oil in a small pan over a low heat and add the onion. Season with salt and pepper, and cook, stirring occasionally, until soft.

Stir the onions, almonds, apricot, mint, rocket, lemon juice and the remaining olive oil through the cooked rice. Taste for seasoning and adjust if necessary. Store in the fridge for up to 2 days.

IN EACH LUNCHBOX

A portion of rice salad.

TO FINISH

Eat.

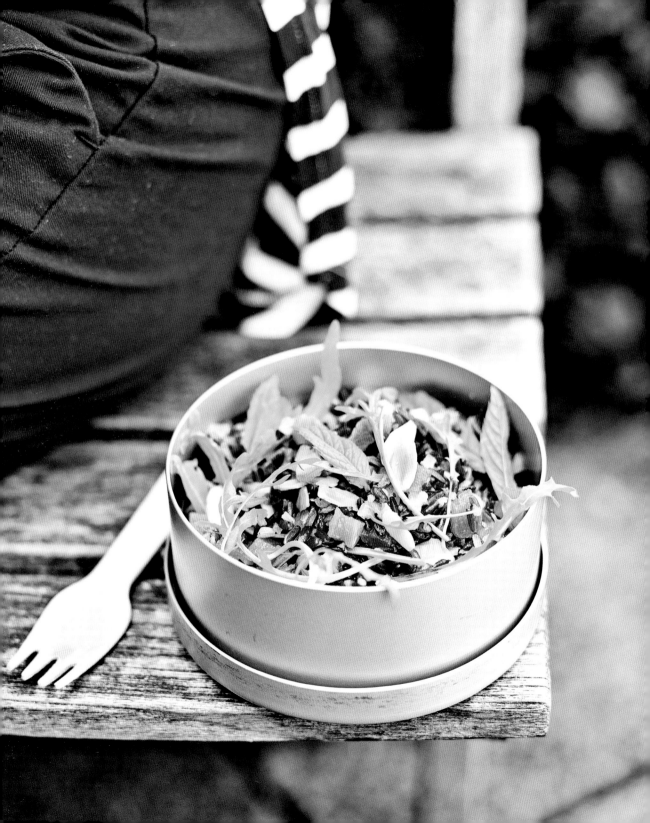

CHILLED CUCUMBER SOUP

There are rich versions of this and there are light versions. A more British affair might – perhaps should – involve butter and cream and chicken stock and all the things that can make life worth living. But on a stinking hot day, or when you're watching the calories, a lighter version such as this can be every bit as satisfying. I won't pretend low-fat yogurt tastes as good as full-fat – it doesn't – but it's a decent enough replacement if you're being strict. Serve with warm pitta bread.

Prep time: 10 minutes
Freezable? Yes

1 shallot, peeled and roughly chopped
1 small garlic clove, peeled and thinly sliced
1 large cucumber, peeled, deseeded,
    roughly chopped
400g/14oz/generous 1½ cups plain yogurt
juice of ½ lemon
salt and pepper
a few sprigs of dill, to serve
2 tbsp olive oil (optional)

AT HOME

Put the shallot, garlic, cucumber, yogurt and lemon juice in a blender. Season with salt and pepper and blend thoroughly until smooth. Taste for seasoning and add a little more salt if necessary.

    Chill and store in the fridge for up to 5 days.

IN EACH LUNCHBOX

A portion of cucumber soup; dill, olive oil (optional).

TO FINISH

Serve the soup with a few sprigs of dill and a drizzle of olive oil if you fancy.

PEARL BARLEY, ARTICHOKE AND FENNEL SALAD

A friend of my parents' stock response to pretty much any food you put in front of him is 'surprisingly good'. This salad, I feel confident in saying, is surprisingly good.

You can find marinated artichokes in most large supermarkets, and certainly in Italian delis.

Prep time: 10 minutes

Cooking time: 45 minutes

Freezable? No

50g/1¾oz/¼ cup pearl barley

salt and pepper

1 fennel bulb, thinly sliced

2 spring onions (scallions), thinly sliced at an angle

150g/5½oz marinated artichokes, roughly chopped

a handful of parsley, finely chopped

juice of 1 lemon

2 tbsp olive oil

a few shavings of Parmesan cheese

AT HOME

Rinse the pearl barley under running water, then boil in a pan of salted water for 45 minutes, until tender. Drain and run under a cold tap again until cool. Shake dry.

Toss together the barley, fennel, spring onions, artichokes and parsley. Season with salt and plenty of pepper, and dress with lemon, olive oil and Parmesan. Store in the fridge for up to 3 days.

IN EACH LUNCHBOX

A portion of pearl barley salad.

TO FINISH

Put in mouth.

GRIDDLED COURGETTE AND HALLOUMI *SALAD* WITH TOASTED QUINOA

Toasted quinoa is an excellent thing to have kicking about. Scattered over salads, tossed through pasta, or whatever, it adds a great nutty crunch to food. This particular recipe makes more than you need – it seemed to me that if you're going to toast quinoa, you may as well do more than a single tablespoon. Store it in a jar.

Prep time: 10 minutes

Cooking time: 25 minutes

Freezable? No

50g/1¾oz/⅓ cup quinoa

2 courgettes (zucchini), sliced thinly on
    the diagonal

2 tbsp olive oil

100g/3½oz halloumi cheese, cut into chunks

2 tbsp vegetable oil

salt and pepper

a good handful of rocket (arugula)

a few mint leaves, shredded

1 red chilli, deseeded and finely chopped

juice of ½ lemon

AT HOME

Boil the quinoa for 12 minutes, until tender. Drain and dry on kitchen paper as thoroughly as you can.

Meanwhile, heat a griddle or frying pan over a high heat. Toss the courgettes in 1 tbsp of the olive oil and griddle for a couple of minutes on each side. Remove the courgettes, add a little more olive oil and the halloumi, and cook for a minute on each side.

Heat the vegetable oil in a non-stick frying pan or sauté pan over a medium-high heat. Add the quinoa and a pinch of salt. Sauté, stirring occasionally, until golden, crisp and toasty, which should take 5 minutes. Set aside to cool.

Toss together the courgettes, halloumi, rocket, mint, chilli and lemon juice, and add a handful of toasted quinoa. Store in Tupperware in the fridge for up to 2 days.

IN EACH LUNCHBOX

A portion of courgette and halloumi salad.

TO FINISH

Eat.

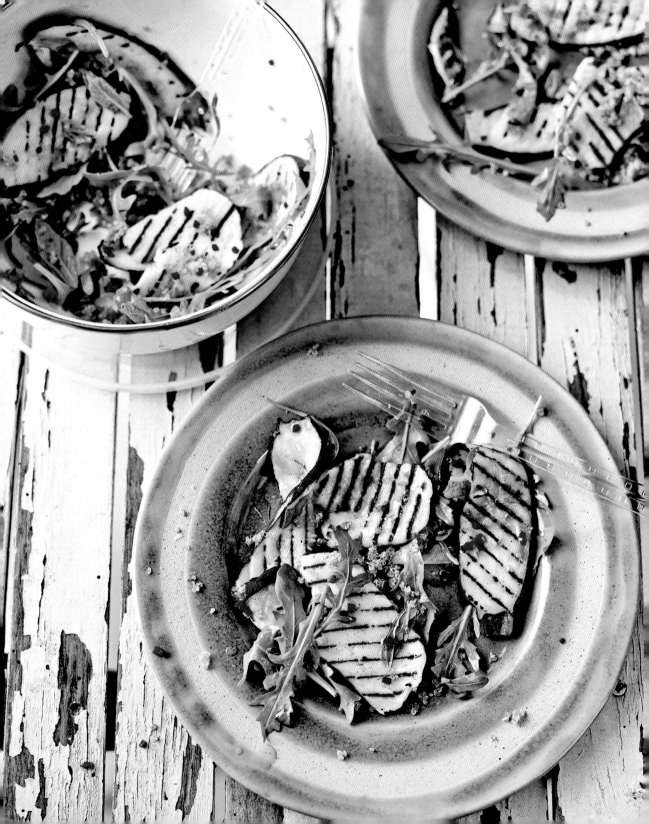

BURNT LEEK AND GOAT'S CHEESE TART

I'm into burning alliums at the moment. Onions baked with sausages that have just caught slightly in the oven, spring onions charred, chopped, and stirred through sour cream (p.61), and leeks, aggressively griddled, hollowed out and stuffed with cheese and herbs. This is a sort of tartish interpretation of the latter dish.

You could replace the goat's cheese with goat's curd (see p.50), but in the interests of speed use a soft goat's cheese.

Prep time: 25 minutes

Cooking time: 30 minutes

Freezable? Yes

200g/7oz puff pastry (shop-bought, obviously)

plain (all-purpose) flour for dusting

200g/7oz leeks, halved down the middle

100g/3½oz soft goat's cheese

1 egg, beaten

4 tbsp finely chopped parsley

2 tbsp finely chopped chives

salt and pepper

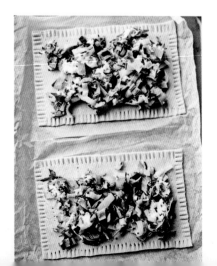

AT HOME

Preheat the oven to 160°C/325°F/Gas mark 3. Divide the pastry in half and roll out into rectangles the size of a paperback book. Prick a few times with a fork, place on a lightly floured baking sheet and chill.

Get a dry frying pan good and hot and add the leeks. Char for a few minutes on each side, until well blackened. Chop finely and beat together with the goat's cheese, most of the egg, and the herbs. Season generously.

Divide this mixture between the pastries, leaving a small border, and crimp around the edges. Brush the pastry with the remaining beaten egg and bake for 20–25 minutes. Leave to cool, cover and store in the fridge for up to 3 days.

IN EACH LUNCHBOX

A leek and goat's cheese tart.

TO FINISH

Serve cold, or reheat in an oven at 180°C/350°F/Gas mark 4 for 7 minutes.

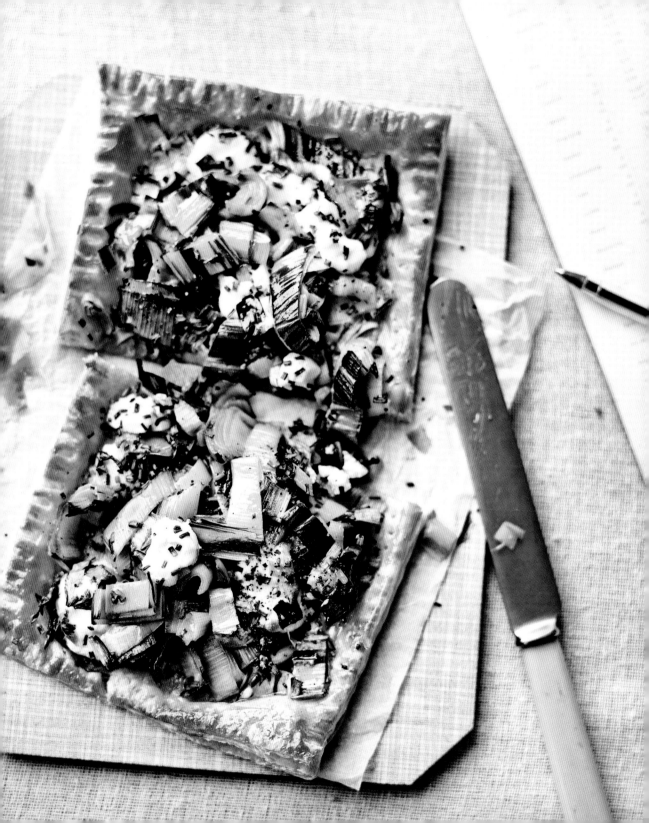

Pea, spring onion and Gruyère frittata

The trick here is having a smallish frying pan (ideally a 16cm/6¼in omelette pan). If the frying pan's too wide, as Joni Mitchell discovered, then there's a risk of overcooking. It also means you don't get the benefit of a lovely fat frittata that's set top and bottom with a slightly wet middle.

Prep time: 10 minutes

Cooking time: 12 minutes

Freezable? No

1 tbsp olive oil

4 spring onions (scallions), roughly chopped

1 tsp finely chopped green chilli

salt and pepper

100g/3½oz/⅔ cup frozen peas

6 eggs, beaten vigorously

50g/1¾oz Gruyère cheese, grated

2 tbsp finely chopped parsley

AT HOME

Preheat the grill to high.

Heat the oil in a small frying pan over a medium heat and add the onions and chilli. Season with salt and pepper, and fry for a couple of minutes until softened, stirring occasionally.

Add the peas and shuggle the pan to separate them, then add the eggs, cheese and parsley. Add a little more salt and pepper, and cook over the lowest heat possible for 10 minutes, until set on the bottom but still runny on top.

Cook under the grill for 2 minutes, until set and a little browned. Leave to cool, then store in the fridge for up to 2 days.

IN EACH LUNCHBOX

Fat slices of frittata.

TO FINISH

Serve cold, with a green salad if you like.

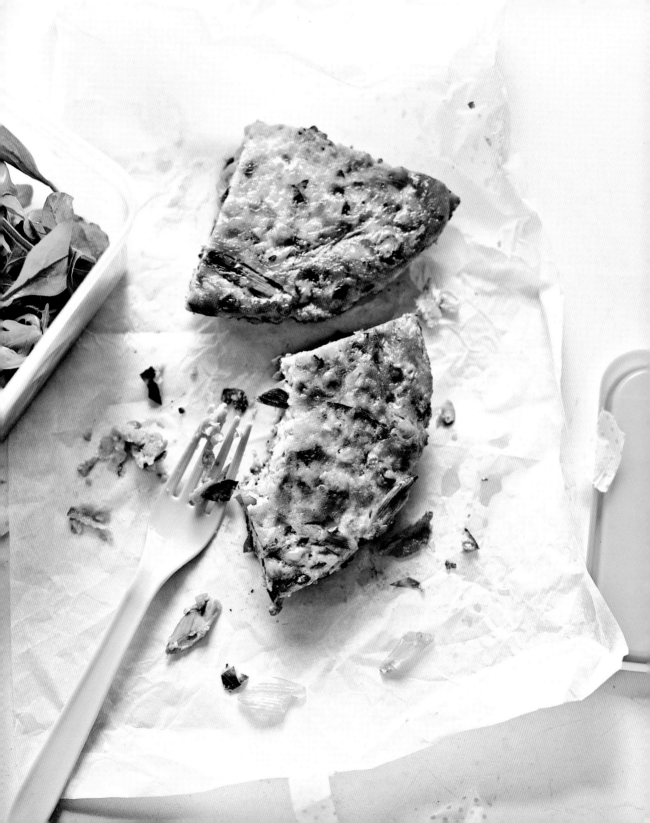

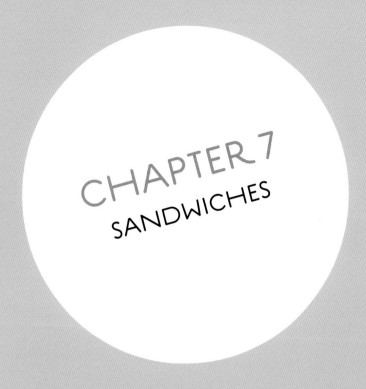

CHAPTER 7
SANDWICHES

The sandwich is surely the quintessential midweek lunch, devoured and adored around the world, from the Franco-Vietnamese *banh mi* to the humble cheese and pickle, from the meatball sub to the endless permutations of the Scandi *smørrebrød*.

Helen Graves, queen of the sandwich as far as I'm concerned, and author of the comprehensive and sensational *101 Sandwiches*, explains it to me thus: The insane popularity of the sandwich is surely owed to its convenience and versatility. A basic sarnie can be fashioned in minutes, but it's also good to put in a little extra effort occasionally. The world boasts some incredibly elaborate sandwich recipes, for example, the French-Viet mash-up that is the *banh mi* (a lesson in the power of contrasts), or the Portuguese *franceshina*, which packs four kinds of meat, cheese and, outrageously, beer sauce. How can you not instantly love anything that's drowned in beer sauce? There are endless combinations of fillings and wrappings to be explored but to be honest, for me, it's very hard to beat a well-cooked ham number with slightly too much nose-searing English mustard.

Can't argue with that, though you don't need me to give you a recipe for ham and mustard sandwiches. Here are 10 of my favourites.

A SANDWICH OF DUBIOUSLY ITALIAN PROVENANCE

When I was 17, I did an Italian exchange to Liguria in north-west Italy. The family I stayed with was lovely and kind and generous and fed me like a soldier. Sending me off on a trip one day, the mother forced a packed lunch of quite extraordinary proportions on me, comprising, among other things, a trio of sandwiches that could each have dispatched a goose. Not wanting to be rude, I gobbled the lot, only to find my hostess lost for words at the gluttony of this strange English boy. I believe she was just trying to give me several options, though my Italian wasn't good enough to be sure.

This sanger is partly based on that sandwich and partly based on *muffuletta*, an Italo-Louisianian sandwich.

Prep time: 10 minutes
Freezable? No

200g/7oz focaccia bread
50g/1¾oz pitted green olives, finely chopped
2 tbsp finely chopped parsley
1 shallot, peeled and finely sliced
½ small garlic clove, peeled and finely chopped
1 tbsp olive oil
salt and pepper
slices of salami
slices of mortadella or other pinkishly
        cured sausage
100g/3½oz mozzarella or provolone cheese, sliced

AT HOME

Cut the focaccia in two and then halve each piece horizontally.

Mix the olives, parsley, shallot, garlic and olive oil. Season with salt and pepper, and spoon over the bottom half of each sandwich-to-be.

Top with salami, mortadella and cheese, add a twist of pepper and a drop of oil, if you like, and finish with the other piece of bread. Press down firmly, then wrap tightly in clingfilm and store in the fridge for up to a day.

IN EACH LUNCHBOX

A sandwich.

TO FINISH

Eat cold, or warm in an oven at 180°C/350°F/ Gas mark 4 for 10 minutes. Come to that, you could also pop it in a toastie maker.

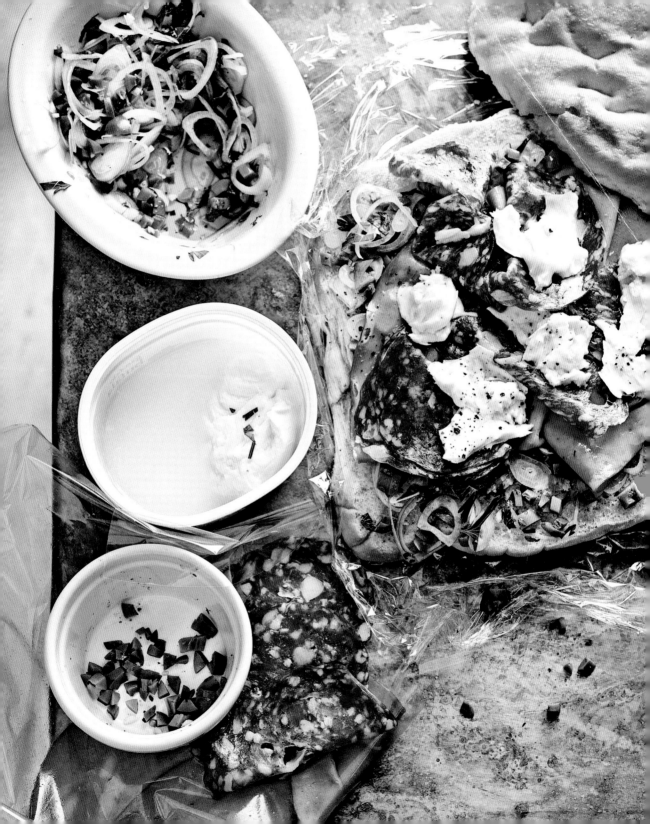

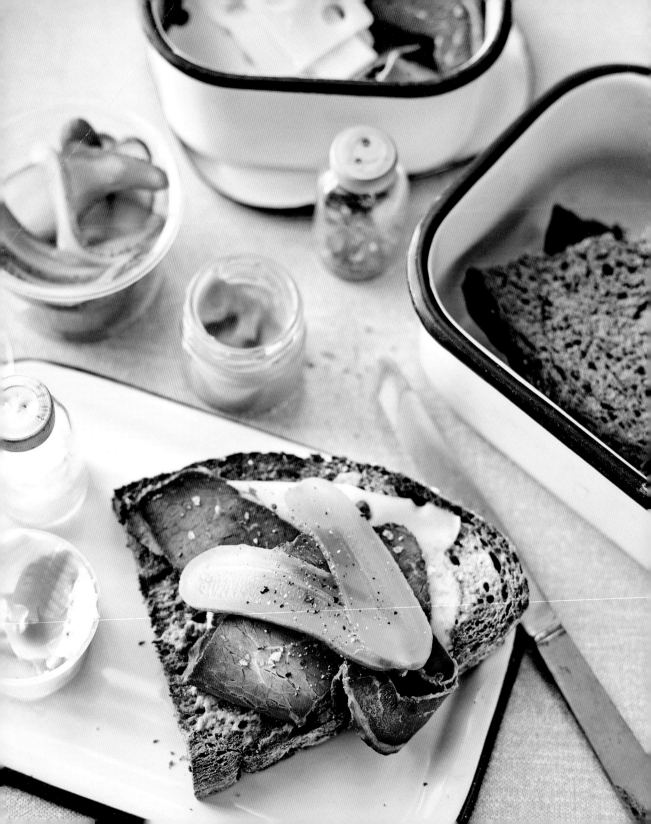

Chapter 13:
Entertaining with Whole Foods 248

Chapter 14:
For the Sweet Tooth **268**

Introduction
Kitchen Confidence

Do you want to know the secret to changing your diet and sustaining a new lifestyle over the long term? Cooking.

Preparing your own meals, in your own kitchen, gives you control over what you eat and a connection to your food choices that is hard to achieve any other way. We've helped guide thousands of patients, Whole Foods Market team members, friends, and family through the transition to a whole foods, plant-based diet, and we've concluded that the willingness and confidence to cook may be the key to success.

If you want to give yourself and your family the best chance of reaping the health benefits of diet change, the revolution needs to start in your kitchen. That's not to say there's anything wrong with having a special dinner out once in a while, or getting takeout on occasion when you're just too tired to do anything else. And, happily, it's getting easier to find healthy, real food on restaurant menus. But if you eat out, order in, or choose premade meals too often, you'll find yourself making countless small compromises that, over time, will add up to poor health. And too many families are doing just that. Research has shown that Americans today spend half as much time cooking as they did fifty years ago, and less time cooking than any other nation in the world.[1] Meanwhile, sales of prepared foods have risen steadily.

If you're someone who loves to cook, and you're blessed with the time to prepare delicious, nutritious meals for yourself and your family, you may not need much encouragement to roll up your sleeves and get cooking. But for many people, it's a daunting prospect. "I'm not much of a cook" is a common reaction. "I don't have time" is another, as are "I'm too tired" and "My kids don't like the food I make."

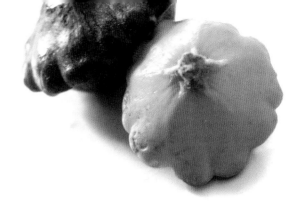

As busy professionals, we sympathize with those sentiments. We know what it's like to come home after a long day at work and feel like the last thing we want to do is put on an apron. We know how picky children can be. And we know how challenging it is to learn new ways of preparing food when we've spent our whole lives doing it the way our parents taught us. But we also know it doesn't have to be as hard as it seems. With some basic techniques, a few simple ingredients, and a dash of creativity, you can prepare meals that will satisfy you and your family without taking too much time out of your day. Cooking doesn't have to be complicated—it just takes a little confidence. And kitchen confidence is developed through rolling up your sleeves and trying new things! The one thing we can tell you without a doubt is that your investment of time and energy in the kitchen will be repaid many times over in the health dividends you'll enjoy every day.

How to Use This Book

Those who are familiar with the principles of whole-food, plant-based eating may be ready to jump ahead and start cooking. If that's you, bon appétit! Jump to part 2, page 24, for recipes. If you're new to this way of eating, or just need a refresher on the basics, read on for a short overview of the Whole Foods Diet. In part 1 of this book, we will:

- Review the key guidelines for the Whole Foods Diet
- Introduce the Essential Eight foods to eat as often as possible
- Share tips and best practices for successfully making the transition and simplifying your day-to-day cooking experience

In part 2, chefs Chad and Derek Sarno of Wicked Healthy, plus a few of our whole foodie friends and family, will present more than 120 carefully designed recipes. Following their simple, step-by-step guidelines will guarantee a delicious result every time. But because you don't want to always be dependent on recipes, they'll also teach you foundational techniques for preparing foods, developing flavor, and constructing your own meals—smoothies, breakfast bowls, soups, salads, sauces, dressings, entrées, and more. You'll learn basic principles for mixing and matching your favorite ingredients and shortcuts for making quick and easy family feasts.

The last thing we expect you to do is get out a recipe book three times a day and make something entirely new. As you gain confidence, you'll find that you can develop plans that allow you to quickly assemble meals to suit your schedule and preferences, using and reusing ingredients you have on hand or have prepared in advance. (See page 21 for more on meal planning and examples of how we plan our weekly menus.) You'll find a few favorite recipes that you can return to again and again, trying variations as you feel inspired. When you have a little more time, you can try a new recipe.

Our intention, in this book, is to equip you with the knowledge, skill, and confidence to create breakfasts, lunches, and dinners that will delight your senses and nourish your body, whether you follow these recipes or come up with your own. We want to make cooking so easy and enjoyable that you'll be inspired to make it part of your everyday routine. So let's get cooking!

Part 1
The Whole Foods Diet at Home

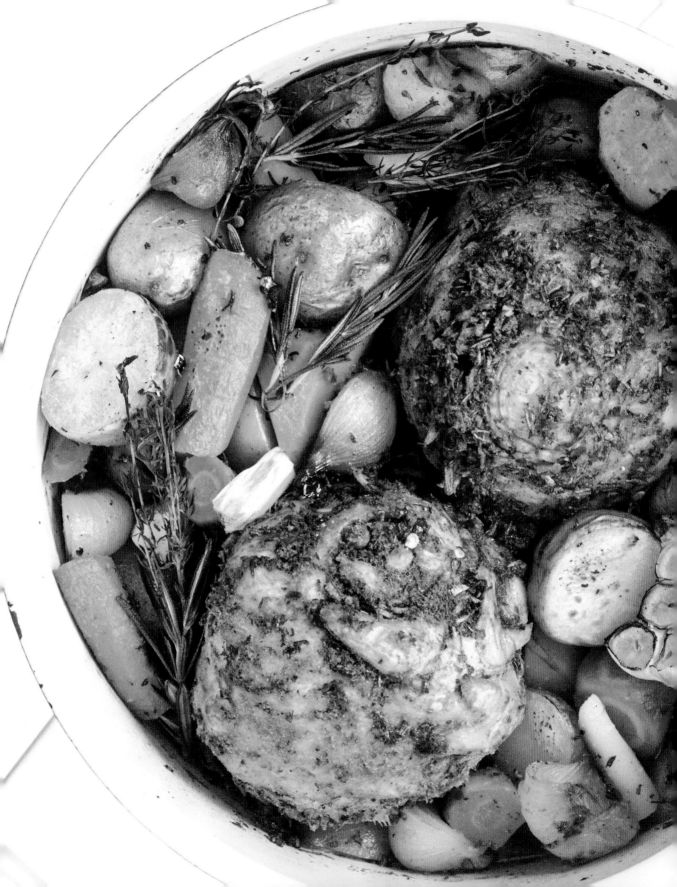

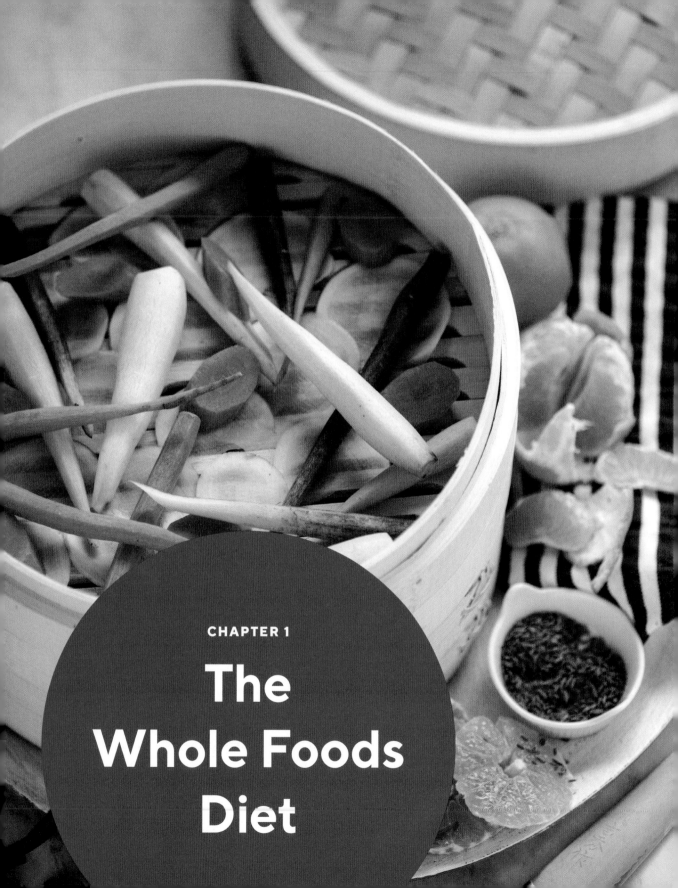

CHAPTER 1

The Whole Foods Diet

What is a whole foods, plant-based diet? Put simply, it's a diet that prioritizes eating whole or unprocessed plant foods; minimizes or eliminates meat, fish, dairy products, and eggs; and eliminates highly processed foods.

The Whole Foods Diet follows two simple guiding principles:

1. **Eat whole foods instead of highly processed foods.**

2. **Eat mostly plant foods (90 to 100% of your daily calories).**

Follow these two rules, and fairly quickly you may notice that you have more energy and youthful vitality. Continue eating this way, and you'll naturally reach and be able to maintain your optimum weight. You may find that existing health complaints resolve themselves and you're able to reduce your dependence on medications and even reverse chronic conditions. And you'll give yourself a much better chance of living a long, healthy, disease-free life.

This dietary pattern reflects the best science available on diet and health and is modeled on the eating habits of some of the world's longest-lived populations.[1] People who eat this way consistently report losing weight and maintaining a healthy weight without portion control or feelings of deprivation. Rigorous laboratory experiments, carefully controlled clinical trials, and long-term observational studies following millions of people over several decades all confirm the wisdom of eating more whole plant foods and minimizing or eliminating highly processed foods and animal products. The research supporting the wisdom of this way of eating, even briefly summarized, is enough to fill several books, and certainly far more than we have time to cover here. Suffice it to say that whole foods, plant-based diets have been shown to prevent and reverse heart disease and type 2 diabetes; lower cholesterol, blood pressure, and body weight; significantly reduce your risk of getting multiple types of cancer; extend your life span; and much more.[2] (For a summary of the key findings on whole foods, plant-based diets and health, with detailed references, we encourage you to read our companion book, *The Whole Foods Diet*.)

We are lucky to live in a time when there is an unprecedented wealth of information available about the relationship between diet, lifestyle, and health. However, many people feel confused and overwhelmed by the conflicting messages promoted by the media, the food industry, and the latest fad diets. Sometimes it can seem like no one agrees on what diet helps humans thrive. But don't be fooled. Yes, there will always be

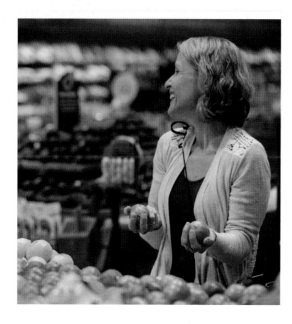

We as authors consider ourselves lifetime students of nutritional science. We have each spent decades studying the topic and continue to seek out the latest studies. But it's our firm conviction that, while new information will continue to inform us, the information we already have is more than enough to ensure that we live long, healthy lives. We just need to act on it! And that means, above all, eating a whole foods, 90 to 100% plant-based diet.

controversies and contradictions, and there is still a lot that science does not yet understand about the interplay between the foods we eat and the systems of our bodies. But there is far more agreement than there is disagreement about the basic themes of a healthy diet.

Dr. David Katz, founding director of the Yale-Griffin Prevention Research Center, puts it bluntly: "We are not, absolutely not, emphatically NOT clueless about the basic care and feeding of Homo sapiens. The fundamental lifestyle formula, including diet, conducive to the addition of years to our lives, and life to our years, is reliably clear and a product of science, sense, and global consensus."[3] What is that formula? In 2014, after carefully comparing the medical evidence for and against each of the major dietary trends in the West today—including Paleo, Mediterranean, low-fat, low-carb, low-glycemic, vegetarian, and vegan—Katz's conclusion was unequivocal: "A diet of minimally processed foods close to nature, predominantly plants, is decisively associated with health promotion and disease prevention."[4]

Is This a Vegan Diet?

The authors of this book eat a 100% plant-based (or vegan) diet, because in addition to its health benefits, we believe from an ethical and environmental standpoint that taking animal lives in order to satisfy our appetites is unnecessary. However, our focus in this book is health, not ethics, and therefore we have based our dietary recommendations on our best reading of nutrition science. Our conclusion, from a health standpoint, is that the optimum diet for general health and longevity is one in which *90 to 100% of calories* are derived from plants—a whole foods, 90 to 100% plant-based diet. This means that if you choose to eat meat, fish, eggs, or dairy products, you keep them to 10% or less of your total calories. And while there's no exact certainty on what percentage is ideal, we believe that less is better.

Did you know that the longest-lived populations on earth—people living in what researcher Dan Buettner calls the Blue Zones—eat diets that are, on average, 90% plant-based? Studies show that people who eat predominantly plant foods have significantly better long-term health outcomes than those who eat a diet heavy in animal foods. And plant-based diets have been shown to not only prevent but even reverse chronic conditions like type 2 diabetes and heart disease.

Furthermore, there is growing evidence for

The Whole Foods Diet at a Glance

Foods to Eat Freely

- Vegetables, fruits, intact whole grains and whole-grain pasta, beans and other legumes, starchy vegetables

Foods to Eat in Moderation
(especially if you're trying to lose weight)

- Whole-grain breads, tortillas, crackers, dry cereals, tofu, tempeh, soy and nut milks, nuts, seeds, avocados, olives, dried fruit
- Meat (unprocessed), fish, eggs, and dairy products (keep animal foods to 10% or less of your caloric intake)

Foods to Avoid

- Refined flours, sugar, oils, baked goods, sweets, junk food, soda
- Lunch meats, bacon, sausages, hot dogs, salami

links between high levels of animal foods and chronic disease. Red meats and processed meats in particular have been connected with greater risk of death from all causes, and high consumption of animal protein has been correlated with higher incidences of cancer and mortality. The links between processed meats and cancer are so concerning that the World Health Organization recently classified them as a Group 1 carcinogen, alongside cigarettes and asbestos.

All this adds up to a conclusive case for *significantly reducing* consumption of animal foods. Some doctors and nutritionists extrapolate that this means we should eliminate animal foods altogether. Perhaps they are right (particularly for those people looking to reverse chronic disease), but the science on this point is not yet definitive. Once again, we personally eat 100% plant-based, and believe it's a very healthy choice, as well as the most compassionate one, but we try not to let our ethical convictions cloud our objectivity when it comes to what the science shows. We remain open-minded as to what future research may tell us about the benefits and risks of including limited amounts of animal products in a healthy diet.

It's also important to understand that merely avoiding animal foods does not make a diet healthy. Plenty of people who choose a vegan or vegetarian diet (perhaps for ethical reasons) end up eating very unhealthy, highly processed foods. Whether you choose to be vegan or not, eating more whole plant foods, in all their wonderful and varied forms, is a clear path to health and longevity. And because health is not the only consideration when it comes to what we eat and do not eat, we encourage you to also consider the impact of your food choices on your fellow creatures and on the planet we all share.

How Animal Foods Are Used in This Book

Since the chefs who created the recipes in this book are vegan, all their recipes are 100% plant-based.

For those readers who are not 100% plant-based, we have included a few recipes created by Whole Foods Market that include animal foods as optional ingredients, with plant-based options for those who are vegan.

If you do choose to eat animal foods, we suggest you think of them as occasional side dishes or condiments—not as the primary calorie source in every meal. This is reminiscent of more traditional diets, in which animal foods were eaten sparingly or occasionally, on particular feast days, not as the centerpiece on the table. We also recommend that you choose grass-fed, organic, antibiotic-free meat and dairy products, pasture-raised chickens and eggs, and wild-caught fish and seafood (where possible), and avoid all processed meats.

Whole Foods vs. Processed Foods

A *whole food* means an unprocessed food—a food that is still close to the form in which it grew. It has not been broken down into its component parts and refined into a different form. None of its essential nutritious parts have been removed, and no unhealthy substances (sugar, salt, oil, or chemicals such as artificial flavors, preservatives, or colors) have been added to it. In short, it's *real* food.

Consider a fresh ear of corn compared to a salty fried corn chip. Or a ripe, juicy bowl of strawberries compared to a bowl of strawberry ice cream. Or a grain of wheat compared to a

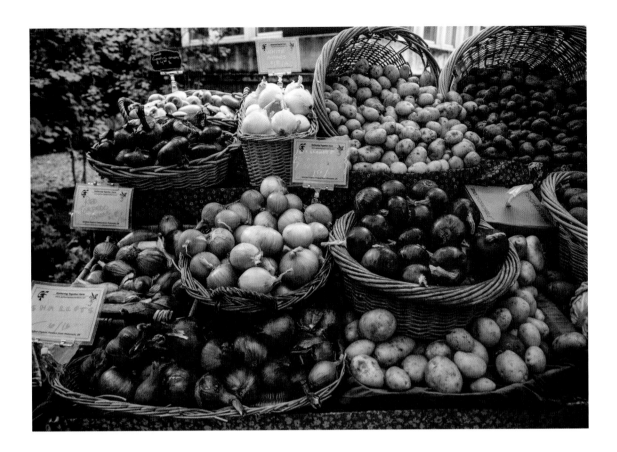

doughnut. In each of these examples, the original whole food gets stripped of fiber and essential nutrients, and then combined with ingredients like oil, salt, sugar, chemical flavorings, and preservatives to create something bearing little resemblance to the original plant.

Does that mean you need to eat your food looking exactly as it did when it was picked from the ground, the vine, or the tree? No. The truth is that almost every food undergoes some form of processing, even if it's simply the process of being harvested and having its stalks, leaves, or inedible husks removed. Processing is best understood as a spectrum. If you take oats and cut them up, you get steel-cut oats. If you press them flat, you get rolled oats. While these forms of oats are

technically not "whole," what matters is that none of their important nutrients have been removed in the process and nothing unhealthy has been added to them—no sugar, salt, oil, chemicals, or preservatives. They are so minimally processed that they fit our favorite definition of a whole food, taken from Dr. Michael Greger: "Nothing bad added, nothing good taken away."[5]

By this definition, you can see why whole wheat pasta, made from ground-up whole grains, is a better choice than white pasta, made from refined flour with most of its fiber removed. You can see why peanut butter that is made from ground-up peanuts is a better choice than peanut butter with added oil, sugar, and salt. And you can see why a fresh orange is a better choice than a glass

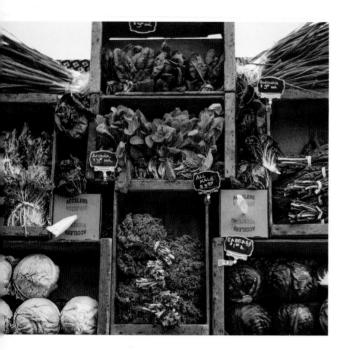

What you'll find, if you do, is that this food loves you right back—nourishing your body, supporting your immune system, and boosting your vitality.

Understanding Calorie Density: The Secret to Weight Loss

Because weight loss is the number one reason people change their diets, and because excess weight plays a part in so many chronic conditions, we'd like to take a moment to share a key concept that can help you reach your ideal weight and feel nourished and well-fed every day. The secret to weight loss is this: *Choose foods that leave you feeling full and satisfied without consuming more calories than you need.*

The last thing we want you to do is spend your life counting calories, and one of the wonderful things about a whole foods, plant-based diet is that once you get the hang of it, you won't have to worry about that. However, understanding how calories work can be helpful as you shift your diet and develop healthy habits. Calories are a measure of the energy contained in a food, and they can come in the form of carbohydrates, protein, or fats. You need a certain number of calories to fuel your daily activity, but if you consistently consume more than

of orange juice, with much of its fiber removed and its sugars therefore concentrated. The bottom line is that real foods, eaten close to their whole and natural state, are optimally beneficial for the body.

To summarize, here's your recipe for health and longevity: Eat lots of fruits, vegetables, whole grains, and legumes, plus some nuts and seeds. Cut out highly processed foods, especially refined flours, sugars, and oils. If you choose to eat animal foods, keep them to 10% or less of your calories—and the less, the better.

The Whole Foods Diet is not a short-term plan—it's a sustainable, healthy lifestyle that we hope you'll never look back from. If you follow the overall pattern described above, you'll ensure that you get all the benefits. Get the big picture right, and there's room to customize the particulars to fit your individual goals, health conditions, and personal preferences.

We hope you'll fall in love with the delicious, life-enhancing foods you'll find in these pages.

How Processing Increases Calorie Density

Corn: 500 calories/pound →
Corn oil: 4,000 calories/pound

Sweet potato: 389 calories/pound →
Sweet potato chips: 2,400 calories/pound

Beets: 200 calories/pound →
Refined beet sugar: 1,800 calories/pound

you need, your body will store them as fat, causing you to gain weight. If you reduce your calorie intake to less than you need, your body will burn stored fat and you'll lose weight. The problem, however, is that many low-calorie diets leave you feeling hungry all the time. Your body sends hormonal signals telling your brain it has not eaten enough. No matter how strong your willpower, it's tough to override those powerful instincts for too long.

To be successful in losing weight (or maintaining a healthy weight), you need to feel satiated by the foods you eat. Satiety is the opposite of hunger, and it's the body's mechanism for telling you when to stop eating. When it comes to satisfying and filling you up, not all calories are created equal. For example, four chicken nuggets contain about 200 calories, but won't make you feel full at all; eat one medium sweet potato, which also contains 200 calories, and you'll start to feel quite satisfied. Therefore, the sweet potato is a much better choice if you want to avoid eating more calories than your body needs.

The technical term for this is *calorie density*. A calorie-dense food contains a lot of calories but has a fairly low bulk or weight (like the chicken nuggets, deep-fried in oil). A less calorie-dense food contains fewer calories relative to its much greater bulk or weight (like the sweet potato). The reason this matters is that your body has several ways to measure the amount of food you eat and tell you when to stop, and one of those is directly related to how much the food you consume "stretches" your stomach. When you eat calorie-dense foods, you confuse your stomach's "stretch receptors" into thinking you're not eating enough, even though you're consuming more calories than you need. When you choose less calorie-dense foods, you'll feel satisfied, because their greater bulk fills you up.

The good news is that almost all whole plant foods are naturally on the lower end of the

Weight Loss Strategies: Working with Calorie Density

If you're trying to lose weight, it's important to learn to spot calorie-dense foods and to limit their place on your plate. That doesn't mean you can't ever eat these foods, but they should be balanced with larger portions of foods that are lower in calorie density, and when possible, play a smaller role in your overall diet. Here are some tips for navigating recipes to ensure you'll feel full without overconsuming calories:

- Focus on fruits and vegetables, whole grains, starchy vegetables, and legumes. Save more calorie-dense plant foods, like nuts, seeds, coconut, avocados, and olives, for special occasions, and avoid eating them in large amounts.

- If a recipe contains nuts, seeds, coconut, or dried fruit, be aware that it's likely to be more calorie-dense. Eat a smaller portion or reduce the quantity of nuts, seeds, coconut, or dried fruit.

- If a recipe calls for a nondairy milk, such as soy, nut, or coconut milk, consider diluting it with water as your palate allows.

- Pay attention to sauces and condiments that contain nuts and seeds. You don't need to use too much to enjoy the flavor.

- Remember that even whole-food desserts tend to be calorie-dense, since they often contain nuts and dried fruit. Keep your portions small and consider fresh fruit before choosing more calorie-dense desserts.

Whole Foods vs. Processed Foods

While these do not apply in every case, here are some general rules you can use to help distinguish between whole and processed foods:

Whole Foods:

- Are close to their original state
- Spoil faster
- Are things your great-grandparents would have recognized as food
- Don't usually have ingredient lists, or, if they do, have short ones
- Are often sold without packaging
- Are often found around the perimeter of the grocery store

Highly Processed Foods:

- Bear little resemblance to their original state
- Do not spoil easily
- Are things your great-grandparents probably wouldn't recognize
- Have (often long) ingredient lists and are packaged or boxed
- Are often found in the center of the grocery store

dramatically. The results are high-calorie foods that take up very little space in your stomach, leaving you feeling hungry even though you've consumed a lot of calories. These unnaturally concentrated foods subvert your natural instincts, confusing your body's regulation systems and tricking you into overeating. Animal foods also contain very little fiber and more calories, especially processed animal foods. When you eat whole plant foods, you can begin to trust the messages your body is giving you, and know when you've eaten enough instead of too much.

With these basic principles in mind, you can start to understand why so many people struggle with weight gain, and why diets that rely on portion control and calorie restriction rarely work. By choosing whole foods, mostly plants, you won't have to obsessively monitor your portion sizes or deny your hunger. In fact, you may need to eat larger meals than you are accustomed to! Don't make the mistake of just eating salads and a few veggies and thinking that's the best way to lose weight. You also need to include highly satiating plant foods like starchy vegetables, whole grains, and legumes to ensure that you meet your energy needs (see page 14 for our list of the Essential Eight foods that together will ensure that you are nourished and satisfied every day).

calorie-density scale. This is because they contain large amounts of fiber and water in addition to carbohydrates, proteins, or fats, which increases the bulk of the food without adding calories. The most calorie-dense plant foods are nuts and seeds, or fatty fruits like olives or avocados.

Processed foods tend to be calorie dense because they have been stripped of fiber and water and have often had fats and sugars added; hence, the number of calories relative to weight increases

Why Are Oils Off-Limits?

The Whole Foods Diet recommends staying away from all refined, extracted oils—including canola oil, olive oil, sunflower oil, corn oil, coconut oil, and more. That may surprise you—especially when it comes to olive oil and coconut oil, which many people consider to be health foods.

Oils are basically empty calories. They are 100% fat and largely devoid of other nutritional value. A single tablespoon of oil contains approximately 120 calories (more calories than an entire pound of many vegetables), making them one of the most calorie-dense foods on the planet. And they won't fill you up at all, because all the fiber has been removed, making them a recipe for weight gain. Oils are processed foods, and although there may be differences between the types of fats they deliver, we don't consider any of them to be "healthy." You're much better off eating the whole plants they came from—olives, corn, nuts, and seeds.

The recipes in this book don't use oil, with the exception of an occasional spray to coat a grill or a pan when needed. You may be surprised how easy it is to cook without oil—you can roast, sauté, and dress salads without reaching for that bottle of empty calories. See page 78 for the Dry Sauté Method and page 153 for salad dressings.

What Sweeteners Should I Choose?

We do not recommend using any extracted or concentrated sweeteners—that includes table sugar, high-fructose corn syrup, and all the so-called "natural" sweeteners like maple syrup, honey, agave nectar, and so on. (One or two recipes in this book use small amounts of date sugar or date syrup, but we don't recommend these as everyday ingredients.) If you have a sweet tooth, see chapter 14 for some guilt-free desserts and learn how to use fruit pastes (page 56) to sweeten parfaits, crumbles, sorbets, and more.

Can I Use Salt?

There is nothing health-promoting about added sodium other than when it helps to encourage you to eat more whole plant foods. That being the case, we recommend using as little added sodium as necessary and learning other ways to make your food taste great (see chapter 6 for tips on maximizing flavor). We've been mindful of not using too much added salt in the recipes in this book, but if you're trying to reduce your sodium intake, you can choose to use even less. We also encourage you to try adding a sprinkle of salt to the food on your plate rather than using it in a recipe; you'll get better bang for your buck because you taste more and use less. Over time you'll find that you need less salt as you stay mindful of it in your diet and your taste buds evolve.

When buying packaged foods, pay particular attention to the sodium content. When possible, choose foods with no added sodium—for example, canned beans or tomatoes are often available in both versions. Choose low-sodium versions of tamari and vegetable broth. If you do buy foods with added salt, use the following handy rule: look for a 1:1 ratio or less of sodium milligrams to calories.

Is It Important to Buy Organic?

The most important dietary change you can make is to eat more fruits and vegetables. Even if they are not organic, the benefits of eating them far outweigh the potential risks of pesticide consumption. However, if you have the option to choose organic, there are many good reasons to do so. You'll be encouraging better farming practices, protecting the environment from toxic chemicals, supporting independent farmers, and ensuring that your food has met stringent quality standards.

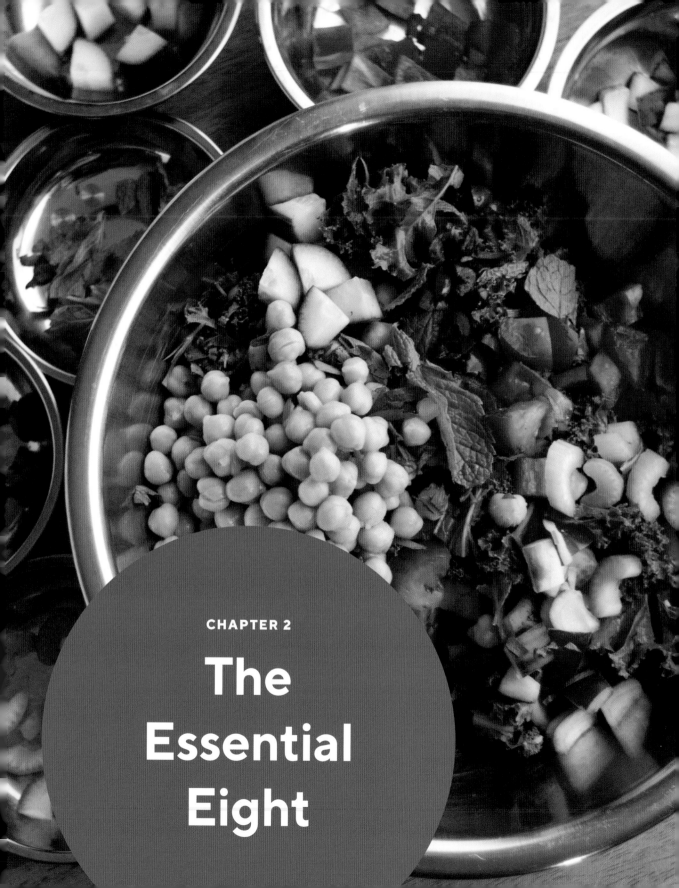

CHAPTER 2

The Essential Eight

Health isn't just about cutting out the "bad" stuff; it's also about loading up on the "good" stuff—the foods that are delicious *and* nutritious! Diet change doesn't have to be a story of deprivation—it can be an experience of abundance and satisfaction. You'll find there is an endless variety of nutrient-rich, health-promoting whole plant foods, and the good news is, they're all good for you! To help you maximize the disease-fighting, life-extending power of your diet, we've come up with a list of food groups we call the Essential Eight. We encourage you to eat these foods as often as possible—ideally, every day.

1. Whole Grains and Starchy Vegetables

Sweet and earthy yams. Hearty winter squashes. Chewy, satisfying grains. Tender, juicy corn. Creamy potatoes. All these comforting carbohydrate-rich foods are central to the Whole Foods Diet. This is great news for many people who have reluctantly adopted the popular "carbs are bad" philosophy and been taught to shun some of our favorite foods.

When it comes to carbohydrates, there's a critical distinction that many popular diets miss: the difference between whole carbohydrates, such as whole grains and starchy vegetables, and highly processed refined carbohydrates, such as white

flours, sugars, and the countless foods made from these ingredients. It's true that highly processed carbs spell disaster for your health, delivering a condensed load of calories with little or no fiber or healthful micronutrients, and leading to weight gain and a host of related problems. But whole grains and starchy vegetables play a key role in an optimum diet. In fact, they should make up the bulk of your calorie intake.

Contrary to popular belief, eating whole grains and starchy veggies can actually help you *lose* weight. Whole-grain consumption has been associated with lower levels of abdominal fat in adults.[1] These hearty foods leave you feeling full and satisfied, which means you are less likely to overeat. Carbohydrates are the best energy

The Essential Eight

1
Whole grains and
starchy vegetables
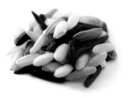

2
Beans and
other legumes
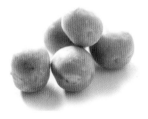

3
Berries
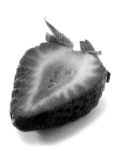

4
Other fruits
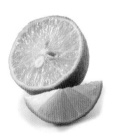

5
Cruciferous
vegetables
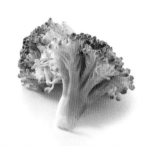

6
Leafy greens
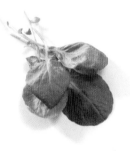

7
Nonstarchy
vegetables
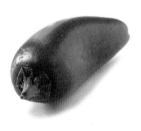

8
Nuts and seeds
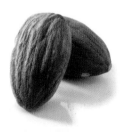

source available for the human body, and starch has formed the basis of human diets for millennia.[2] Whole grains also provide fiber, protein, essential fatty acids, vitamins, minerals, and numerous phytochemicals. They have been linked to a reduction in heart disease, cancer, respiratory disease, infectious disease, and mortality from all causes,[3] and have been associated with lower risk of type 2 diabetes.[4]

Eating whole grains is also beneficial for bowel health and promotes the growth of healthy gut bacteria.

Whole grains and starchy vegetables can be added to your daily menu in any number of ways.

Keep some cooked grains in the fridge or freezer for adding to salads or building quick and easy grain bowls (see chapter 5 for basic instructions on cooking grains). Steel-cut oats, buckwheat, and amaranth make warming, nutty breakfast cereals. Potatoes and sweet potatoes can be topped with chili or other sauces. Whole-grain pastas can be served with lots of fresh, vibrant vegetables.

Note: In this category we also include grainlike seeds (or "pseudograins")—such as quinoa, millet, amaranth, buckwheat, and teff—which are nutritionally similar to grains.

TRY THIS...

Spring Risotto with Peas & Mint (page 37)

"Fried" Farro with Caramelized Fennel & Tofu (page 173)

Spiced Sweet Potatoes with Green Onion Vinaigrette (page 77)

2. Beans and Other Legumes

Wholesome, satisfying, and bursting with health benefits, the legume family—which includes beans, lentils, and peas—plays a starring role in a whole foods, plant-based diet. Look beyond the two or three familiar beans and lentils you typically encounter, and you'll be amazed at the incredible variety and versatility of the legume.

Most legumes are low-fat, high-protein, starchy foods packed with vitamins, minerals, antioxidant compounds, and dietary fiber. Almost all varieties provide iron, zinc, B vitamins, magnesium, and potassium, among many other nutrients. They also contain significant amounts of fiber and resistant starch, which helps to regulate bowel movements, remove toxins, and keep blood sugar levels in check.[5] Beans have been found to lower blood pressure[6] and reduce cholesterol.[7]

A love of legumes is a common denominator among all the world's longest-lived cultures. According to Blue Zones researcher Dan Buettner, beans are a "cornerstone of every longevity diet."[8] An average of 1 cup per day is associated with a four-year increase in life expectancy, and scientists have pointed to legume consumption as "the most important dietary predictor of survival in older people of different ethnicities."[9]

Try dried or canned beans such as black, pinto, navy, cannellini, and kidney beans, as well as chickpeas (garbanzo beans) and black-eyed peas. Soybeans and foods made from them, such as tempeh, tofu, soy milk, and miso, are also a healthy choice (although we advise you to be aware of their higher fat content and avoid highly processed soy products such as fake meats). Peas and lentils come in many colors. Some varieties of legume, like fava beans, lima beans, English peas, and soybeans (edamame), are eaten fresh.

We love to cook up a batch of beans once a week and add them to salads or grain bowls (see instructions, page 41). The possibilities for eating these nutritious and delicious foods are endless, and you can find inspiration for legume-based meals from around the globe.

Note: Green beans and snow peas are legumes, but because the whole pod is eaten, we group them with nonstarchy vegetables. Peanuts are classified as legumes, but nutritionally behave more like nuts, so we group them with nuts and seeds.

TRY THIS...
Wicked Good Pot of Cassoulet Beans (page 46)
Ethiopian Lentils (page 49)
Thai Curry Chickpeas, Collards, & Rice (page 196)

3. Berries

Plump blackberries. Zesty raspberries. Succulent strawberries. Juicy blueberries. Berries are like nature's candy—and they're good for you as well.

There is a growing body of scientific evidence for the health benefits of berries. They have been shown to potentially protect against cancer and inhibit the formation of tumors,[10] and protect against cognitive decline.[11] Consuming berries daily raises "good" HDL cholesterol and lowers blood pressure, both factors associated with a lower risk of cardiovascular disease.[12] Berries contain more antioxidants per serving than any other food except spices, which may account for their outsize health benefits.[13]

You can eat berries any time of the day! They make a great topping for a breakfast bowl, add a burst of zesty sweetness to a salad, or satisfy your sweet tooth in (or as) a dessert. Choose organic berries when possible—conventional varieties often receive a large dose of pesticides. Frozen berries are a healthy and convenient choice, retaining all the benefits of the fresh fruit. If you're trying to lose weight, be careful with dried berries, such as raisins, dates, currants, goji berries, or cranberries; although they're still a healthy choice, dehydration concentrates their natural sugars, making them more calorie-dense foods.

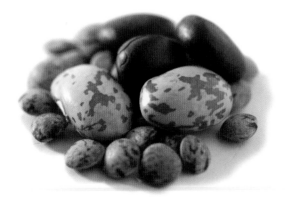

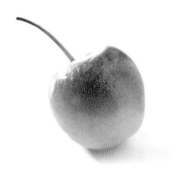

Note: We use the term *berry* in its colloquial rather than its scientific form, so we include cherries, grapes, cranberries, currants, and so on in this category.

TRY THIS...

Cherry Cocoa Kicker Smoothie (page 111)

Dark Chocolate Pudding Parfaits with Berries & Cacao Nibs (page 270)

Berry Port Compote (page 273)

than fruit juice, which has lost its essential fiber and many other nutrients along with it, and will deliver a highly concentrated dose of sugar to your bloodstream.

Note: The only exceptions to our wholehearted encouragement to eat as much fruit as you like are avocados and olives—both are technically fruits, but are also high in fat, so they're best consumed in limited quantities, especially if you're trying to lose weight.

TRY THIS...

Mango Millet with Raspberries & Toasted Pistachios (page 116)

Roots & Fruits Pad Thai Salad (page 143)

Riesling & Orange Poached Pears (page 277)

4. Other Fruits

Crisp apples, creamy bananas, tangy mangoes, succulent peaches, zesty citrus, juicy melons—nature's sweet bounty offers you so many options to choose from. Fruits are high in fiber and boast hundreds of beneficial nutrients. They're truly one of the healthiest foods you can eat. It's not surprising that humans evolved to be drawn to sweetness—when fruits were the only sweet choice (besides wild honey), that instinct served our ancestors well. Unfortunately, today that instinct often leads us to less healthy choices, like cookies, chocolate, or candy, but you can learn to redirect it.

You can eat fruit for breakfast, in smoothies, in salads, or in desserts. Choose organic where possible, especially for varieties where you eat the skin. Whole fruit is always a better choice

Don't Fear the Fruit!

There's a common concern that fruits are a sugary food and should be avoided, especially by those suffering from diabetes or trying to lose weight. These fears are misguided, and unfortunate, because they lead people to shun one of the healthiest foods on the planet. It's true that fresh fruit contains high levels of fructose. However, when fructose comes in the form of a whole fruit (rather than in its processed forms, such as high-fructose corn syrup), it's combined with plentiful fiber, water, and other nutrients that change the way it affects the body. Numerous studies have confirmed that eating fruit is hugely beneficial to health and has no negative effects, even for diabetics.[14] So don't fear the fruit!

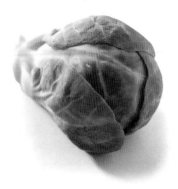

5. Cruciferous Vegetables

What do broccoli, radishes, cabbage, collard greens, Brussels sprouts, cauliflower, artichokes, arugula, and kale have in common? Not only are these diverse foods all part of the cruciferous (or brassica) family, they also share extraordinary health benefits, especially when it comes to preventing cancer.[15] In fact, Dr. Joel Fuhrman calls them "the most powerful anticancer foods in existence"—a distinction that may be attributable to a group of substances called glucosinolates that give these foods their pungent aroma.[16]

If your mom always told you to eat your broccoli, she was right! The good news is, there are numerous creative and delicious ways to eat cruciferous vegetables that your mom may not have known about.

TRY THIS...
**Roasted Brussels Sprouts & Shallots
(page 92)**
Whole Roasted Spiced Cauliflower (page 94)
**Wild Mushroom & Kale Ragout over Soft Polenta
(page 194)**

6. Leafy Greens

Leafy greens are a nutritional powerhouse. In fact, they hold the distinction of being the most nutrient-dense foods you can eat.[17] Spinach, chard, and romaine are packed with fiber, protein, and micronutrients, as are many leafy greens that also

fall into the cruciferous category, such as kale, collards, arugula, and bok choy. Greens were found by Harvard researchers to be the food most highly associated with protection from major chronic diseases and cardiovascular disease.[18] In addition, they have been associated with a reduced risk of developing diabetes.[19]

You can eat greens raw as a salad, blended in a smoothie, steamed, or wilted in a soup or stew. Greens are so extraordinarily healthful that we recommend adding them to the dishes you cook whenever possible.

TRY THIS...
**Spinach Gomae with Toasted Sesame Seeds
(page 77)**
Green Energy Smoothie (page 107)
Moroccan Kale & Hemp Seed Salad (page 145)

7. Nonstarchy Vegetables

If there's one piece of advice that nutritionists and dietary experts seem to universally agree upon, it's this: *eat more vegetables!* Yet shockingly few Americans—a mere one in ten, according to a recent government report—eat even the minimal recommended amount daily.[20] If you follow a whole foods, plant-based diet, you'll be safely part of

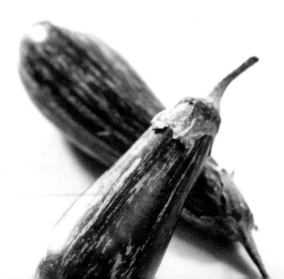

that minority, and your body will thank you for it. It has been estimated that if Americans ate just one more serving of fruits and vegetables daily, it would save more than thirty thousand lives and billions of dollars in medical costs annually.[21]

In addition to the specific categories of vegetables already discussed, there are countless others you can try, including zucchini, carrots, peppers, mushrooms, green beans, onions, eggplants, celery, asparagus, and many, many more. Each of these vegetables has its own list of health benefits, and eating a wide variety of vegetables regularly will ensure optimum nourishment for your body. Learn foundational techniques for grilling, roasting, steaming, and slow cooking your favorites in chapter 7. Add them to salads, soups, or pasta dishes. However you enjoy them, eat them. Then eat some more!

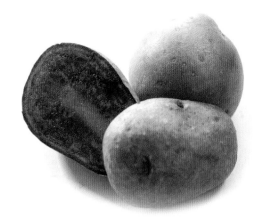

TRY THIS…
Vibrant Veggie Gado Gado (page 138)
Summer Chopped Bowl (page 179)
Very Veggie Pizza (page 240)

8. Nuts and Seeds

If you want to add years to your life, there's good reason to add nuts and seeds to your diet. Consumption of nuts and seeds has been associated with reduced risk of heart disease and diabetes, as well as an increased life span.[22] The centenarians living in the Blue Zones consume a handful (around 1 to 2 ounces) of varying types of nuts per day, and in the Adventist Health Studies (a series of long-term studies exploring the relationship between diet, lifestyle, and disease among the Seventh Day Adventists, who have a significantly lower risk of several chronic diseases than other Americans), nut-eaters were shown to live a couple of years longer than those who did

not eat nuts.[23] The nutritional power of these foods is not surprising when you consider that each nut or seed contains the makings of an entire plant or tree.

One particularly important feature of nuts and seeds is that they are some of the most concentrated plant sources of omega-3 fatty acids. The body can't make these essential fats, which support brain function, among other things, so we have to get them from food or supplements. Flaxseeds, chia seeds, hemp seeds, and walnuts are especially rich in omega-3s.

Some people raise concerns about the relatively high calorie density of nuts; however, studies have generally *not* associated them with a significant increase in weight or BMI, perhaps because they are a naturally filling food.[24] If, however, you're trying to *lose* weight, limit your nut and seed intake to less than a handful per day.

Nuts and seeds make great toppings for breakfast bowls or salads, and they can be blended into creamy sauces for your favorite grains and vegetables.

TRY THIS…
Steamed Kale with Toasted Seeds (page 76)
Almond-Chile Sauce (page 158)
"Supercede" Bars (page 272)

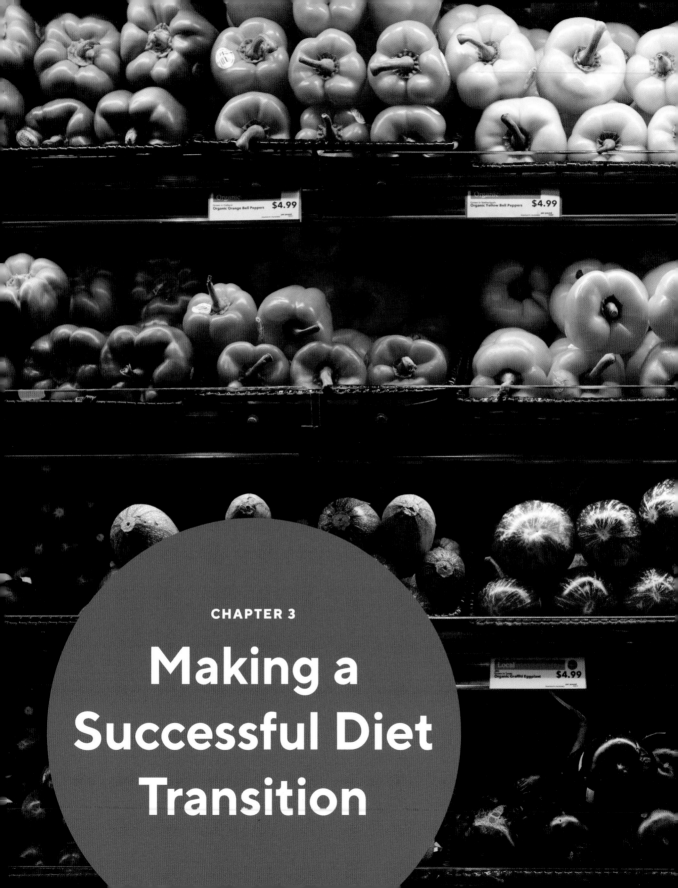

CHAPTER 3

Making a Successful Diet Transition

The Whole Foods Diet is a fundamental change in your habits around eating and preparing food. Once you become accustomed to the new routine, it will become easier and easier. You don't need to become a gourmet chef or rely on recipes every day to be a happy, healthy Whole Foodie.

If you enjoy getting creative in the kitchen, by all means, entertain yourself with elaborate new meals. But if you're pressed for time, don't be afraid to keep it simple. In the midst of our busy lives, the last thing most of us need is an overly complicated diet. Get the basics right, learn to cook a few meals you love, and eat plenty of them. Once you become accustomed to the whole foods, plant-based lifestyle, you'll quickly gain the confidence to create your own variations. Check out our favorite time-saving strategies below.

Meal Planning and Batch Cooking: Keys to Success

If you want to take the stress out of day-to-day eating, we highly recommend that you get in the habit of making a weekly meal plan. This can allow you to think ahead, be prepared, and make your ingredients multitask. For example, you might plan several meals that use similar ingredients so you don't end up with half-used bags of produce, bunches of herbs, cans of beans, or jars of condiments.

If you work Monday to Friday, you might do your planning Friday evening or Saturday morning, including making a shopping list, so you can use some time on the weekend to shop and prepare. Here's how we approach our weekly meal planning:

Breakfasts: Pick one or two simple favorites for weekdays (a breakfast bowl, oatmeal, or a smoothie, for example) and plan to eat these every day, varying the fruit or other toppings if you want to mix it up. On weekends, if you feel like eating something different, pick a brunch dish like pancakes or a savory hash.

Lunches: If you've cooked a nice dinner the night before, you might plan on leftovers for lunch. Otherwise, go with a simple salad, wrap, sandwich, and/or soup.

Dinners: Once or twice a week, you might choose a new recipe and cook enough for dinner and leftovers. For the other nights, plan on putting together simple bowl or salad meals that include a grain or starchy vegetable, some kind of bean or other legume, some vegetables, and a sauce or dressing. (See chapter 9 for how to create hearty main-dish salads and chapter 11 for how

Trust That Your Tastes Will Evolve

When you shift to a new way of eating, the tastes, smells, and textures may be unfamiliar at first. It's natural to long for the familiar flavors you've eaten all your life. If you find yourself struggling with the experience of new foods, here's the good news: Tastes are not innate; they are acquired. You've developed them over a lifetime of eating certain types of food—particularly the salty, fatty, or sugary variety. And if they've developed, that means they can change (a process called neuroadaptation).

You're not condemned to crave salty, fatty, sugary foods forever—in fact, you may be surprised to find that before long, you don't even miss them. But because these foods have drug-like properties, you've probably become addicted to the "high" they provide. Therefore, it will take some time for your palate to readjust and your taste buds to become resensitized. Soon you'll come to appreciate subtleties you might not have noticed before—the delicate nuances of different herbs, the fresh flavors of fruits and vegetables, the textures of grains and nuts, the earthy pungency of spices. (See chapter 6 to learn the chefs' secrets to building flavor.)

When it comes to diet change, the journey is as much a psychological one as it is a physical one. Don't be too hard on yourself, and give yourself the time you need to make the transition. If you're interested in reading more about the psychology of eating, we highly recommend *The Pleasure Trap* by Douglas Lisle, PhD, and Alan Goldhamer, DC.

to construct bowl meals.) You can prep the key ingredients in advance so you have them ready in the fridge. One night per week, you might decide to eat out or order in.

Snacks: It's a good idea to plan healthy snacks and have them on hand for moments when you need a little something extra. Fresh fruit or raw vegetables, whole-grain crackers and hummus, dried fruit or frozen fruit with a little nut butter—all of these make quick and nutritious snacks.

The key to making this kind of plan work is **batch cooking**. This means preparing certain staple foods in larger quantities so you have them on hand when you need to throw together a quick meal. It may take a little extra planning at first, but soon it will become part of your routine. Most people will set aside a couple of hours to do this on the weekend. For example:

Pick your grains: Choose one or two whole grains and/or starchy vegetables (like yams or potatoes) that will be your staples for the week.

Pick your legumes: Choose one type of beans or lentils (you can also use canned if you prefer).

Choose a couple of sauces and/or dressings: These can go in jars in the fridge and be ready for use. (You can also buy ready-made oil-free sauces and dressings—we like Dr. Fuhrman, Engine 2, and Forks Over Knives brands.)

Choose one or two main dishes: Pick a new recipe or return to a family favorite, and plan to make enough for at least two meals.

Choose a soup: Something hearty with beans or lentils is ideal so that it makes a satisfying lunch paired with salad or whole-grain bread. Make enough for several meals.

During your weekly batch-cooking session, in addition to preparing your staples, you might:

* Make sandwich or wrap fillings (hummus, baked tofu, etc.).

- Steam or grill a big batch of mixed vegetables—they'll keep for a few days in the fridge and add substance to salads. Grilled veggies make great sandwich fillings.
- Wash and prep your fruits and vegetables.
- Wash and dry your greens.
- Cut carrots, celery, and peppers into snack-size sticks.
- Blend up a jar of no-oil salad dressing (see page 153).
- Make homemade nut milk (see page 104).

If you don't have time to do all this, or just don't feel like spending the time in the kitchen, consider buying ready-washed, cut, or prepared versions of these foods. It may also come in handy to have a good supply of frozen vegetables and cooked grains to pick from when you need them quickly.

Getting the Family on Board

Matt & Alona: Changing your own diet and lifestyle is one thing, but getting your family on board is another thing altogether. Many people can't imagine how they'll get their kids to eat kale, cauliflower, or tempeh. As the parents of two girls, we understand and we've developed strategies to keep our kids happy *and* healthy.

Kids have simple palates. Figure out the foods they like, and don't be afraid to repeat. Our girls eat the same buckwheat pancakes for breakfast most days (we cook up a big batch and then reheat). They love them! They really like potatoes and sweet potatoes, so those will be the basis of their dinner several nights a week.

Kids are more likely to eat food they've had a hand in making. You may not want to do this on a busy weeknight (it takes double the time and makes double the mess!), but getting children involved in the kitchen is a great way to increase their enthusiasm for home-cooked food.

Kids love an adventure. Take them with you to the grocery store or the farmers' market, and make it fun. Challenge them to find items on your shopping list, and get them to choose a vegetable they've never eaten for the whole family to try.

Kids like fun shapes and colors. Cut fruits and veggies into interesting shapes, and make a smiley face on a pancake, or stir berries into oatmeal to turn it pink or purple.

Kids want to grow strong and run faster. Children may not think about "health" the way adults do, but it matters to them, too. For them, it means being able to run fast, play with friends, feel energetic, and excel at sports. Connect their food choices to these outcomes and you'll build motivation that will last them a lifetime.

A Day on the Plate

John Mackey: I keep my breakfasts simple. Sometimes I make oatmeal overnight in a rice cooker, which I eat with berries. Other days, I have a smoothie. I travel a lot, so I even carry my small rice cooker and a blender—that's how much I care about starting my day off right.

For lunch, I'll eat leftovers, or a salad with some whole grains and beans. If I'm home, I love to cook dinners. Indian food is one of my favorites, and I've learned to make some classic dishes without using oil. (See page 215 for a recipe I love, Saag & Tofu Paneer, from my friend Dan Marek.) If I'm pressed for time, my go-to dinner is a bowl meal. I'll use a whole grain or sweet potatoes, steamed veggies, beans, and a sauce. There are so many variations on this simple meal, it never gets boring!

Part 2
The Recipes

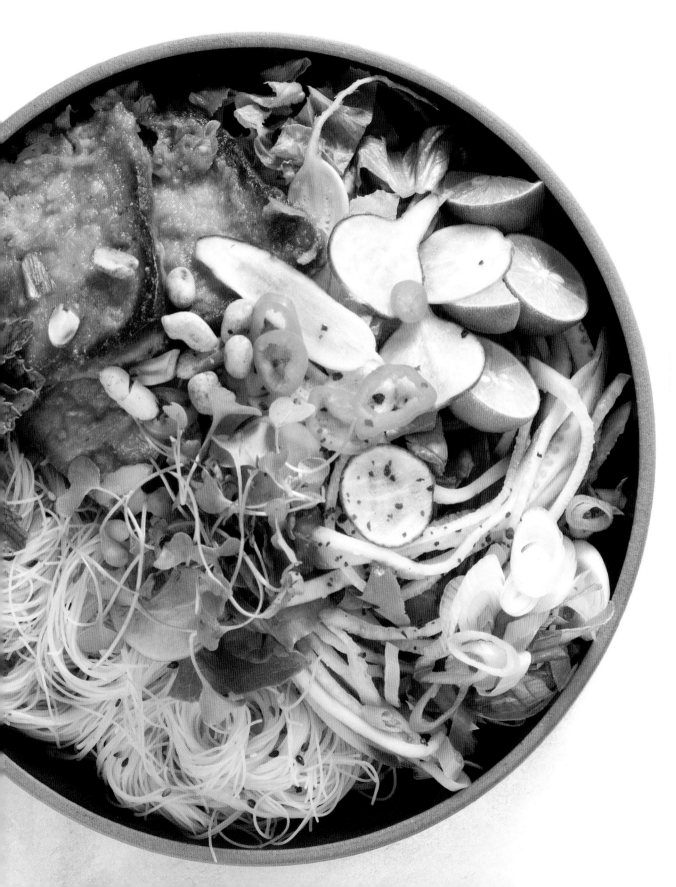

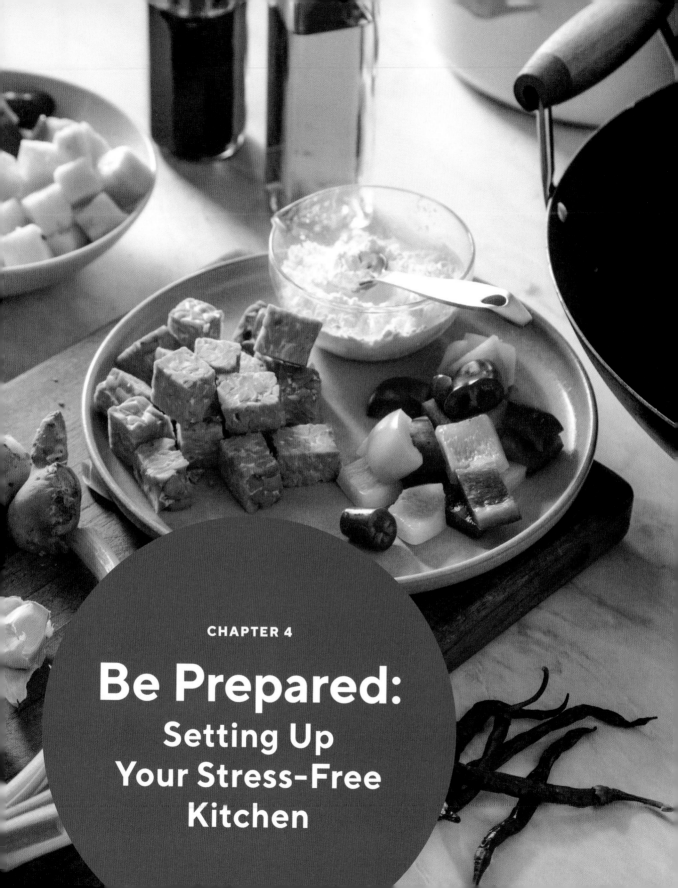

CHAPTER 4

Be Prepared:
Setting Up Your Stress-Free Kitchen

Are you ready to cook? In this chapter and those that follow, you'll learn core techniques of whole foods, plant-based cooking and explore more than 120 original recipes—from quick bites to family favorites to dinner party sensations. Taking control of your health starts in the kitchen!

Cooking should be fun, creative, and satisfying on multiple levels. To help take the stress out of the kitchen, in this chapter we'll offer guidance on how to ensure you're well prepared, including a list of **essential tools**, a **shopping list**, and some tips on **choosing the best ingredients**. But first, we'd like to take a moment to share one simple concept that could transform your experience of cooking.

The Value of *Mise en Place*

Mise en place (pronounced *MEEZ ahn plahs*) is a French term that literally means "setting in place." In culinary circles, it's used to describe the process of gathering and prepping all your ingredients, tools, and utensils before you begin cooking so you'll be organized during the process. For many chefs, however, *mise en place* is not just the act of getting ready; it's a state of mind that symbolizes focus, ease, and presence in the kitchen. If you're familiar with mindfulness practices, you might think of this as a meditative approach to cooking.

In a busy restaurant, *mise en place* is a critical part of every day's work. Long before the orders start coming in and the menu items are cooked, plated, and served, each station must be set up with all the necessary ingredients sliced, diced, and chopped. This allows the activity of a busy kitchen to flow rather than descend into chaos. Next time you dine out at a trendy restaurant with an open kitchen or a "chef's table," take a look at how carefully the ingredients are laid out.

If you're a naturally organized person, you may already know the value of prepping and laying out your ingredients in advance. But many of us tend to just start a recipe and prepare the ingredients as we go. Before you know it, you've overcooked one vegetable while you're hurrying to chop another. You're scrambling to wash the pan you need for the next stage, waiting impatiently while something reaches the required room temperature, or running to the corner store to pick up an essential ingredient.

Mise en place not only saves time, it relieves stress. It can help you relax as you cook, knowing you have everything you need on hand. In some dishes, timing is critical, so having the ingredients lined up and ready to go will ensure you add them in the right order and at the right time to get the desired result.

Essential Cooking Tools

Knives: For the home chef, a large set of knives is not necessary, but make sure you have a good **8-inch to 10-inch chef's knife**, a **serrated knife**, a **paring knife**, and **a honing steel.** Invest in the best quality your budget allows, and sharpen them regularly.

Pots and Pans: For the recipes in this book, you'll need a variety of pots and pans, including a **large stockpot**, a **skillet**, and a **large sauté pan** or **wok.** Stainless steel is a great cooking surface, and many chefs swear by pans with a copper core or coating for its superior heat distribution. Heavier cast-iron pans also offer excellent heat distribution. If you use nonstick pans, avoid Teflon, and be sure to choose pans coated with 100% PFOA and PTFE free, nontoxic, and natural substances, such as ceramic. You'll also want a **steamer basket**—a stackable bamboo steamer is our favorite; a collapsible metal steamer is fine as well. In addition, you might consider investing in a **pressure cooker**, which significantly cuts cooking times for grains and beans. Other great tools are a **rice cooker** and a **slow cooker.**

Blenders/food processors: A **high-speed blender** is an essential tool in a healthy kitchen, and will allow you to make your own nondairy milks, smoothies, soups, and creamy sauces. If you can afford a Vitamix or Blendtec model, they are well worth the investment. The smaller and more affordable NutriBullet is a great option, particularly for making dressings and sauces. A basic **food processor** is also useful for making dips, spreads, sauces, and desserts. A **stick blender**, also known as an immersion blender, is a great tool for blending sauces or soups directly in a pan or dressings in a jar.

Other

- Baking sheets
- Box grater
- Citrus squeezer
- Cutting board
- Heat-resistant rubber or silicone spatulas
- Large colander
- Mandoline (either an affordable, smaller Japanese model or a larger French one)
- Measuring cups (dry and liquid) and measuring spoons
- Mesh bag/cheesecloth (for making nut milk)
- Microplane rasp grater (essential for grating citrus zest and fresh ginger)
- Mixing bowls (various sizes)
- Mixing spoons (slotted, regular, wooden)
- Peeler
- Pizza peel
- Pizza stone
- Rectangular roasting pan or casserole dish
- Salad spinner (the stainless steel OXO version is one of our favorites)
- Silicone baking mats (a reusable substitute for parchment)
- Small bowls for ingredient prep, *mise en place*, and spices
- Storage containers (glass), mason jars, freezer bags
- Tongs and ladles
- Whisk

Chef's Tip

"An organized cook is a successful cook. At Rouxbe Online Culinary School, the largest online culinary school, I helped launch a plant-based certification course and the Forks Over Knives course. The concept of *mise en place* is drilled into every course. *Mise en place* is truly a state of mind, and it will change the way you look at and prepare your meals."—**Chad Sarno**

Tips for Stress-Free Cooking

- **Keep a well-stocked fridge and pantry** (see page 30 for a shopping list).

- **Read through the entire recipe ahead of time** and make sure you have all the ingredients you need and are doing all the prep necessary to execute the recipe correctly. If you're not using a recipe, make yourself a list.

- **Note whether anything needs to be prepared in advance.** Does any ingredient require toasting, soaking, marinating, defrosting, warming, or chilling?

- **Make sure your space is clear and you have your tools and utensils clean and ready** (see opposite page for a list of essential tools).

- **Keep a shopping list on hand** so you can make a note to restock if you run out of any pantry or fridge staples while you're cooking.

- **Invest in a set of bowls of varying sizes** so you can organize your chopped vegetables and herbs.

- **Prep all your ingredients before you begin** (this includes measuring, washing, chopping, blending, etc.).

- **Clean up as you go.** This may be the most important piece of advice we can give! If you're waiting for something to boil or cook, use those few minutes to keep your space clean and tidy.

Shopping List

Fresh, healthy food is getting easier to find, and the variety of options available seems to increase every day. The following list offers suggestions for foods you should be able to find in your local supermarket, Whole Foods Market, or any natural foods store. You don't need to always have all these things on hand, particularly the fresh and perishable produce, but having a variety at your reach will inspire you to prepare healthier options during the week. If you're planning to cook specific recipes, check the ingredient lists and use them to make your shopping list each week, in addition to keeping your staples stocked.

Fresh Vegetables

There are so many varieties of vegetable to choose from. Here are some suggestions—at the store, pick whatever looks fresh and appealing to you.

Starchy Vegetables

- Butternut squash
- Parsnips
- Potatoes (red, Yukon Gold, russet, purple)
- Sugar pumpkins
- Yams or sweet potatoes

Leafy Greens

You can buy many of these prewashed for convenience.

- Arugula
- Bok choy
- Chard (Swiss, rainbow)
- Collard greens
- Kale
- Lettuce (romaine, butter, oak leaf, etc.)
- Mixed greens
- Spinach
- Sprouts/microgreens

Other Produce

- Asparagus
- Beets (red, yellow)
- Bell peppers (red, yellow, green)
- Broccoli
- Brussels sprouts
- Cabbage (napa, red, green)
- Carrots
- Cauliflower
- Celery
- Chiles (jalapeños, red, green, serrano)
- Corn
- Cucumbers
- Daikon radishes
- Fennel
- Green beans
- Green onions (scallions)
- Leeks
- Mushrooms (button, cremini, oyster, portobello, shiitake)
- Onions
- Radishes
- Shallots
- Snow peas
- Tomatoes (cherry, Roma or plum, vine)
- Yellow squash
- Zucchini

Fresh Fruits

- Apples
- Apricots
- Avocados
- Bananas
- Black cherries
- Blueberries
- Cantaloupe
- Clementines
- Grapefruit
- Lemons
- Limes
- Mangoes
- Nectarines
- Oranges
- Papaya
- Peaches
- Pears
- Pineapples
- Raspberries
- Strawberries
- Watermelon

Fresh Herbs and Spices

- Basil (regular, Thai)
- Chives
- Cilantro
- Dill
- Garlic
- Ginger
- Horseradish root
- Lemongrass
- Mint
- Oregano
- Parsley
- Rosemary
- Sage
- Tarragon
- Thyme

Frozen Foods

Be sure these contain no added oil or sugar.

- Frozen cooked grains and beans
- Frozen fruits (berries, mangoes)
- Frozen vegetables (corn, peas, edamame, mixed green veggies, and any other favorites)
- Frozen veggie burgers

Whole Grains

- Brown rice (short- and long-grain)
- Brown rice noodles
- Buckwheat (soba) noodles
- Millet
- Oats (old-fashioned rolled and steel-cut)
- Pasta (Whole-grain or legume-based;

whole wheat, brown rice, quinoa, spelt, farro, corn, lentil, chickpea)
- Quinoa (white, red, black, mixed)
- Wild rice

Beans

- Dried beans (black, pinto, cannellini, kidney beans; chickpeas; black-eyed peas)
- Dried lentils (red, green, brown, French, beluga)
- Dried split peas (green, yellow)

Bulk

- Almond flour
- Arrowroot powder
- Baking powder
- Cacao nibs
- Cocoa powder (unsweetened)
- Cold cereals (puffed corn, rice, millet, Kamut; no added sugar or refined grains)
- Cornstarch
- Muesli (no added sugar)
- Nutritional yeast
- Sun-dried tomatoes (dry, no oil)
- Whole wheat or other whole-grain flour

Jarred and Canned Foods

Choose brands with no added salt, oil, or sugar. Choose jars, non-BPA cans, or cartons.

- Applesauce (unsweetened)
- Artichoke hearts
- Beans (black, cannellini, kidney; chickpeas)
- Capers
- Hearts of palm
- Marinara sauce (no oil or sugar added)
- Mustards (Dijon, whole-grain)
- Nut and seed butters (almond, sesame, cashew, peanut; no added oil, salt, or sugar)
- Olives
- Roasted red peppers (in water, not oil)
- Sriracha or your favorite hot sauce
- Tabasco sauce
- Tomato paste
- Tomatoes (no salt added)

Nuts, Seeds, and Dried Fruit

For nuts and seeds, choose raw, no-added-oil, unsalted varieties.

For dried fruits, choose unsulfured, no-added-oil, no-added-sugar varieties.

- Almonds
- Cashews
- Chia seeds
- Coconut (unsweetened flakes)
- Dates
- Dried fruit (apples, apricots, figs, mangoes, goji berries)
- Hazelnuts

- Hemp seeds
- Macadamia nuts
- Peanuts
- Pecans
- Pine nuts
- Pistachios
- Pumpkin seeds (pepitas)
- Sesame seeds
- Sunflower seeds
- Walnuts

Liquids

- Bragg Liquid Aminos
- Coconut water (unsweetened)
- Nondairy milk (unsweetened; almond, soy, rice, oat)
- Spray oil
- Tamari or soy sauce (low-sodium)
- Vegetable broth (low-sodium)
- Vinegar (apple cider, balsamic, white balsamic, champagne, red wine, sherry, umeboshi, unseasoned rice)

Dried Herbs, Spices, and Seasonings

Choose spices with no added ingredients and pure extracts.

- Almond extract
- Bay leaves
- Caraway seeds
- Cayenne pepper
- Chili powder
- Chipotle powder
- Cinnamon (ground and sticks)

- Coriander seeds
- Cumin (ground and seeds)
- Curry powder
- Fennel seeds
- Garlic (granules and powder)
- Ginger (ground)
- Mustard seeds
- Nutmeg (whole seeds, for grating)
- Onion granules
- Oregano
- Paprika (sweet and smoked)
- Parsley
- Peppercorns (whole black and Sichuan)
- Red pepper flakes
- Saffron threads
- Sea Salt (good-quality fine for general use, flaky for finishing)
- Star anise pods
- Turmeric (ground)
- Vanilla extract, vanilla beans, and vanilla bean paste

Chilled

- Fermented veggies (kimchi, sauerkraut)
- Fresh salsa (no oil)
- Hummus (no oil)
- Miso (dark and white)
- Tempeh
- Tofu (extra-firm, silken)
- Tortillas (whole wheat or corn)
- Whole-grain bread
- Whole-grain wraps

Spring Risotto with
Peas & Mint, page 37

Spring Risotto with
Peas & Mint, page 37

CHAPTER 5

Working with Beans & Grains

Cooking Whole Grains

Hearty, satisfying whole grains are both delicious and nutritious—no wonder humans have been cultivating and eating them for tens of thousands of years. There are at least nineteen varieties of whole grain to choose from, including several varieties of rice; ancient forms of wheat such as farro, spelt, and Kamut; and gluten-free options like quinoa, buckwheat, and amaranth. Each grain has its own unique flavors, textures, and nutritional benefits.

There are many ways to cook grains, but the two most common are the **steaming method** and the **boiling method**. In the steaming method, the grain is combined with a precise amount of liquid, the liquid is brought to a boil, then the pot is covered and the heat is lowered to maintain a slow simmer until all the liquid has been absorbed, leaving the tender cooked grains. In the boiling method, the grain and a larger (usually not precise) quantity of liquid are combined, the liquid is brought to a boil and kept at a high simmer until all the grains are cooked, then the excess liquid is drained off.

The list that follows (see page 36) gives estimated ratios of grains to liquid and times for cooking common grains using the steaming method. In general, larger, harder grains will cook more slowly than smaller grains or those that have been milled. Presoaking, where applicable, will shorten the cooking time, as noted for some of the grains. Some grains, such as quinoa, millet, and buckwheat, benefit from being toasted before they're cooked, which gives them a slight nuttiness. Also, note that altitude may affect cooking times. Last, be sure to double or triple your batches—grains are one of the easiest items to batch cook and keep in the fridge for easy use in multiple menus.

Seasoning and Finishing Your Grains

Grains should not be plain! There are many ways to infuse flavor into your grains during and after cooking. You can add aromatics such as diced onion or chopped garlic or your favorite herbs and spices to the pot. You can cook grains in vegetable broth instead of water. Top them with a favorite sauce or stir in a dressing and some chopped vegetables, raw or cooked. Two particularly flavorful grain-based dishes are pilaf and risotto. We've designed whole foods, plant-based versions of these dishes that avoid the oil and dairy products used in traditional recipes but retain the flavors and textures of the originals. Try the recipes in the pages ahead, and then use the same formula to experiment with different combinations of vegetables, herbs, and spices.

Gluten Free?

You still have plenty of whole-grain options. Rice, in all its varieties, is gluten-free—try brown, red, black, or wild rice. Oats are also gluten-free (be sure they are produced in a GF facility—check the label for this info), as are millet, quinoa, buckwheat, corn, teff, sorghum, and amaranth.

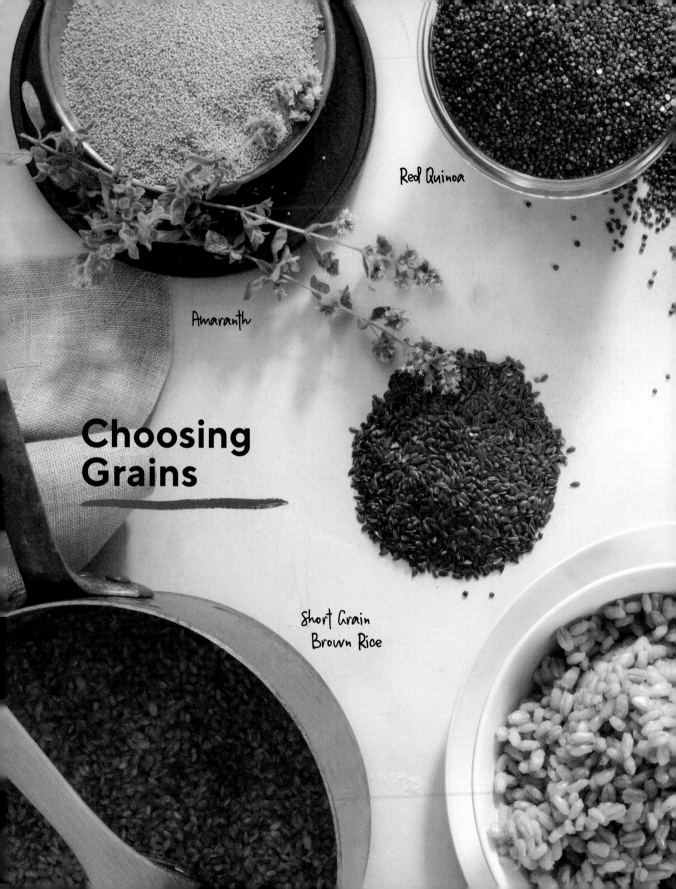

Red Quinoa

Amaranth

Choosing
Grains

Short Grain
Brown Rice

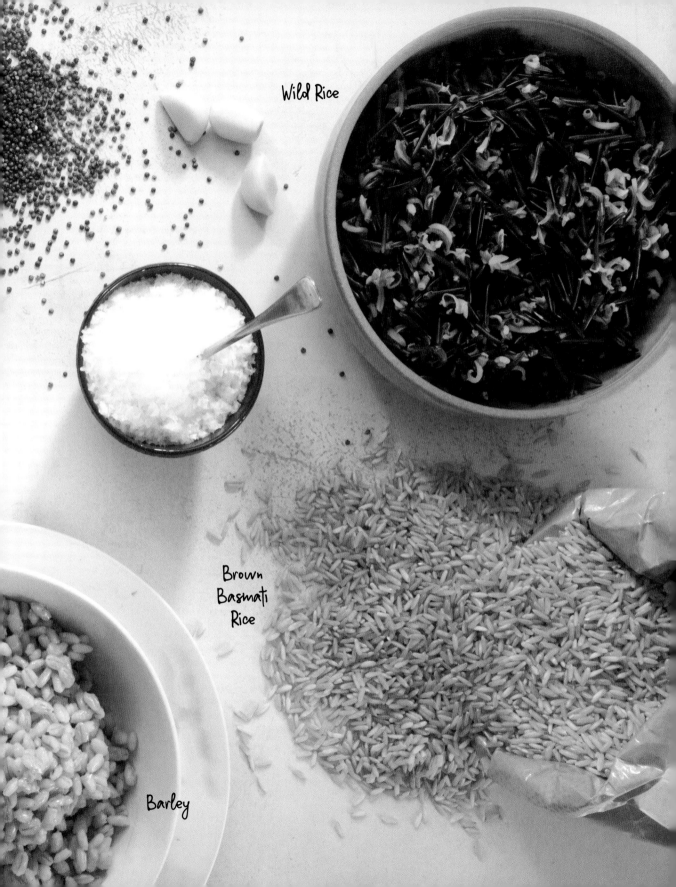

Wild Rice

Brown
Basmati
Rice

Barley

Whole Grains: Ratios & Cooking Times

Amaranth

1 cup dry amaranth:
2 cups water

Cooking time:
25 minutes

Yield: 2½ cups
cooked amaranth

Barley (hulled)

1 cup dry barley:
3 cups water

Cooking time:
45 to 60 minutes

Yield: 3½ cups
cooked barley

Black Japonica rice

1 cup dry rice:
2 to 2½ cups water

Cooking time:
45 minutes

Yield: 2½ cups
cooked rice

Brown rice (long-grain)

1 cup dry rice:
2 to 2½ cups water

Cooking time: 35 to
45 minutes

Yield: 3½ cups cooked
rice

Brown rice (short-grain)

1 cup dry rice:
2 to 2½ cups water

Cooking time: 35 to
45 minutes

Yield: 3¾ cups
cooked rice

Buckwheat (kasha)

1 cup dry buckwheat:
2 cups water

Cooking time:
15 to 20 minutes

Yield: 4 cups
cooked buckwheat

Cornmeal (Polenta)

1 cup dry cornmeal:
2½ cups water

Cooking time:
30 to 40 minutes

Yield: 3½ cups
cooked polenta

Farro

1 cup dry farro:
2 cups water

Cooking time:
30 to 40 minutes

Yield: 2 cups
cooked farro

Kamut (presoaked)

1 cup dry Kamut:
3½ to 4 cups water

Cooking time:
10 to 15 minutes

Yield: 3 cups
cooked Kamut

Millet

1 cup dry millet:
2½ cups water

Cooking time:
45 to 60 minutes

Yield: 4 cups cooked
millet

Oats (steel-cut)

1 cup dry oats:
4 cups water

Cooking time:
25 minutes

Yield: 3 cups
cooked oats

Quinoa

1 cup dry quinoa:
2 cups water

Cooking time:
30 minutes

Yield: 3 cups
cooked quinoa

Sorghum

1 cup dry sorghum:
4 cups water

Cooking time:
15 to 20 minutes

Yield: 3 cups
cooked sorghum

Spelt (presoaked)

1 cup dry spelt:
4 cups water

Cooking time:
45 to 60 minutes

Yield: 3 cups cooked
spelt

Teff

1 cup dry teff:
3 cups water

Cooking time:
45 to 60 minutes

Yield: 2½ cups
cooked teff

Wheat berries (presoaked)

1 cup dry wheat berries:
2 cups water

Cooking time:
30 to 40 minutes

Yield: 2½ cups cooked
wheat berries

Wild rice

1 cup dry rice:
3 cups water

Cooking time:
45 to 50 minutes

Yield: 3½ cups
cooked rice

Spring Risotto with Peas & Mint

Serves 4

Risotto is a northern Italian dish, in which rice (usually Arborio rice) is cooked with aromatics in a flavorful broth, which is added slowly while the risotto is stirred continuously. This continuous stirring agitates the outer starch of the rice and creates a very creamy consistency. While the traditional risotto method involves sautéing the rice in butter or oil, our easy-to-prepare, oil-free *à la minute* formula achieves a similar creaminess through the addition of cashew cream sauce. You can use precooked brown rice or any other larger whole grain (try farro, barley, or spelt). This recipe captures the youthful flavors of spring with green peas, zesty lemon, and fresh mint. Once you master the technique, try swapping out the peas for fresh asparagus, or adding earthy morel mushrooms to soak up the sauce.

1½ cups Basic Cashew Cream Sauce (page 165)

1½ cups thawed frozen peas

¼ cup chopped fresh mint

2 lemons

½ cup chopped leeks (see Note)

¼ cup low-sodium vegetable broth, plus more as needed

½ cup cubed zucchini

½ cup asparagus tips

¼ cup dry white wine

3 cups cooked grain (see page 36), such as short-grain brown rice

¼ cup minced fresh parsley

Freshly ground black pepper

Flaky sea salt, to finish (optional)

Fresh summer truffle (optional)

In a blender, combine the cashew cream sauce, ½ cup of the peas, 2 tablespoons of the mint, and the zest and juice of 1 lemon. Blend until smooth, 2 to 3 minutes. Set aside.

Heat a deep sauté pan over medium heat. Add the leeks and dry sauté, stirring often, until the leeks begin to stick, 2 to 3 minutes. Add the broth and stir to deglaze the pan. Add the remaining 1 cup peas, the zucchini, and the asparagus tips. Cook, stirring occasionally, until the vegetables are tender, 3 to 4 minutes. When the zucchini begins to stick, add the wine and stir to deglaze the pan again. Simmer until the liquid has evaporated.

Reduce the heat to medium and stir in the cooked grain, parsley, and remaining 2 tablespoons mint. Cook until the grain is reheated, 2 to 4 minutes. If the grain begins to stick, add a splash of broth to loosen it.

Pour the cashew cream mixture over the grain mixture and reduce the heat to medium-low. Cook, stirring continuously, until the sauce thickens, about 5 minutes. Remove from the heat and season with pepper.

To serve, spoon a generous amount of risotto on each plate and sprinkle with flaky salt. Grate the zest from the remaining lemon over the risotto and shave fresh truffle on top, if desired.

Note: Leeks grow in sandy soil, and often have grit between their layers. To clean them, trim both ends, slice lengthwise, and wash thoroughly under running water.

Per serving: 337 calories, 7 g total fat, 1 g saturated fat, 0 mg cholesterol, 196 mg sodium, 62 g total carbohydrate (8 g dietary fiber, 7 g sugar, 0 g added sugars), 10 g protein, 4 mg iron

Wild Rice Pilaf with Squash, Pears, & Herbs

Serves 4

Pilaf is traditionally made by sautéing aromatics, then adding rice and vegetables and cooking them in a seasoned broth. Variations on this dish are common to many global cuisines. Wild rice has a pleasing nutty flavor, nicely complementing the sweetness of the zucchini and pears in this recipe. You can use all wild rice or a wild rice–brown rice mix.

1 cup wild rice, soaked overnight and drained

2 cups low-sodium vegetable broth

1 onion, finely chopped

4 garlic cloves, minced

1 cup small-diced yellow squash

1 cup small-diced zucchini

2 Bartlett pears, cored and cut into small wedges

3 tablespoons thinly sliced green onion

¼ cup chopped fresh parsley

2 tablespoons minced fresh oregano

2 tablespoons nutritional yeast

1½ tablespoons grated lemon zest

¼ teaspoon sea salt

¼ teaspoon freshly ground black pepper

½ teaspoon thinly sliced red Fresno chile (optional)

Put the rice in a medium saucepan, add 1¾ cups of the broth, and bring to a simmer over medium-high heat. Cover, reduce the heat to low, and cook until the rice is tender, 18 to 20 minutes. (If you didn't presoak the rice, increase the cooking time to 35 to 40 minutes and stir the rice occasionally.)

Heat a large sauté pan over medium heat. When hot, add the onion and garlic and dry sauté, stirring, until the onion begins to stick to the pan, 3 to 4 minutes. Add the remaining ¼ cup broth and stir to deglaze the pan. Add the squash and zucchini and cook, stirring, until slightly softened, about 4 minutes.

When the rice is cooked, add it to the pan with the squash and stir to combine. Remove from the heat and stir in the pears, green onion, parsley, oregano, nutritional yeast, lemon zest, salt, pepper, and chile (if using). Mix well.

Serve immediately, or cover and refrigerate for up to 1 day and serve as a cold salad.

Per serving: 274 calories, 2 g total fat, 1 g saturated fat, 0 mg cholesterol, 244 mg sodium, 55 g total carbohydrate (7 g dietary fiber, 13 g sugar, 0 g added sugars), 9 g protein, 2 mg iron

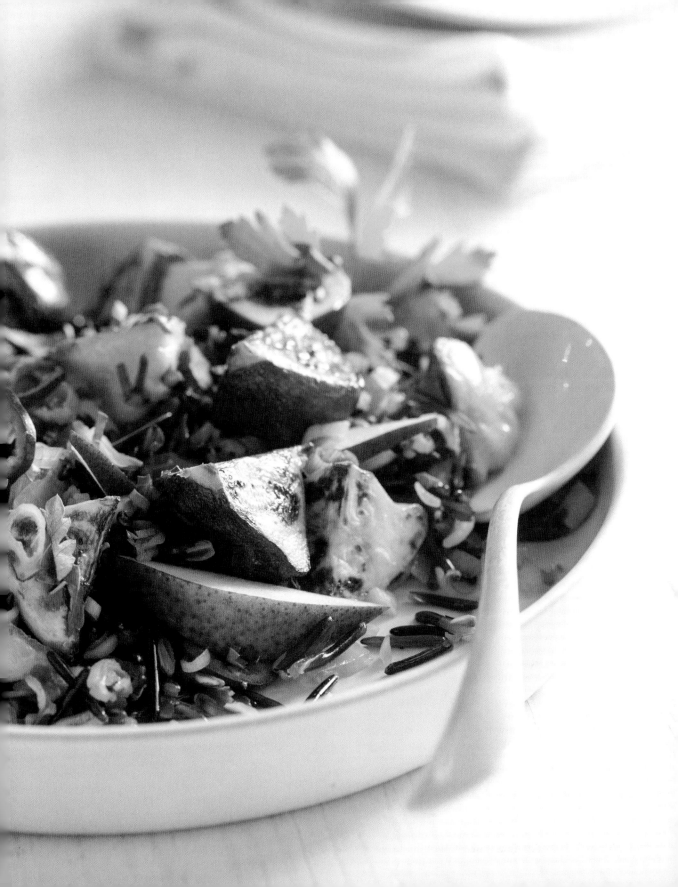

Winter Risotto with Butternut Squash

Serves 4

This warming risotto is perfect for those cooler days when winter squashes are available. The *à la minute* formula uses cashew cream sauce to mimic the creaminess traditionally created by Arborio rice. Fresh horseradish adds a finishing kick. Add a few slices of roasted chestnut on top to give this dish a holiday character.

2½ cups ¼-inch cubes peeled butternut squash

1½ cups Basic Cashew Cream Sauce (page 165)

Juice of ½ lemon

½ teaspoon ground cinnamon

½ cup chopped onion

½ cup low-sodium vegetable broth, plus more as needed

¼ cup white wine

3 cups cooked grain (see page 36), such as short-grain brown rice

3 tablespoons minced fresh parsley

1½ teaspoons minced fresh sage

Freshly ground black pepper

Flaky sea salt, for finishing (optional)

Fresh horseradish, peeled, for grating

Steam 1½ cups of the butternut squash in a covered steamer basket over gently simmering water until soft, 8 to 10 minutes. Transfer to a (preferably high-speed) blender such as a Vitamix. Add the cashew cream sauce, lemon juice, and cinnamon and blend until smooth, about 1 minute in a high-speed blender or a few minutes in a standard blender.

Heat a deep medium sauté pan over medium heat. When hot, add the onion and dry sauté, stirring often, until it begins to stick, 3 to 4 minutes. Add the broth and stir to deglaze the pan. Add the remaining 1 cup butternut squash and simmer, stirring occasionally, until the squash is tender and liquid has evaporated, 4 to 5 minutes. When the squash begins to stick to the pan, add the wine and stir to deglaze the pan.

Stir in the grain, parsley, and sage and cook for 2 to 3 minutes. If the grain begins to stick, add a splash more broth.

Pour the butternut–cashew cream mixture over the grain mixture and reduce the heat to medium-low. Cook, stirring often, until the sauce thickens, about 5 minutes. Remove from the heat and season with pepper.

Serve with a sprinkling of flaky salt and grated fresh horseradish.

Note: If you can't find fresh horseradish root, stir about 1½ teaspoons prepared horseradish into the pan along with the butternut–cashew cream sauce.

Per serving: 439 calories, 14 g total fat, 2 g saturated fat, 0 mg cholesterol, 441 mg sodium, 70 g total carbohydrate (10 g dietary fiber, 7 g sugar, 0 g added sugars), 11 g protein, 4 mg iron

Risotto Flavor Combinations

The *à la minute* risotto method used in the recipes above lends itself to endless flavorful combinations of vegetables, herbs, and spices. Here are a few you can try:

- Steamed asparagus and roasted garlic
- Wild mushrooms and thyme
- Roasted beets and tarragon
- Spinach and caramelized onion
- Roasted Cherry Tomatoes & Garlic (page 88) and fresh basil

Cooking Beans & Other Legumes

Beans and other legumes proudly take center stage in a whole foods, plant-based diet. With over eight hundred varieties of beans, lentils, and peas to choose from, this versatile food group has been a staple of traditional cultures around the world; in fact, beans are one of humanity's oldest cultivated crops. They are hearty, satisfying foods that offer an excellent source of protein, dietary fiber, and complex carbohydrates.

When using dried beans, soak larger varieties overnight (soaking is not necessary for smaller legumes such as lentils). This will reduce cooking time by up to 25% or more, and some people strongly believe it makes the beans easier to digest. Adding some kombu (seaweed) when cooking beans is said to aid digestion as well. Beans should be simmered in a covered pot, and more water should be added as needed during the cooking process to ensure they stay submerged. Cooking times vary depending on type and size—some lentils take only twenty minutes to cook, whereas larger beans can take more than a couple of hours. Altitude may also affect cooking times. Want to cook your beans faster? Try a pressure cooker—it cuts the cooking time in half. And always make a big pot—beans are a great food to batch cook and keep in the fridge for easy addition to soups, salads, and more.

Working with Frozen and Canned Beans

If you're using canned beans, be sure to choose a high-quality brand with no added salt, packaged in BPA-free cans or, better yet, cartons. You can also buy frozen precooked beans—these just need to be simmered or steamed for a few minutes to be ready to serve.

Chef's Tip

NEVER COOK BEANS BY THEMSELVES!

Don't miss the opportunity to add flavor to your beans during the cooking process. Try vegetable broth instead of water, and add your favorite aromatics—sliced onion or garlic, hearty herbs, and chiles will all impart their flavors to the beans as they cook. Save the salt for after cooking, though—it can alter the texture of the beans if it's added while they're cooking.

Dried Legumes: Ratios & Cooking Times

The list that follows shows estimated ratios and cooking times for some common bean varieties. Add more water as needed.

Note: This list assumes that beans have been presoaked for at least 4 hours.

Adzuki (aduki)
1 cup dry: 4 cups water
Cooking time: 45 to 55 minutes
Yield: 3 cups

Black beans
1 cup dry: 4 cups water
Cooking time: 1 to 1¼ hours
Yield: 3 cups

Black-eyed peas
1 cup dry: 3 cups water
Cooking time: 1 hour
Yield: 2 cups

Cannellini beans
1 cup dry: 3 cups water
Cooking time: 45 minutes
Yield: 2½ cups

Cassoulet beans
1 cup dry: 3 cups water
Cooking time: 45 minutes
Yield: 2½ cups

Chickpeas (garbanzo beans)
1 cup dry: 4 cups water
Cooking time: 1½ to 2 hours
Yield: 2 cups

Cranberry beans
1 cup dry: 3 cups water
Cooking time: 40 to 45 minutes
Yield: 3 cups

Great northern beans
1 cup dry: 3½ cups water
Cooking time: 1½ hours
Yield: 2⅔ cups

Kidney beans
1 cup dry: 3 cups water
Cooking time: 1 hour
Yield: 2¼ cups

Lentils (black)
1 cup dry: 4 cups water (it's also good to use more water since this cooking liquid is delicious once lentils are cooked. See recipe on page 61)
Cooking time: 45 to 55 minutes
Yield: 2 to 2½ cups

Lentils (brown)
1 cup dry: 2¼ cups water
Cooking time: 45 to 60 minutes
Yield: 2¼ cups

Lentils (green)
1 cup dry: 2 cups water
Cooking time: 30 to 45 minutes
Yield: 2 cups

Lentils (split red)
1 cup dry: 3 cups water
Cooking time: 20 to 30 minutes
Yield: 2 to 2½ cups

Lima beans (large)
1 cup dry: 4 cups water
Cooking time: 45 to 60 minutes
Yield: 2 cups

Mung beans
1 cup dry: 2½ cups water
Cooking time: 1 hour
Yield: 2 cups

Navy beans
1 cup dry: 3 cups water
Cooking time: 45 to 60 minutes
Yield: 2⅔ cups

Pinto beans
1 cup dry: 3 cups water
Cooking time: 1 hour
Yield: 2⅔ cups

Soybeans
1 cup dry: 4 cups water
Cooking time: 2 to 3 hours (black soybeans have a shorter cooking time)
Yield: 3 cups

Split peas (green)
1 cup dry: 4 cups water
Cooking time: 45 to 60 minutes
Yield: 2 cups

Split peas (yellow)
1 cup dry: 4 cups water
Cooking time: 45 to 60 minutes
Yield: 2 cups

Gallo Pinto (Simple Beans & Rice)

Serves 2

If you ever visit Costa Rica—home to one of the world's "Blue Zones," or areas with the longest-lived populations—you won't leave the country without tasting *gallo pinto*. The country's national dish, this simple combination of black beans and rice is eaten with just about everything and at every meal, including breakfast.

This recipe comes straight from centenarian Panchita Castillo's kitchen. Be careful with habanero chiles—they are incendiary. Start with a small amount; you can always add more. Avoid touching the cut chiles themselves, because their capsaicin, the compound in chiles that gives them their heat, will transfer to your fingers and from there could get into your eyes or other sensitive parts and cause irritation or worse. Serve this dish with guacamole for a satisfying small plate or alongside a more substantial recipe. **Recipe by Dan Buettner**

1 small onion, chopped

2 teaspoons minced garlic

2 cups cooked black beans (see page 42) or no-added-sodium canned black beans, drained and rinsed

3 cups cooked long-grain rice (see page 36)

½ teaspoon sea salt

¼ teaspoon freshly ground black pepper

2 tablespoons chopped fresh cilantro

1 to 2 teaspoons minced seeded habanero chile (optional)

Heat a large saucepan over medium heat. When hot, add the onion and cook, stirring often, until it begins to stick to the pan and lightly brown, about 4 minutes. Add the garlic and cook until fragrant, about 20 seconds. Add ¼ cup water and stir to deglaze the pan.

Stir in the beans and another ¾ cup water. Raise the heat to medium-high and bring to a simmer. Gently stir in the rice, salt, and pepper and cook until heated through, about 2 minutes.

Stir in the cilantro and habanero (if using). Serve hot.

Per serving: 603 calories, 2 g total fat, 0 g saturated fat, 0 mg cholesterol, 584 mg sodium, 128 g total carbohydrate (22 g dietary fiber, 2 g sugar, 0 g added sugars), 22 g protein, 5 mg iron

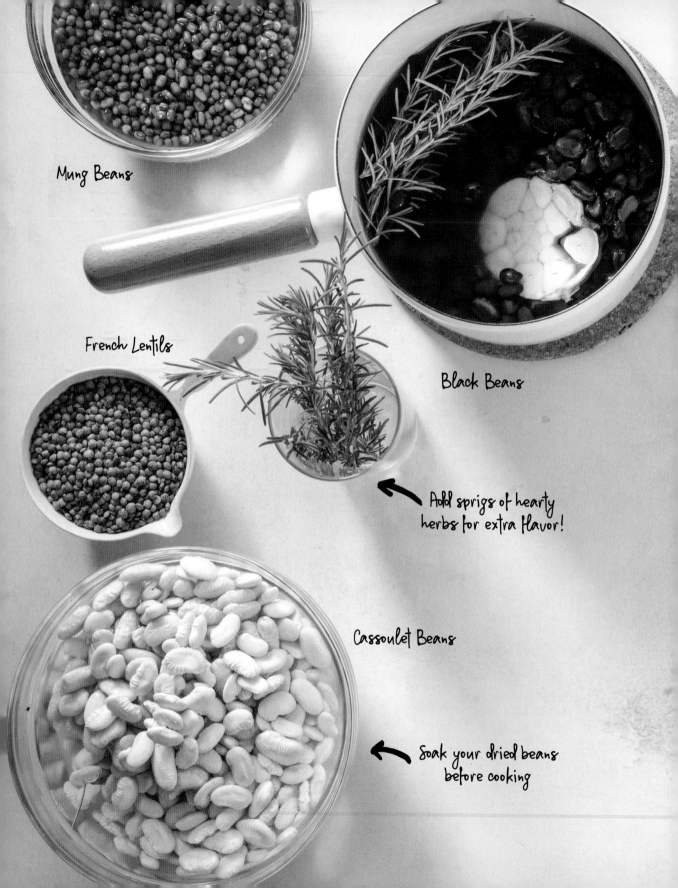

Mung Beans

French Lentils

Black Beans

Add sprigs of hearty herbs for extra flavor!

Cassoulet Beans

Soak your dried beans before cooking

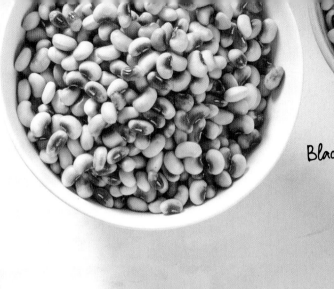

Black-Eyed Peas

Adzuki Beans

Cooking beans & other legumes

Add aromatics such as garlic, onions, and chiles to bump up flavor

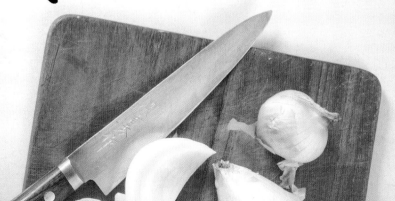

Wicked Good Pot of Cassoulet Beans

Serves 8 as a side dish

This is a simple pot of beans with classic flavors that is easy to make in a big batch for use in multiple meals. Cassoulet beans are a creamy, buttery French variety and are delicious served with toasted whole-grain bread. You can also substitute cannellini or navy beans in this recipe.

1 pound dried cassoulet beans, such as Tarbais, or cannellini beans, soaked overnight

8 cups low-sodium vegetable broth

1 white onion, cut into small cubes

4 garlic cloves, minced

2 bay leaves

½ teaspoon freshly ground black pepper

Drain and rinse the beans, then place them in a large (at least 3-quart) soup pot. Add the remaining ingredients, cover, and bring to a boil over medium-high heat. Uncover, reduce the heat to medium, and simmer until the beans are tender, 40 to 45 minutes. If the liquid level drops below the beans, add just enough water to keep the beans covered.

When the beans are tender, remove the bay leaves and serve.

Serve with seeded whole-grain bread.

Per serving: 218 calories, 1 g total fat, 0 g saturated fat, 0 mg cholesterol, 142 mg sodium, 40 g total carbohydrate (20 g dietary fiber, 4 g sugar, 0 g added sugars), 12 g protein, 5 mg iron

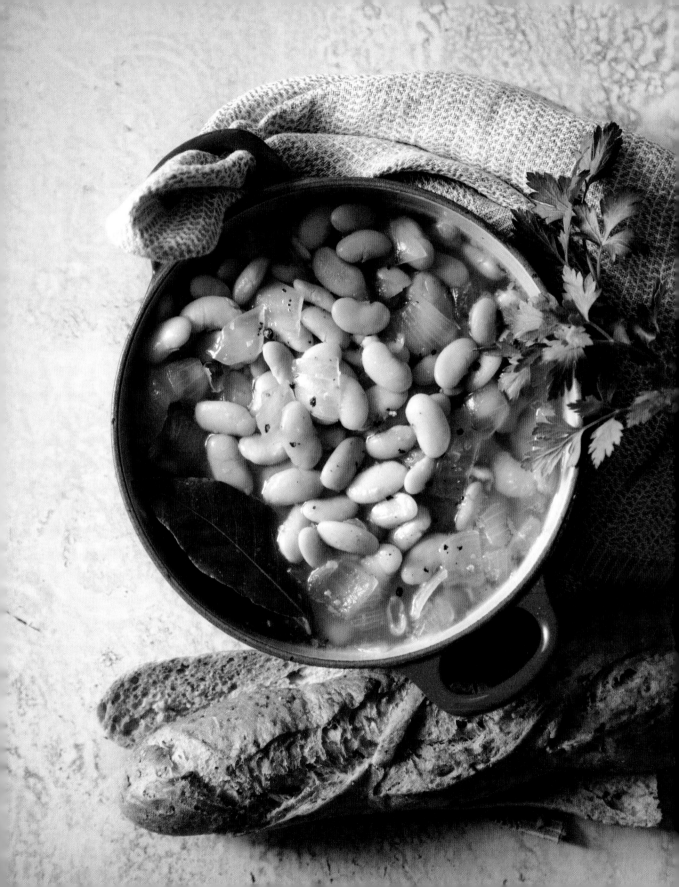

"Refried" Cumin Black Beans

Serves 4

These creamy beans make a perfect addition to taco night. You can eat them on the side or use them as a filling, paired with salsa, guacamole, and rice.

8 ounces dry black beans, soaked overnight

3 cups low-sodium vegetable broth

1 tablespoon smoked paprika

2 tablespoons ground cumin

6 garlic cloves

1 onion, chopped

½ jalapeño, chopped

Drain and rinse the beans and place them in a medium pot.

Add the broth, paprika, cumin, garlic, onion, and jalapeño and bring to a boil over high heat. Reduce the heat to medium-low, cover, and simmer until the beans are tender, 45 to 55 minutes.

Remove from the heat and let cool slightly. Use an immersion blender to puree the mixture directly in the pot until still chunky and not completely broken down. (Alternatively, transfer half the bean mixture and cooking liquid to a food processor or upright blender and blend until nearly smooth. Pour the blended mixture into a bowl and repeat with the remaining bean mixture and cooking liquid, then return the pureed bean mixture to the pot.)

Cook the pureed beans over medium-low heat until slightly thickened, about 5 minutes. Serve hot or warm.

Per serving: 251 calories, 2 g total fat, 0 g saturated fat, 0 mg cholesterol, 117 mg sodium, 46 g total carbohydrate (11 g dietary fiber, 4 g sugar, 0 g added sugars), 14 g protein, 5 mg iron

Ethiopian Lentils

Serves 6

Taste the flavors of North Africa in this fragrantly spiced lentil dish. Berbere is the signature spice blend of Ethiopia, containing ground chiles, cardamom, coriander, and other spices. Look for it in the spice aisle. For an authentic marriage of taste and texture, serve atop Ethiopian *injera* bread, made from fermented teff. It also works well in a tortilla or over rice. If you have leftovers, you can thin these lentils out with some vegetable broth and serve as a soup.

1 cup chopped onion

10 garlic cloves, minced

¼ teaspoon minced seeded serrano chile

1½ tablespoons minced fresh ginger

1 tablespoon berbere spice mix

2½ cups low-sodium vegetable broth

1½ cups dry brown lentils

1 (14-ounce) can no-added-sodium crushed tomatoes

Juice of 1 lemon

1 teaspoon grated orange zest

½ teaspoon sea salt

2 tablespoons minced fresh parsley

Heat a soup pot over medium-high heat. Add the onion and dry sauté, stirring often, until it begins to stick to the pan and lightly brown, 3 to 4 minutes. Reduce the heat to medium-low, add the garlic, chile, ginger, and berbere spice and cook, stirring frequently to prevent burning, until fragrant, about 2 minutes.

Add a splash of broth and stir to deglaze the pan. Add the lentils and the remaining broth and bring to a simmer. Reduce the heat to medium-low and simmer until the lentils are tender and most of the liquid has been absorbed, 15 to 18 minutes.

Add the tomatoes, lemon juice, orange zest, and salt and simmer, 4 to 5 minutes. Stir in the parsley, reserving a pinch for garnish, if desired.

Serve hot, garnished with the parsley.

Per serving: 217 calories, 1 g total fat, 0 g saturated fat, 0 mg cholesterol, 261 mg sodium, 40 g total carbohydrate (10 g dietary fiber, 6 g sugar, 0 g added sugars), 12 g protein, 4 mg iron

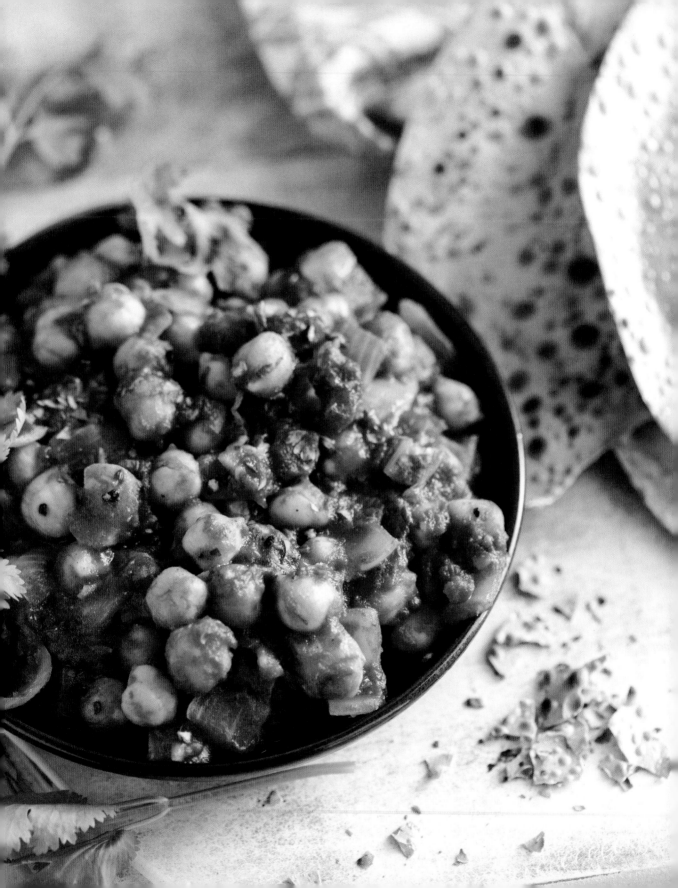

Indian Chickpeas

Serves 4

This whole foodie take on the traditional Indian dish *chana masala* features chickpeas cooked in a tomato-based sauce infused with aromatics and spices. Serve with brown rice and *papadum*.

2 cups chopped onions

½ teaspoon minced seeded serrano chile

6 garlic cloves, minced

2 tablespoons minced fresh ginger

1½ teaspoons cumin seed

1¼ teaspoons ground coriander

1 teaspoon ground turmeric

3½ cups cooked chickpeas (see page 42) or no-added-sodium canned chickpeas, drained and rinsed

1 cup low-sodium vegetable broth

1 (15-ounce) can no-added-sodium crushed tomatoes

1½ tablespoons apple cider vinegar

1 tablespoon date paste (see page 56)

½ teaspoon sea salt

½ cup chopped fresh cilantro

Heat a soup pot over medium-high heat. When hot, add the onions and dry sauté, stirring often, until they begin to stick to the pan and lightly brown, 3 to 4 minutes. Add the chile, garlic, ginger, cumin, coriander, and turmeric and cook until fragrant, 2 to 3 minutes.

Stir in the chickpeas, broth, tomatoes, vinegar, date paste, and salt and bring to a simmer. Reduce the heat to medium-low and simmer, stirring frequently to prevent scorching, 8 to 10 minutes.

Remove from the heat and stir in all but a pinch of the cilantro. Garnish with the reserved cilantro and serve.

Per serving: 339 calories, 2 g total fat, 0 g saturated fat, 0 mg cholesterol, 386 mg sodium, 59 g total carbohydrate (13 g dietary fiber, 12 g sugar, 0 g added sugars), 16 g protein, 5 mg iron

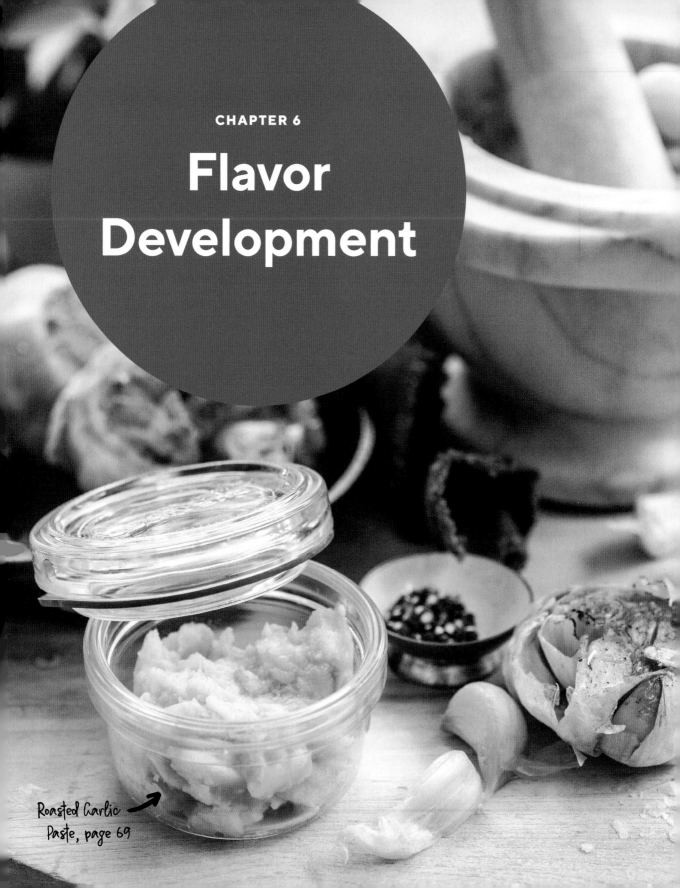

CHAPTER 6

Flavor Development

Roasted Garlic
Paste, page 69

Cooking is an art and a science. Great cooks—whether they are dazzling diners at celebrated restaurants or feeding a happy family around the kitchen table—have mastered both the science of good technique and the subtle art of building flavor.

While the best cooks will tell you they are always still learning about the mysteries of pleasing the human palate, it's also true that a little knowledge will take you a long way. So don't be intimidated: in this chapter we'll be sharing a few simple principles of flavor development that can take any dish from dull to delightful.

There are two essential ways to build flavor in the kitchen: through ingredients and through cooking technique. We'll discuss techniques in the next chapter; here we will focus on ingredients. Preparing your own meals with fresh, high-quality ingredients, or "scratch cooking," is a wonderful opportunity to build flavor throughout the cooking process. If you choose premade foods, there's little you can do to alter the flavor, short of adding a favorite hot sauce or drowning them in other condiments. But when you start with a blank slate, each step of the cooking process is a chance to build flavor from the ground up, in layers, so that it is infused into the food.

Modern processed foods usually rely on large quantities of fat, salt, and sugar to give them flavor. Our palates become accustomed to these concentrated taste sensations and dulled to the subtleties of more natural flavors. If you're trying to change your eating habits and reduce your intake of these unhealthy substances, it's essential to learn how to make your food tasty in other ways, rather than reaching for these addictive ingredients. It may take a little more attention at first, but you'll soon fall in love with the variety of sensory experiences you can create with the right combinations of herbs, spices, acids, and whole-food fats and sweeteners.

As you work—and play!—in the kitchen, ask yourself, *How can I infuse as much flavor as possible with every ingredient I'm using?* You'll need to focus your attention on the experience of flavor as you're cooking—bringing mindfulness to the aromas, textures, and tastes of the food. Notice how flavors combine, layer, and build on one another. Being well prepared and organized will help free up your attention for this task (see page 27 to learn about the secret to stress-free kitchens: *mise en place*).

Familiarity with seasonings and flavorings liberates the cook. As you gain more confidence with the basic ingredients, you'll feel less constrained by recipes and better equipped to cook creatively and intuitively with what you have on hand.

The Five Flavors

The experience of flavor is made up of two components: taste and aroma. While there are an infinite number of aromas, taste can be broken down into just five categories:

1. Sweet

Sweet is one of the easiest tastes to discern—it's found naturally in fruits and some vegetables, and in syrups like maple syrup and agave nectar. Refined sugars are more intensely sweet. White sugar lacks any aroma to give it a more definitive character; it is a neutral sweetness. The beauty of using dried and fresh fruits for sweetness is that you get other notes of flavor, such as citrus, tropical, or caramel, with your sweet. Using a sweet will help tone down bitterness and sour tastes.

2. Sour

Sour is the taste we associate with acidic foods like citrus fruits and vinegars. Fermented foods also have a sour flavor. Adding a touch of citrus to your salads and sauces will add brightness and a light finish to your dishes.

3. Bitter

Bitter is a flavor found in many leafy green vegetables such as arugula, chicory, and escarole. Some herbs and spices are also bitter, as are hops, coffee, and horseradish.

4. Salt

Salty is the familiar taste created by the presence of sodium. Naturally high-sodium vegetables include celery and chard. Besides sea salt, you can find saltiness in condiments and foods that are preserved with salt, such as tamari, soy sauce, shoyu, miso, many prepared mustards, seaweeds, and some pickles. Salt is not technically considered a flavor in itself; rather, it enhances the expression of other flavors.

5. Umami

Umami has long been recognized as a flavor in Eastern cuisines, but is a recent addition to Western culinary parlance. It refers to a particular pungent savoriness commonly found in mushrooms and soy. Try our Umami Spice Blends on page 68.

Working with Whole-Food Sweeteners

It's no secret that humans love sweet foods. Indeed, scientists suggest that our love of sweets is an evolutionary predilection that once helped to ensure we'd consume plenty of fruits, with all their natural health benefits—hence, the abundance of sweet receptors found on the human tongue. But while the simple sugars in whole fruit support human health, the refined, extracted sugars found in so many foods today do quite the opposite. And with such a readily available array of highly processed sugary confections, our sweet tooth tends to lead us astray.

The good news is that there are plenty of ways to create the desired sense of sweetness without adding refined sugars. From comforting baked goods to delectable desserts, you can use whole-food sweeteners to pamper your palate without sacrificing your health. In this book, we use only whole-fruit-based sweeteners, such as whole fresh fruits, blended fruits, dried fruits, and fruit pastes. Try some of the recipes in chapter 14; you'll be amazed at how good they taste!

Sweetness is not just for dessert. Sometimes the right touch of sweet can add depth to a savory dish or balance the acidity in a dressing. You'll see examples of this throughout this book, and if you pay attention to the effect of adding those ingredients, you'll develop your own sense of when and how much sweetness is called for.

START WITH FRESH INGREDIENTS FOR OPTIMUM FLAVOR!

Before you even start adding seasonings, the foundations of flavor come from your core ingredients—fruits, vegetables, grains, beans, and so on. Choosing foods in their highest state of freshness will give you optimum flavor. If you've ever picked a ripe tomato from your own backyard, you'll know it's dramatically more flavorful than the anemic tomatoes you find at the grocery store. You may not always be able to grow your own fruits and veggies, but you can buy them ripe, fresh, and in season at your local store or farmers' market.

Fruit Pastes

Makes about 2 cups

An easy way to create a whole-food sweetener is to make a paste using dried fruit. Try dates, figs, mangoes, apricots, or tart cherries—but any type of fruit will work, depending on the flavor profile you're looking for. For example, in a sweet-and-sour sauce you might want more tropical notes, so you could choose mango. For a darker, more caramelized flavor, dates might be appropriate. Apricots have a citrusy tang that works well in dressings. Use fruit paste as a topping for morning grains, as a sweet component in sauces and marinades, or to make a simple parfait by layering with fresh fruit and Vanilla Coconut Cream (page 271).

1 cup unsulfured no-added-sugar dried fruit of choice

Place dried fruit and 2 cups water in a medium bowl (add more water if needed to cover the fruit) and soak for at least 1 hour or up to overnight.

Use a slotted spoon to transfer the rehydrated fruit from the soaking water to a (preferably high-speed) blender. Blend, adding just enough of the soaking water to get the fruit moving, until smooth and broken down to a paste the consistency of thick honey, about 2 minutes. For a thinner paste, add more water. For a thicker, more concentrated paste, add less water.

Use immediately or scrape into an airtight container and refrigerate for up to 1 week or freeze for up to 4 months.

Per serving (2 tablespoons): 23 calories, 0 g total fat, 0 g saturated fat, 0 mg cholesterol, 1 mg sodium, 6 g total carbohydrate (1 g dietary fiber, 4 g sugar, 0 g added sugars), 0 g protein, 0 mg iron

Health Tip

When using dried fruit, always choose unsulfured varieties without added sugar. Since the natural sugars in dried fruits are more concentrated due to loss of water, they are a calorie-dense food, so if you're trying to lose weight, be aware of your portion sizes.

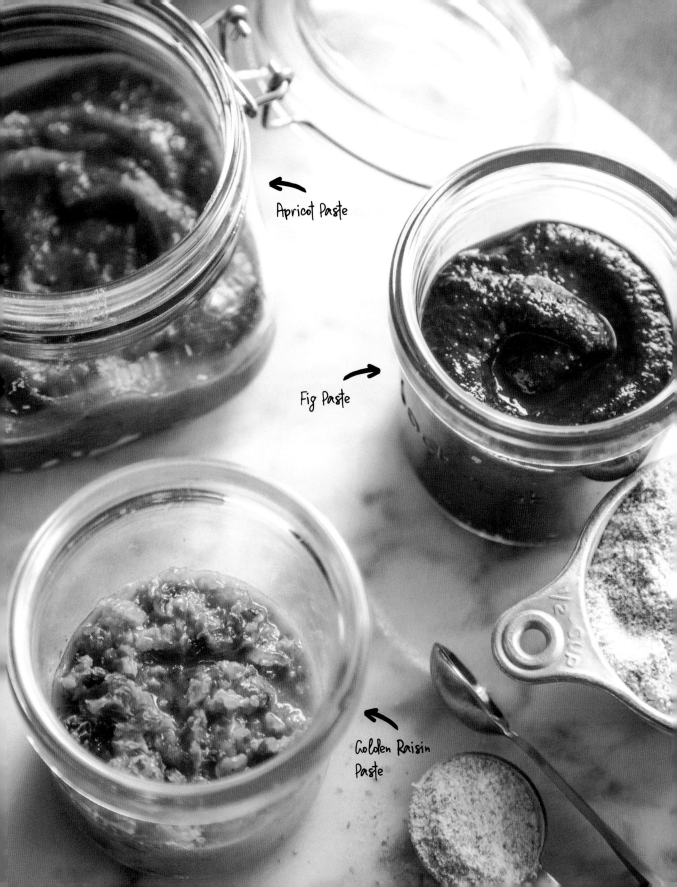

Apricot Paste

Fig Paste

Golden Raisin
Paste

Choosing Whole-Food Fats

In a whole foods, plant-based diet, the majority of calories come from starchy foods such as whole grains, starchy vegetables, beans, and other legumes. Fat plays a smaller role than it does in the standard American diet, and when it is consumed, it's in the form of whole foods such as nuts, seeds, olives, and avocados, rather than extracted oils (see page 10 for more on the health concerns related to oils, and page 78 for tips on cooking without oil).

Many culinary schools teach that "Fat is flavor!" In fact, there are plenty of ways to build flavor without fats, as you'll see in these pages. However, fat has a key role to play in some recipes and is often used as a vehicle to carry other flavors smoothly over the palate. Just a small amount of whole-food fat can transform dressings, sauces, and desserts, allowing you to achieve a rich flavor, texture, and "mouthfeel." When it comes to flavor-building, fats balance sharper tastes like acidity, salt, or bitterness, and provide that creaminess that is essential to many dishes. Here are some of the most common whole-food fats:

- **Nuts and seeds** are wonderfully versatile. You can use them raw, toasted, or dry roasted; whole or ground; in salads and vegetable dishes. You can soak and blend them to make rich, creamy sauces, dressings, and desserts.

- **Avocado** can be blended into creamy dressings or even used in desserts (you'll never even know it's there!).

- **Olives** have a bold, salty flavor paired with a rich texture. Try adding just a few to salads, sauces, dressings, or pasta dishes for a pop of flavor.

- **Coconut**, used sparingly, adds authentic flavor and texture to Asian dishes, soups, and sauces. Fresh or unsweetened flaked coconut can also be added to salads or used in desserts or as a garnish.

Health Tip

Whole plant foods that are higher in fat tend to be more calorie-dense foods, so those trying to lose weight should be mindful of portion sizes when eating foods such as nuts, seeds, coconut, avocados, and olives.

Sodium Reduction

No discussion of flavor would be complete without mentioning salt. Humans love salt, and have for millennia. In fact, some cultures prized it so highly that they used it as a form of currency. Once a rare delicacy, salt is readily available today, and many of us suffer adverse health effects from consuming too much.

If you want to reduce your sodium consumption, the simplest and most important step you can take is to stop eating processed foods and instead choose whole foods and prepare them yourself. Most of the sodium we consume comes from packaged, processed foods and fast food.

In your own kitchen, you have control over how much salt you use. For many of us, it's second nature to salt dishes liberally. In order to reduce your reliance on sodium without sacrificing flavor, you need to ensure that all the other ingredients in a dish are playing their part in making the food taste balanced and delicious. Salt may play a role in enhancing the flavors of food, but should not be used to compensate for blandness. Focus first on building flavor with acid, spices, and sweetness.

Tips for Reducing Salt

1. **Finish with salt.** If you add salt to your food as you cook, it's easy to oversalt without realizing it. A good alternative is to "finish" with salt, which means sprinkling just a small amount of salt onto your food right before eating it. Because the salt hits your taste buds directly, you'll experience it more intensely than if you added a much larger amount to the dish during cooking. For best results, choose a high-quality flaky sea salt.

2. **Stimulate your senses in other ways!** Tantalize your taste buds with herbs and spices. A little hot pepper, like cayenne or red pepper flakes, goes a long way toward boosting flavor without the need for salt. Toasted seeds and spices (see page 61) give recipes a kick. Onion and garlic are intensely flavorful, either fresh, concentrated into pastes for what we call flavor bombs (see page 69), or in the form of dried granules or powder.

3. **Try a salty alternative.** Some foods, including sea vegetables (try kelp or dulse flakes) and celery or celery powder, have a naturally salty flavor. While these do contain sodium, they also contain many other micronutrients not found in salt, so you can use less and get more nutritional value.

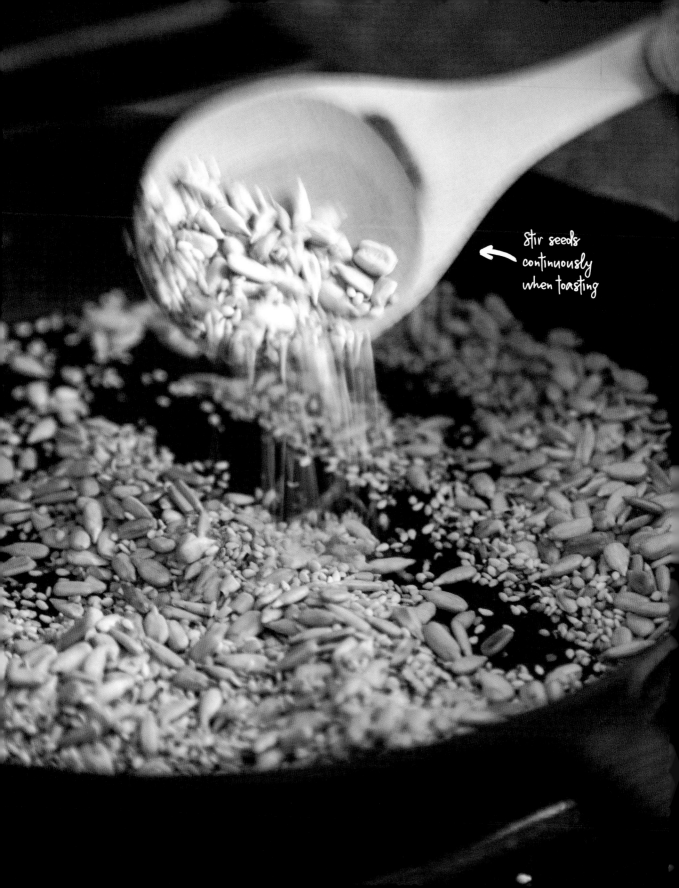

Stir seeds continuously when toasting

Toasting Seeds and Spices

Here's a simple experiment you can try. Take a handful of seeds—for example, sesame seeds—and eat half of them raw. Now, take a hot skillet, throw in the remaining seeds, and toast them for a few minutes over medium heat, until golden brown. Can you taste the difference? Toasting seeds brings out wonderful nutty flavors and enhances the seeds' satisfying crunchiness, making them a great alternative to salt. You can use toasted seeds whole or grind them into powder—the recipe that follows uses both techniques. Try them as a topping for steamed vegetables, as we do in Steamed Kale with Toasted Seeds (page 76), or salads.

To toast seeds or spices, heat a skillet over medium to high heat, add the seeds or spices and cook, moving them continuously (with a spoon or by shaking the pan), for 2 to 3 minutes, until golden. Smaller seeds, such as sesame, will "pop" when done. Transfer them to a plate to cool, then grind them using a spice grinder and use them in your dishes as you like. Freshly toasted spices will make a huge difference in your cooking.

Spicy Seed Blend

Makes about ⅔ cup

Put this flavor-packed blend in a shaker and have it on hand to use as a topping for rice, pastas, salads, or any other savory dishes.

2 tablespoons sunflower seeds, toasted (see directions at left)

¼ cup sesame seeds, toasted (see directions at left)

2 tablespoons hemp seeds, toasted (see directions at left)

2 tablespoons finely ground nutritional yeast

1½ teaspoons onion granules

½ teaspoon jalapeño powder or hot pepper of your choice

Pour the toasted sunflower seeds into a spice grinder and grind to a coarse meal. Transfer the meal to a small bowl and stir in the remaining ingredients.

Transfer the blend to a shaker or spice jar and store at room temperature away from heat and light for up to 3 weeks.

Per serving (1 tablespoon): 39 calories, 3 g total fat, 0 g saturated fat, 0 mg cholesterol, 2 mg sodium, 1 g total carbohydrate (1 g dietary fiber, 0 g sugar, 0 g added sugars), 2 g protein, 1 mg iron

The World of Herbs and Spices

Pungent, exotic, fragrant, and distinctive, herbs and spices capture the culinary character of the world's diversity of cultures. They have been used for thousands of years not just for cooking but for healing, ceremonial purposes, and trading.

What distinguishes an herb from a spice? Herbs are the leaves and stalks of a plant, and are generally best used fresh, although they can also be used dried. Spices are made from the roots, bark, seeds, fruits, buds, or flowers of a plant and are typically used dried.

Choosing Herbs

You'll notice a lot of fresh herbs in the recipes in this book. When possible, always choose fresh herbs over dried. If you do use dried herbs, keep them in your cupboard for no longer than six months; after that, buy a new jar, as their flavors will have dissipated. Sometimes you might want to combine several herbs, like basil, thyme, and oregano, creating complementary layers of flavor. Other times, you might want to highlight the distinctive flavor of a single herb, like tarragon or cilantro. Every herb has a unique fragrance and flavor, but they can be broadly divided into two categories: hearty and delicate.

Chef's Tip

DO YOU HAVE EXTRA FRESH HERBS?

Vacuum seal them and freeze them, or blend them with a touch of water to make a paste and freeze the paste in ice cube trays; pop a cube into a soup or sauce any time you want a touch of fresh flavor.

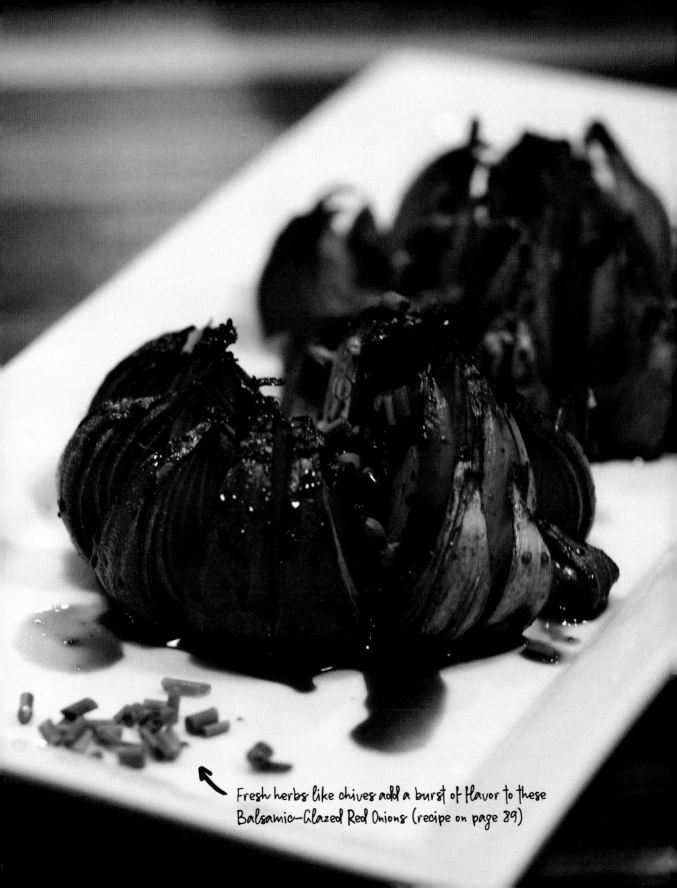

Fresh herbs like chives add a burst of flavor to these
Balsamic-Glazed Red Onions (recipe on page 89)

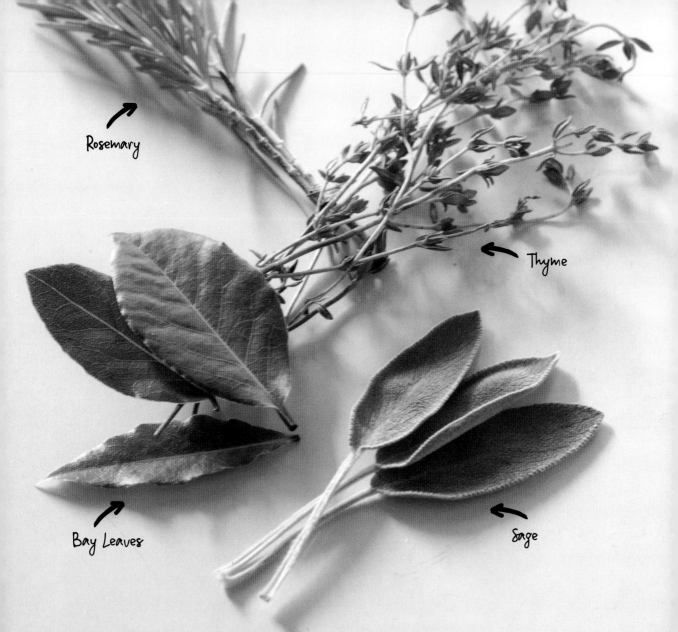

Rosemary

Thyme

Bay Leaves

Sage

Hearty Herbs

Hearty herbs include bay leaf, sage, thyme, and rosemary, and are best added earlier in a recipe so the cooking process brings out their essential oils. For this reason, you'll often see them used on roasted vegetables, as in our Classic Celeriac Pot Roast (page 99), where thyme is used in the coating so it releases its flavors slowly as the dish roasts. Hearty herbs are also used in gravies and soups.

Delicate Herbs

Delicate herbs include basil, cilantro, dill, parsley, tarragon, chives, and mint. These are best added at the end of the cooking process, so that they release their fresh, distinctive flavors directly onto your palate, adding an extra layer to the experience of eating the dish. For example, if you're making tomato sauce, don't cook the basil in the sauce; tear the leaves and add them at the end. This will give you bursts of freshness as you enjoy the sauce.

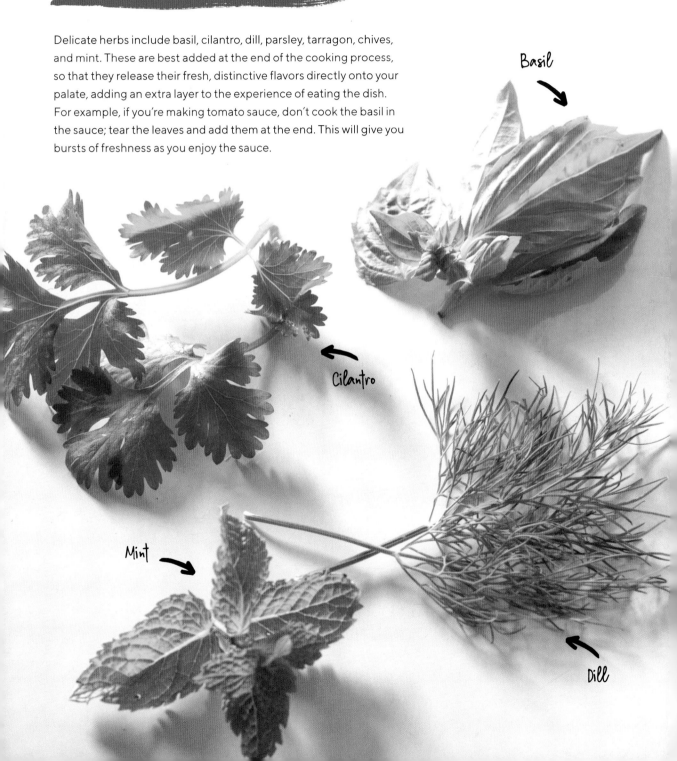

Basil

Cilantro

Mint

Dill

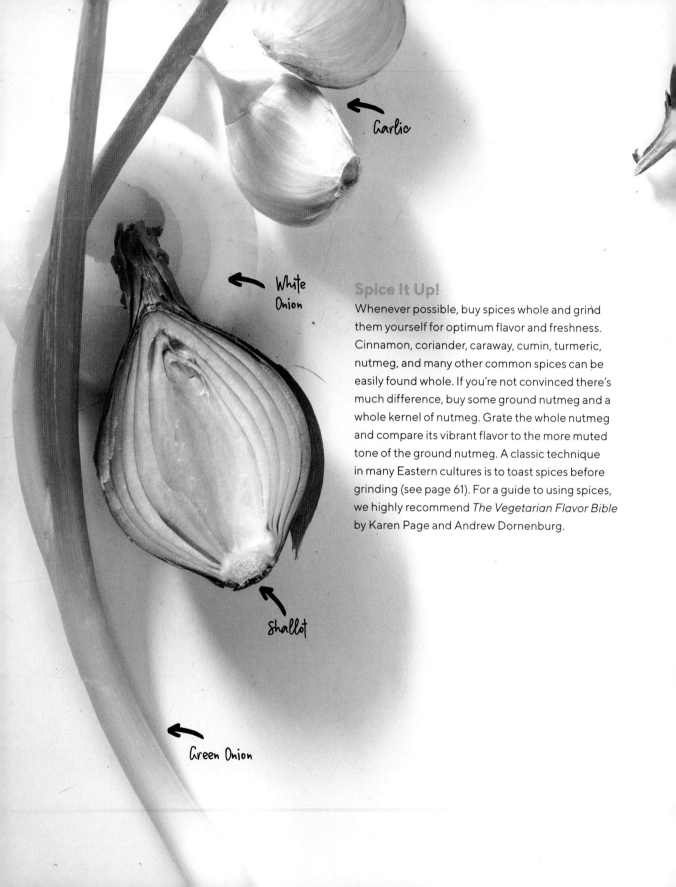

Garlic

White
Onion

Shallot

Green Onion

Spice It Up!

Whenever possible, buy spices whole and grind them yourself for optimum flavor and freshness. Cinnamon, coriander, caraway, cumin, turmeric, nutmeg, and many other common spices can be easily found whole. If you're not convinced there's much difference, buy some ground nutmeg and a whole kernel of nutmeg. Grate the whole nutmeg and compare its vibrant flavor to the more muted tone of the ground nutmeg. A classic technique in many Eastern cultures is to toast spices before grinding (see page 61). For a guide to using spices, we highly recommend *The Vegetarian Flavor Bible* by Karen Page and Andrew Dornenburg.

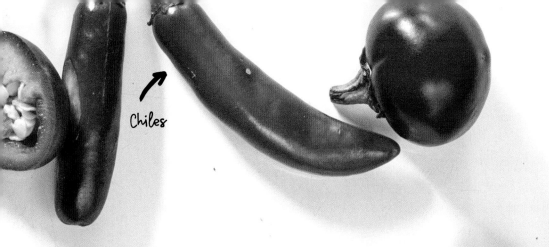

Chiles

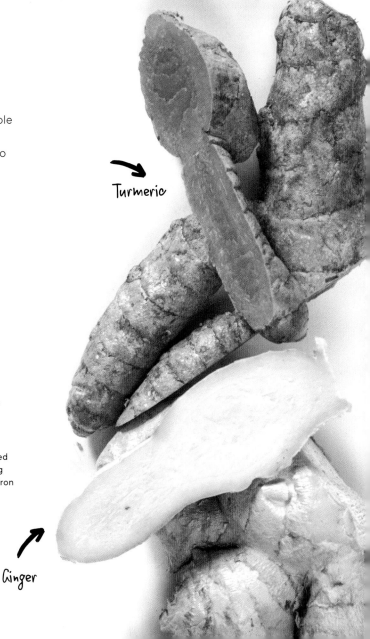

Turmeric

Mum's Spice Blend

Makes about ¾ cup

In this vibrant and umami-rich spice blend, multiple spices complement one another beautifully. Use this whenever you find yourself reaching for salt to add a well-rounded flavor bomb to your dishes.

2 tablespoons smoked paprika

2 tablespoons garlic powder

1 tablespoon onion powder

1 tablespoon dried parsley

1 tablespoon dried basil

1 tablespoon dried oregano

1 tablespoon dried thyme

1 teaspoon cayenne pepper

⅛ teaspoon dried lemon peel

1 teaspoon sea salt (optional)

Combine everything in a small airtight container, cover, and shake well. Store at room temperature away from heat and light for up to 4 months.

Per serving (1 teaspoon): **4** calories, **0** g total fat, **0** g saturated fat, **0** mg cholesterol, **1** mg sodium, **1** g total carbohydrate (**0** g dietary fiber, **0** g sugar, **0** g added sugars), **0** g protein, **0** mg iron

Ginger

Asian Umami Spice Blend

Makes about ⅔ cup

Asian cultures have long prized umami flavors. Use this blend for stir-fries, to top noodles, in sauces, or to garnish steamed greens and rice.

½ cup dried mushrooms, such as shiitake or portobello

¼ cup sesame seeds, toasted (see page 61)

2 teaspoons ground ginger

2 tablespoons garlic granules

2 tablespoons onion granules

1 teaspoon cayenne pepper

1 teaspoon nori or kelp granules or powder

In a spice grinder, grind the mushrooms to a fine powder (you should have about ¼ cup). Transfer the mushroom powder to a small bowl.

Pour the toasted sesame seeds into the grinder and grind to a coarse powder. Transfer to the bowl with the mushroom powder.

Stir in the remaining ingredients and transfer the blend to a shaker or spice jar. Store at room temperature away from heat and light for up to 3 weeks.

Per serving (1 tablespoon): 51 calories, 2 g total fat, 0 g saturated fat, 0 mg cholesterol, 4 mg sodium, 4 g total carbohydrate (1 g dietary fiber, 0 g sugar, 0 g added sugars), 2 g protein, 2 mg iron

Italian Umami Spice Blend

Makes about ½ cup

Try this sprinkled over steamed vegetables, or add it to sauces or pasta.

½ cup dried mushrooms, such as porcini or portobello

2 teaspoons dried rosemary

1 teaspoon dried thyme

1 teaspoon salt-free lemon pepper seasoning

1 tablespoon garlic granules

1 tablespoon onion granules

½ teaspoon red pepper flakes

½ teaspoon freshly ground black pepper

In a spice grinder, grind the mushrooms to a fine powder (you should have about ¼ cup). Transfer the powder to a small bowl.

Put the rosemary, thyme, and lemon pepper seasoning in the grinder and grind to a fine powder. Transfer to the bowl with the mushroom powder.

Stir in the remaining ingredients and transfer the blend to a shaker or spice jar. Store at room temperature away from heat and light for up to 3 weeks.

Per serving (1 tablespoon): 39 calories, 0 g total fat, 0 g saturated fat, 0 mg cholesterol, 3 mg sodium, 5 g total carbohydrate (1 g dietary fiber, 0 g sugar, 0 g added sugars), 2 g protein, 2 mg iron

Flavor Bombs

Chefs have long known that onions and garlic add a concentrated boost of flavor to a dish—that's why they form the starting point for so many recipes. Another way to capture and condense the aromatic intensity of these vegetables is to turn them into pastes (pictured on page 52). Just stir a small amount of these simple pastes into your dishes and you'll be amazed at their powerful impact—that's why we call them flavor bombs!

Roasted Garlic Paste

Makes about ½ cup

By roasting the garlic, this recipe adds more depth of flavor, thanks to the slight caramelization of the juices. Store it in the fridge as an easy addition to most savory dishes.

4 whole heads garlic	**¼ teaspoon sea salt**
Spray oil	**½ teaspoon freshly ground black pepper**

Preheat the oven to 400°F.

Slice off the top of each head of garlic just enough to expose the very tops of the garlic cloves. Place each head of garlic cut-side up on a piece of foil. Very lightly spray the exposed garlic cloves with spray oil to help prevent scorching. Loosely wrap each bulb in the foil. Place the foil packets on a rimmed baking sheet and roast until the garlic cloves are fork-tender, 25 to 35 minutes. Remove them from the oven and let cool in the foil.

When cool enough to handle, unwrap the heads of garlic. Holding one over a small bowl, squeeze the entire head of garlic to force the individual cloves from their papery skins into the bowl (or a mortar). Repeat with the remaining heads of garlic. Add the salt and pepper and mash with a fork (or the pestle) until very smooth. Spoon into an airtight container and store in the refrigerator for up to 1 week.

Per serving (1 teaspoon): 4 calories, 0 g total fat, 0 g saturated fat, 0 mg cholesterol, 24 mg sodium, 1 g total carbohydrate (0 g dietary fiber, 0 g sugar, 0 g added sugars), 0 g protein, 0 mg iron

Poached Garlic Paste

Makes about ½ cup

Garlic pastes are a flavor-building secret weapon. This is the lighter of two versions. Store it in the fridge as an easy addition to most savory dishes.

½ cup garlic cloves

¼ teaspoon sea salt

½ teaspoon freshly ground black pepper

Bring 1 cup water to a boil in a small saucepan. Add the garlic and simmer until soft, about 4 minutes. Remove from the heat.

Drain the garlic and transfer it to a small bowl or a mortar. Add the salt and pepper and mash with a fork or the pestle until very smooth. Spoon into an airtight container and store in the refrigerator for up to 1 week.

Per serving (1 teaspoon): 4 calories, 0 g total fat, 0 g saturated fat, 0 mg cholesterol, 25 mg sodium, 1 g total carbohydrate (0 g dietary fiber, 0 g sugar, 0 g added sugars), 0 g protein, 0 mg iron

Chef's Tip

When making these pastes, freeze them in ice cube trays until solid, then pop them out and store them in a freezer bag for quick and easy use in your next soup, sauce, or dressing.

Onion Buttah

Makes about 3 cups

This flavor bomb leaves dairy butter in the dust! Use it any time you want to bump up the flavor of your soups or sauces.

½ cup raw cashews

4 cups quartered shallots or white onions

2 cups water or low-sodium vegetable broth

Soak the cashews in water to cover for at least 3 hours or up to overnight. Drain and rinse.

Meanwhile, preheat the oven to 375°F.

Place the shallots in a shallow medium baking dish and add just enough water or broth to barely cover them. Roast until most of the liquid has evaporated and the shallots are golden brown with slight charring on the tips, 20 to 25 minutes.

Transfer the roasted shallots to a (preferably high-speed) blender, leaving any remaining liquid in the baking dish. Add the drained cashews and puree to the texture of a loose paste or jam, 1 to 2 minutes.

Use immediately, or transfer to an airtight container and refrigerate for up to 1 week. You can also scrape the mixture into ice cube trays and freeze until solid, then transfer the cubes to a freezer bag and store them in the freezer for up to 2 months.

Per serving (2 tablespoons): 39 calories, 1 g total fat, 0 g saturated fat, 0 mg cholesterol, 4 mg sodium, 6 g total carbohydrate (1 g dietary fiber, 3 g sugar, 0 g added sugars), 1 g protein, 1 mg iron

Garlic Bread: Having Italian night? Grab a loaf of your favorite 100% whole-grain bread, slice it in half horizontally, and spread a generous amount of Onion Buttah (page 71, at left) and Poached or Roasted Garlic Paste (pages 70 and 69) over the cut side of each half. Top with sliced fresh tomatoes, some minced fresh parsley, and lots of black pepper. Sandwich the two halves together, wrap the loaf in foil, and bake in a preheated 375°F oven for 10 to 12 minutes.

Concentrating Flavors Through Reductions

When you "reduce" a liquid like vinegar or wine—cooking it so some of its water content evaporates—you concentrate the sweetness of its natural sugars. For example, taste some white balsamic vinegar and then reduce it using the following recipe and taste it again—you'll notice that it gets thicker, stickier, and sweeter. The resulting syrup can be used in both savory dishes and desserts; we use this syrup as a topping for roasted vegetables in our Autumn Veggie Bowl (page 172) *and* as a topping for our Grilled Pineapple dessert (page 278). You can use the same process to make syrups from other vinegars or wine; store them in an airtight container in the fridge for up to several weeks. Note that the higher the sugar content, the faster a liquid reduces.

White Balsamic Syrup

Makes ⅓ to ½ cup

This sweet, tangy syrup is a great topping for savory dishes or desserts, or try it drizzled over nondairy cheeses.

2 cups white balsamic vinegar

Pour the vinegar into a small pot and bring to a simmer over medium heat. Reduce the heat to medium-low and cook until the vinegar has thickened to the consistency of a syrup. Use a fan during this process, because the aroma is strong. Store in an airtight container in the refrigerator for up to several weeks.

Per serving (1 tablespoon): 128 calories, 0 g total fat, 0 g saturated fat, 0 mg cholesterol, 0 mg sodium, 32 g total carbohydrate (1 g dietary fiber, 26 g sugar, 0 g added sugars), 0 g protein, 0 mg iron

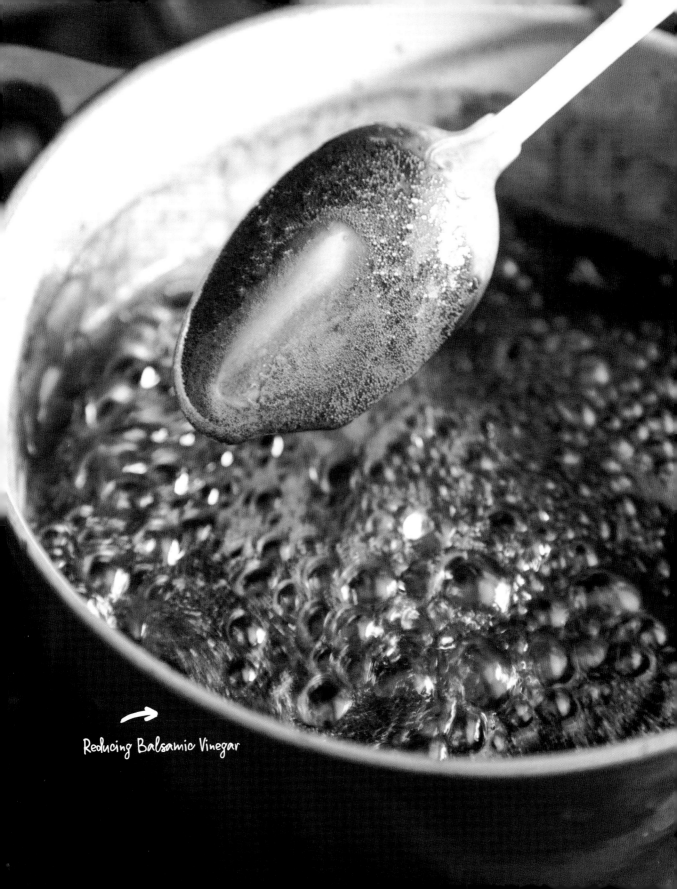

Reducing Balsamic Vinegar

Steaming is one of the easiest and healthiest cooking methods

CHAPTER 7

Core Plant-Based Cooking Methods

Humans are astonishingly inventive when it comes to the ways we apply heat to our food and transform it from raw to cooked. Cooking methods affect the texture of a food, and they also fundamentally alter its flavor and appearance. Consider a raw carrot, a lightly steamed carrot, and a slow-roasted carrot: even without the addition of herbs, spices, condiments, or sweeteners, those three will taste strikingly different. A good cook understands the role of cooking techniques in flavor development, and chooses the right method to get the desired taste, texture, and appearance.

Understanding a few foundational techniques will empower you to be creative in the kitchen. In this chapter, we're going to focus on some of the core methods used in whole foods, plant-based cooking: **steaming**, **sautéing**, **grilling**, **roasting**, **combination cooking**, **slow cooking**, and **salt baking**. You may be familiar with the traditional meaning of many of these terms, but here you'll learn how to adapt them to a diet that doesn't include refined oils. For each cooking method, we'll share some simple, delicious recipes that will allow you to practice the skills and experience the particular flavors that cooking method creates.

The Art of Steaming

Some cooking techniques employ dry heat; others employ moist heat. Steaming is one of the most common and healthiest methods for cooking with moist heat. Food is placed in a basket set over boiling water and covered with a lid, so that the steam is trapped, surrounding the food. While boiling may overcook vegetables quickly if you're not paying attention to timing, steaming preserves their nutrients and often enhances their taste and color, making it a popular choice for cooking vegetables. Most vegetables need only a few minutes of steaming to reach optimum texture and taste.

We recommend using a traditional stackable bamboo steamer, which allows you to steam multiple layers of vegetables. Put those with the highest density, such as potatoes, carrots, and hard squashes, closest to the steam, followed by those with medium density, such as broccoli or cauliflower, and save zucchini or leafy greens for the top layer. They'll be exposed to different intensities of steam so they'll cook at the same time.

Once you have steamed your vegetables, you can finish them by adding new layers of flavor—a squeeze of citrus or splash of vinegar, fresh herbs, toasted spices or seeds. Experiment with different combinations—the recipes on the pages that follow will give you some suggestions to spark your creativity with your next batch of steamed veggies.

Steamed Kale with Toasted Seeds

Serves 4 as a side dish

Kale boasts deep, earthy flavors, and can be rich and hearty and slightly bitter at times. A punchy spice blend stands up to this nutrient dense leafy green, and a splash of lemon juice adds just the right amount of acid to brighten up the dish. See page 61 for instructions on toasting spices.

1½ tablespoons white sesame seeds, toasted

½ teaspoon fennel seeds, toasted

⅛ teaspoon cumin seeds, toasted

⅛ teaspoon caraway seeds, toasted

2 tablespoons sunflower seeds, toasted

1 bunch kale, stemmed, leaves torn into bite-size pieces

1 tablespoon fresh lemon juice

2 tablespoons nutritional yeast

Combine the sesame, fennel, cumin, and caraway seeds in a spice grinder and grind to a coarse powder. Transfer to a medium bowl and mix in the sunflower seeds.

Steam the kale in a covered steamer basket over gently simmering water until vibrant and tender, about 3 minutes.

Transfer the steamed kale to the bowl of seeds, then add the lemon juice and nutritional yeast. Stir to combine, and serve warm.

Note: Add chopped onion and minced garlic to the steaming water for extra flavor. You can also try balsamic vinegar instead of lemon juice.

Per serving: 77 calories, 5 g total fat, 1 g saturated fat, 0 mg cholesterol, 41 mg sodium, 3 g total carbohydrate (1 g dietary fiber, 1 g sugar, 0 g added sugars), 5 g protein, 2 mg iron

Spinach Gomae with Toasted Sesame Seeds

Serves 2

This traditional Japanese side dish pairs perfectly with your favorite vegetable sushi, or try serving it over brown rice. Be sure to press as much liquid out of the spinach as you can before topping it with the rich simple sesame sauce.

1 tablespoon tahini

1 tablespoon unseasoned rice vinegar

1 teaspoon low-sodium tamari

1 pound baby spinach

2½ teaspoons sesame seeds, toasted (see page 61)

In a small bowl, whisk together the tahini, vinegar, and tamari until smooth. Set aside.

Heat a large deep sauté pan over medium heat. Add the spinach and 1 teaspoon water. Cover and cook just until spinach wilts, 1 to 2 minutes, stirring once or twice. Drain and let cool. When cool enough to handle, squeeze out every last bit of liquid from spinach.

Break up spinach in a bowl and toss with the dressing. Top with the sesame seeds.

Per serving: 121 calories, 6 g total fat, 1 g saturated fat, 0 mg cholesterol, 300 mg sodium, 10 g total carbohydrate (6 g dietary fiber, 0 g sugar, 0 g added sugars), 8 g protein, 8 mg iron

Spiced Sweet Potatoes with Green Onion Vinaigrette

Serves 4 as a side dish

The sweetness of the potatoes perfectly complements this punchy green onion dressing. Serve as a side, on top of greens, or tossed with your favorite whole-grain pasta for a delicious pasta salad.

2 sweet potatoes, peeled and cut into 1-inch cubes

2 tablespoons champagne vinegar

2 tablespoons white wine

1 teaspoon Dijon mustard

1 green onion, trimmed and sliced

1 tarragon sprig, minced

1 small garlic clove, cut into thin strips

1 teaspoon Mum's Spice Blend (page 67) or other spice blend of your choice

Parsley sprigs, for garnish

Steam sweet potatoes in a covered steamer basket over gently simmering water until tender, 8 to 12 minutes.

In a medium bowl, whisk together the vinegar, wine, mustard, green onion, tarragon, garlic, and spice blend. Add the sweet potatoes and toss gently to coat. Garnish with parsley.

Note: To crisp up the potatoes, line a baking sheet with parchment and spread the dressed potatoes on the sheet. Broil until crispy, about 10 minutes.

Per serving: 94 calories, 0 g total fat, 0 g saturated fat, 0 mg cholesterol, 64 mg sodium, 20 g total carbohydrate (3 g dietary fiber, 6 g sugar, 0 g added sugars), 2 g protein, 1 mg iron

Sautéing Without Oil

One of the biggest shifts for people adopting a whole foods, plant-based diet is learning to cook without oil. Once you learn a few simple techniques, it's really not that difficult—and you'll remove significant amounts of extra fat and empty calories from your diet (see page 10 for more on why oil is avoided in these recipes).

One of the most common uses of oil in everyday cooking is to sauté aromatics (onions and garlic being the most common) before starting a dish. The Dry Sauté Method can be used instead, and it will work for other vegetables as well. You'll see this method called for in numerous recipes in the pages ahead.

A note about garlic: It burns much faster than onions, so when you're not using oil, it's wise to wait to add your minced garlic until the onions have begun sticking, right before you deglaze the pan.

Dry Sauté Method

Whenever the recipes ahead call for a dry sauté, these are the steps you need to take to start the dish.

1. Heat the pan until very hot. (Use the "water test," a great trick taught by the Rouxbe Online Culinary School, to test if the pan is hot enough: a drop of water should roll around the pan like a mercury ball as soon as it touches the surface.)

2. Add chopped onions, shallots, or leeks to the hot pan.

3. Cook until they begin to color and stick slightly to the pan. You will start to see some speckles around the pan. The browning is important for building flavor. The onions are caramelizing—releasing, concentrating, and bringing their sugars to the surface. If using garlic, add it at this stage.

4. Add a splash of flavorful liquid, such as low-sodium vegetable broth or wine, and stir to deglaze the pan and loosen the onions, scraping up the browned bits on the bottom of the pan.

5. Reduce the heat from medium to low and proceed with the recipe or remove the pan from the heat and add the contents to other dishes.

DON'T PASS UP AN OPPORTUNITY TO BUILD FLAVOR!

Chef's Tip

Some people use just water for a no-oil sauté, but using a flavorful liquid instead allows you to add another layer to the flavor profile of your dish. Every chance you can get, add flavor! Try red or white wine, broth, coconut water, the juice from a can of tomatoes, or the soaking water from dried mushrooms or chiles—each will infuse your dish with a distinct and delicious character.

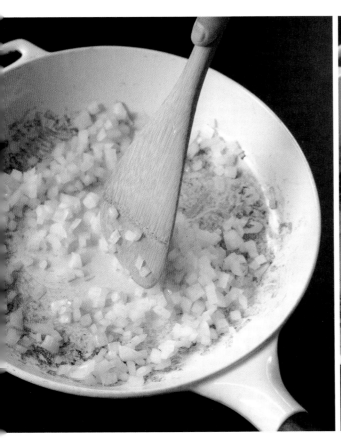

Allow the onions to stick and begin to brown

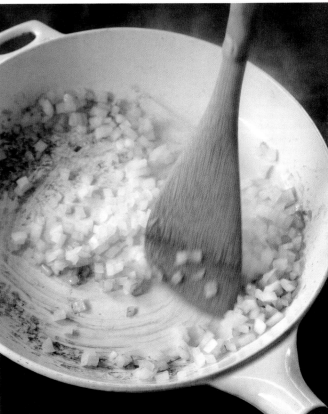

Add a splash of liquid and stir to deglaze the pan

Building Flavor on the Grill

For many of us, the word *grilling* conjures up the smell of charcoal smoke and burgers, the taste of cold beer, the warmth of a summer afternoon. But grilling doesn't have to be about meat. As a cooking technique, it's wonderful for all kinds of vegetables (especially mushrooms), lending them a distinctive sweet, charred flavor.

Technically, grilling means any form of cooking that applies dry heat directly to the surface of a food, usually from flames or coals below. It's the original cooking technique—our ancestors grilled their food over open fires. These days, we have the choice of wood, charcoal, or gas grills, cast-iron grill pans on the stovetop, or electric grills. Each of these will create different flavors in the food, with wood and charcoal adding a smokiness that you won't get from gas or electric.

The act of grilling builds a foundation of flavor, charring, smoking, and caramelizing the vegetables. You may want to enjoy these flavors just as they are, or you may want to add additional layers of flavor by rubbing the vegetables with herbs and spices or basting them with sauces or marinades. As you cook your vegetables, you can continue to add the sauce, concentrating and deepening the flavors.

Always start by heating the grill well. If you're grilling indoors, make sure you have a good fan, as there will be smoke. Have a pair of tongs handy for moving things around on the grill. While we don't encourage cooking in oil, we do advise that you lightly spray the grill grates with spray oil, or the food will stick.

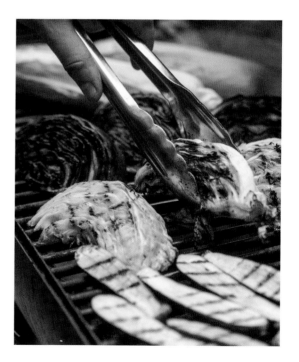

Greek Vegetable Kabobs with Tzatziki

Serves 4 as an appetizer

Who doesn't love eating off a skewer? This combination of marinated and grilled Mediterranean veggies is a perfect recipe for summer backyard eating or picnic food. The tzatziki sauce cools the spices and balances the charred flavors from the grill. You can make the tzatziki with any nondairy yogurt, but we like the clean creaminess of the Kite Hill brand almond milk yogurt. **Recipe by Whole Foods Market**

TZATZIKI
1 cup plain unsweetened Kite Hill almond milk yogurt

1 cucumber, peeled and finely chopped

2 tablespoons minced fresh dill

1 garlic clove, minced

1 tablespoon red wine vinegar

Pinch of sea salt

Freshly ground black pepper

MARINADE
¾ cup red wine vinegar

½ cup chopped fresh parsley

2 garlic cloves, minced

2 teaspoons Dijon mustard

1 teaspoon dried oregano

½ teaspoon freshly ground black pepper

¼ teaspoon sea salt

KABOBS
1 zucchini, halved lengthwise and cut into half-moons

1½ cups cremini (baby bella) mushrooms, stems trimmed

1 red bell pepper, cut into 1-inch squares

1 red onion, cut into 1-inch squares

Shrimp, whole, or chicken or tofu, cut into 1-inch squares (optional)

For the tzatziki, combine everything in a medium bowl and stir well. Cover and refrigerate until ready to use, up to 1 day.

For the marinade, whisk everything together in a large bowl or zip-top bag. Set aside 3 tablespoons of the marinade in a small bowl.

For the kabobs, put all the vegetables (and protein, if using) in the large bowl or bag with the marinade and toss to coat. Cover or seal and marinate at room temperature for about 30 minutes, tossing occasionally.

Heat a grill to high. Thread the vegetables (and protein, if using) onto the skewers, alternating 2 pieces each of zucchini, mushroom, peppers, and onions. Grill until the vegetables are tender and slightly charred, 4 to 6 minutes (or until the protein, if using, is cooked through), turning for even cooking. Remove the kabobs from the grill, set them on a platter, and drizzle with the reserved marinade.

Serve with the tzatziki.

Per serving: 112 calories, 5 g total fat, 1 g saturated fat, 0 mg cholesterol, 329 mg sodium, 12 g total carbohydrate (3 g dietary fiber, 5 g sugar, 0 g added sugars), 5 g protein, 1 mg iron

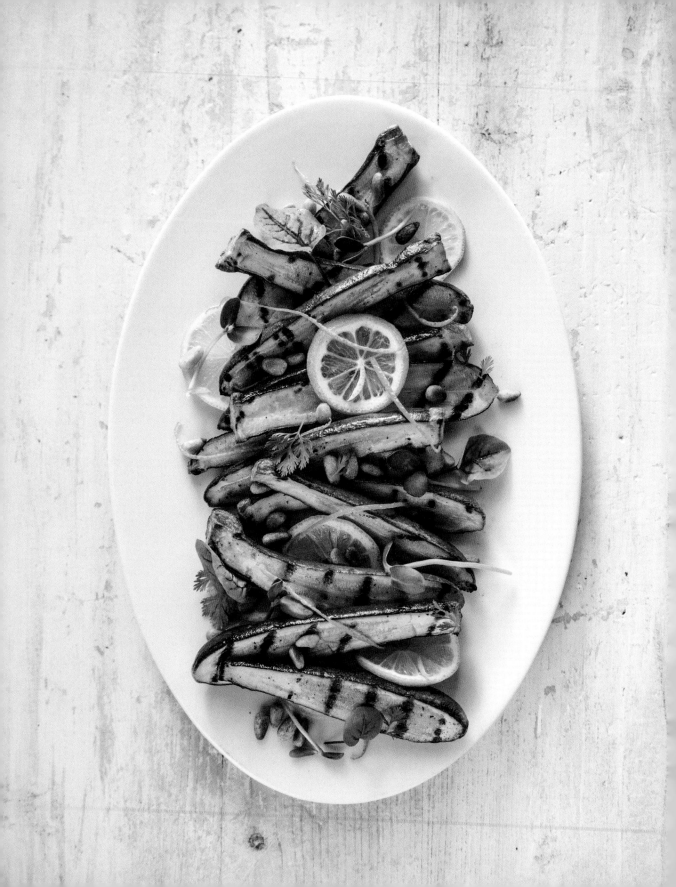

Grilled Zucchini with Lemon & Herbs

Serves 4 as a side dish

This simple, elegant grilled vegetable dish features the classic Italian flavors of herbs, citrus, and toasted pine nuts.

Spray oil (for grill)

¼ teaspoon freshly ground black pepper

10 to 12 baby zucchini, halved, or 2 mature zucchini, cut into long planks

6 thin lemon slices

1 orange wedge

1 teaspoon grated orange zest

1 teaspoon grated lemon zest

3 tablespoons pine nuts, toasted

2 tablespoons mixed chopped fresh herbs (such as oregano, basil, and parsley)

¼ teaspoon flaky sea salt, such as Maldon (optional)

Heat grill to high or heat a grill pan over high heat. Reduce the heat to medium-high, then spray the grill grate or pan lightly with oil.

Sprinkle the black pepper all over the zucchini. Place the zucchini cut-side down on the grill or pan and grill until browned on each side, 2 to 3 minutes per side. Transfer to a small platter, arranging the pieces decoratively on the platter.

Place the lemon slices among the grilled zucchini pieces. Squeeze the juice from the orange wedge over the top and finish with the orange and lemon zests, pine nuts, fresh herbs, and salt (if using).

Per serving: 66 calories, 4 g total fat, 0 g saturated fat, 0 mg cholesterol, 8 mg sodium, 7 g total carbohydrate (3 g dietary fiber, 4 g sugar, 0 g added sugars), 2 g protein, 1 mg iron

Chipotle Grilled Corn

Serves 4

Looking for that picnic side that packs a punch? Look no further. This Mexican-inspired grilled corn has it all: flavor, heat, color, and texture. This recipe showcases the power of garlic paste—a game-changer when it comes to building flavor.

Juice of 2 limes

2 tablespoons Poached or Roasted Garlic Paste (page 70 or 69)

1 tablespoon tomato paste

1 teaspoon paprika

1 teaspoon chipotle powder

¼ teaspoon sea salt

4 ears fresh corn, shucked

½ cup chopped fresh cilantro

Heat a grill to medium-high.

In a small bowl, stir together the lime juice, garlic paste, tomato paste, paprika, chipotle powder, and salt to make a paste. Using a brush or spoon, coat each ear of corn all over with a thin layer of the paste. Wrap each ear of corn individually in foil.

Grill the corn directly over the heat until tender, 5 to 6 minutes, turning a few times for even cooking.

Remove from the grill, open the foil, and garnish with the cilantro. Serve the corn in the foil or on a platter.

Per serving: 164 calories, 1 g total fat, 0 g saturated fat, 0 mg cholesterol, 217 mg sodium, 39 g total carbohydrate (5 g dietary fiber, 5 g sugar, 0 g added sugars), 5 g protein, 1 mg iron

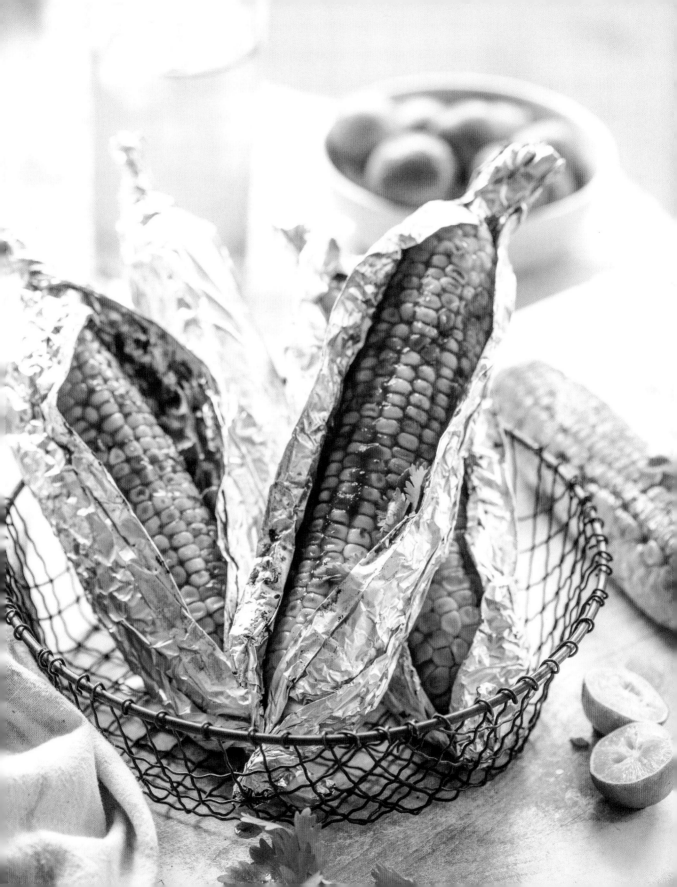

Roasting for Flavor

Roasting is a wonderful method for bringing out the natural sweetness in vegetables and building complex, earthy, umami flavors. Dry heat envelops the food from all sides, creating a crispy outer layer and a soft inside. Traditional roasting involves coating the food with fat or oil to seal in its natural moisture and prevent it from drying out. When cooking without oil, the key is to add flavorful liquid, such as low-sodium vegetable broth or wine, during the cooking process to compensate for what's lost. Just splash a little of the liquid over the roasting vegetables once or twice as they cook. This is also an opportunity to build flavor. Throw in some hearty herbs, such as rosemary or thyme, or some chopped onion or whole garlic cloves for an added boost. Alternatively, coat the roasted vegetables with a sauce or dressing when they come out of the oven.

Chef's Tip

YOU DON'T NEED OIL TO ROAST

The secret to roasting without oil is getting the right combination of timing and heat, and being mindful of adding back some moisture. As a general rule of thumb, for smaller pieces, you want to use higher heat—these will cook quickly from the outside in and be crispy on the outside. For larger pieces, you'll want to use lower heat—these will cook more slowly, from the inside out.

Common Vegetables for Roasting and Estimated Cooking Times

The cooking temperature is 400°F, unless otherwise noted. If the pieces are larger than indicated, the oven temperature will need to be lowered, and vice versa. Roast the vegetables on a baking sheet lined with parchment paper or a silicone baking mat, or on nonstick roasting pans.

Vegetable	Prep	Estimated Roasting Time	Notes
Beets	Cut into 1-inch pieces or wedges	15 to 18 minutes; flip halfway	Use a sharp knife to check if they are tender
Broccoli	Cut into florets (about 1½ inches)	5 to 8 minutes, flip, then 3 to 5 minutes (8 to 13 minutes total)	Be consistent with floret sizes for even cooking
Brussels sprouts	Halve lengthwise	10 to 12 minutes	Trim off wrinkled or older leaves
Butternut squash and most winter squashes	Peeled and cut into roughly 1-inch pieces	8 to 10 minutes, until browned on the bottom, flip, then 5 to 8 minutes (13 to 18 minutes total)	Splash with a flavorful low-sodium vegetable broth or white wine while roasting
Carrots	Cut into 1-inch pieces	8 to 10 minutes, flip, then 3 to 5 minutes more (11 to 13 minutes total)	Finish with a squeeze of orange juice, minced fresh chives, and a dash of ground cumin
Cauliflower	Cut into florets (about 1½ inches)	4 to 6 minutes, until brown, flip, then 3 to 5 minutes (7 to 11 minutes total)	Finish with a drizzle of White Balsamic Syrup (page 72), dried currants, and mint leaves
Fennel	Cut through the core into 1-inch-wide wedges	12 to 15 minutes; flip halfway	Toss with thin slices of apple and lemon juice and zest
Green beans	Trim stem end	5 to 8 minutes	Should be tender and look somewhat shriveled
Mushrooms—button, cremini (baby bella), or any wild mushroom	Wipe off dirt with a lightly damp paper towel, trim stems, and halve	Stem-side down for 8 to 10 minutes, until browned, flip, then 5 minutes, until browned (13 to 15 minutes total)	Drizzle with tamari or balsamic vinegar while roasting; toss with sliced green onion and toasted sesame seeds to finish
Potatoes	Cut into roughly 1-inch pieces; halve baby potatoes	10 to 12 minutes, until browned on the bottom, flip, then 5 to 8 minutes more, or until browned (15 to 20 minutes total)	Toss with chopped fresh rosemary and thyme before roasting; sprinkle with sea salt and black pepper to finish
Sweet potatoes	Cut into roughly 1-inch pieces	8 to 10 minutes, until browned on the bottom, flip, then 5 minutes or until tender (13 to 15 minutes total)	Serve with a drizzle of tahini sauce, or a drizzle of white balsamic vinegar and a sprinkle of ground cinnamon
Tomatoes	Cut into wedges; larger cherry tomatoes cut in half; small cherry tomatoes left whole	12 to 15 minutes (best if roasted at 350°F for a longer time to achieve caramelization)	Finish with a drizzle of aged balsamic vinegar and some fresh basil
Zucchini or summer squash	Cut into 1½-inch cubes	4 to 6 minutes, flip, then 3 to 5 minutes (7 to 11 minutes total)	Finish with a squeeze of lemon juice, flaky salt, and herbs

Roasted Cherry Tomatoes & Garlic

Serves 4

A favorite, simple recipe to have on hand for sandwiches, pasta, or pizza or to jazz up your next slice of avocado toast. This works best when cherry tomatoes are in season and at their peak of sweetness.

1 pint cherry tomatoes, halved lengthwise

10 garlic cloves, smashed

Freshly ground black pepper

Leaves from 1 large sprig thyme

Preheat the oven to 375°F. Line a rimmed baking sheet with parchment paper.

Spread the tomatoes, cut-sides up, over the baking sheet and scatter the garlic cloves among them. Sprinkle everything with pepper and the thyme leaves.

Roast until the tomatoes collapse and char a bit on the edges, about 20 minutes. Use immediately, or let cool and refrigerate in an airtight container for up to 2 days.

Per serving: 46 calories, 0 g total fat, 0 g saturated fat, 0 mg cholesterol, 7 mg sodium, 10 g total carbohydrate (1 g dietary fiber, 2 g sugar, 0 g added sugars), 2 g protein, 1 mg iron

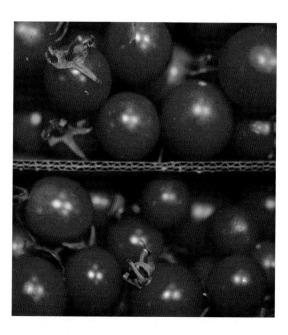

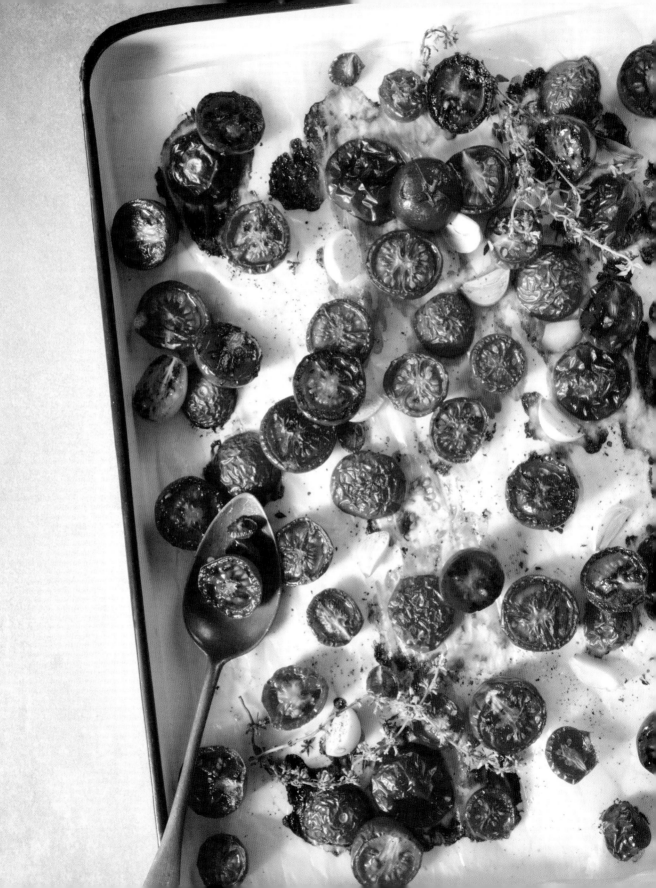

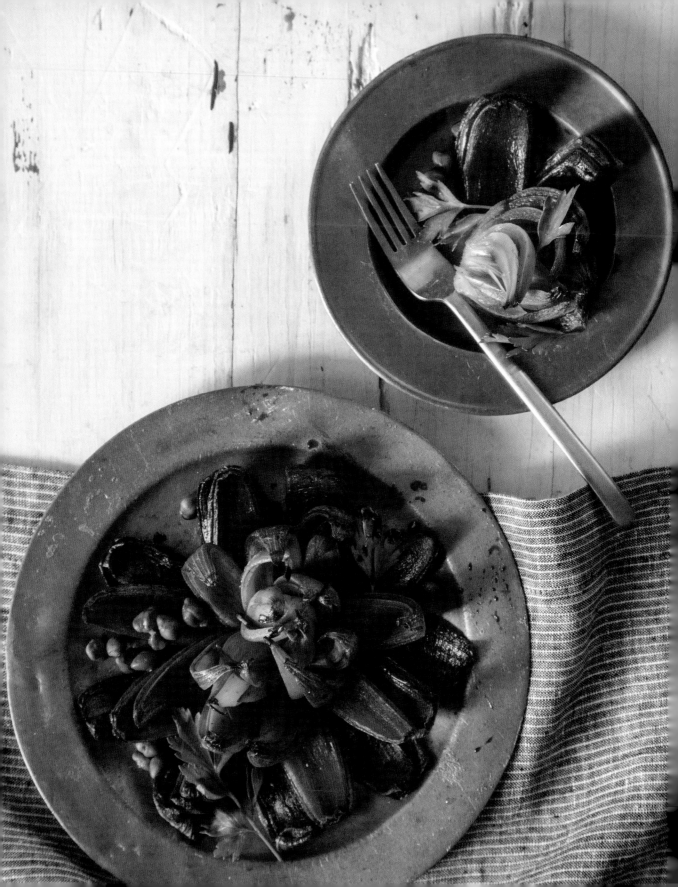

Balsamic-Glazed Red Onions

Serves 4 as a side dish

You'll be surprised how simple these roasted onions are to prepare—and how deliciously sweet they turn out! With their crispy exterior and soft, caramelized interior, they make a nice side dish or a flavorful addition to a pasta salad.

2 red onions, unpeeled

½ cup balsamic vinegar

1 tablespoon white wine

½ teaspoon Mum's Spice Blend (page 67) or your favorite spice blend

1 tablespoon drained and rinsed small capers

2 tablespoons chopped fresh parsley

Preheat the oven to 400°F. Line an 8-inch square baking dish with parchment paper.

Cut the tops off the onions and remove their skins. Slice the onions lengthwise into eighths but leave the root end intact to hold the onion together.

Place the onions in the prepared baking dish and pour ¼ cup of the vinegar and the wine over the top. Sprinkle with the spice blend. Cover with foil and bake for 30 minutes.

Remove from the oven and carefully remove the foil. Rearrange the onion slices so each resembles a flower that has opened up. Spoon any juices in the bottom of the pan over the onions. Pour the remaining ¼ cup vinegar over the onions and bake, uncovered, until the onions are tender and the flower shapes open up completely and crisp a little at the edges, about 10 minutes.

Transfer to a serving dish and scatter the capers and parsley over the onions. Spoon any pan juices over the top and serve.

Note: As a variation, use white or yellow onions and white balsamic vinegar.

Per serving: 55 calories, 0 g total fat, 0 g saturated fat, 0 mg cholesterol, 61 mg sodium, 11 g total carbohydrate (1 g dietary fiber, 7 g sugar, 0 g added sugars), 1 g protein, 1 mg iron

Roasted Brussels Sprouts & Shallots

Serves 2

Brussels sprouts are on the comeback. If they are sautéed or roasted correctly, they make a great addition to any plant-packed meal. This version takes some inspiration from kimchi, a spicy fermented Korean kraut. *Togarashi* is a Japanese seven-spice blend, which you can find in most Asian markets. Serve this as a side dish with brown rice and baked tofu.

1 pound Brussels sprouts, quartered or shaved on a mandoline

1 cup quartered or shaved shallots

½ teaspoon cracked black pepper

¼ teaspoon sea salt

3 tablespoons unseasoned rice vinegar

¼ teaspoon togarashi (see headnote)

¼ cup chopped green onion

1 small red Thai chile or other hot pepper, thinly sliced

In a medium bowl, combine the Brussels sprouts, shallots, black pepper, salt, vinegar, and togarashi. Toss until sprouts are evenly coated, then cover the bowl and let rest at room temperature for 1 hour.

Preheat the oven to 400°F. Line a rimmed baking sheet with parchment paper.

Spread the sprouts over the prepared pan in a single layer and pour any liquid from the bowl over the sprouts. Roast until tender, 15 to 20 minutes.

Transfer to a serving bowl and fold in the green onion and chile.

Per serving: 145 calories, 0 g total fat, 0 g saturated fat, 0 mg cholesterol, 356 mg sodium, 31 g total carbohydrate (11 g dietary fiber, 10 g sugar, 0 g added sugars), 8 g protein, 4 mg iron

Combination Cooking Methods

Combination cooking methods, such as braising or stewing, utilize both dry and moist heat to create tender, juicy, flavor-rich dishes. Traditional combination methods for animal foods often involve starting with dry heat and browning the food, then cooking it in liquid. For plant foods, the opposite approach is more effective: first, infuse the food with moisture, then cook it in dry heat. For example, you can steam tempeh before panfrying it (we use this technique for the kung pao recipe on page 221).

An effect similar to traditional braising can be achieved by roasting semi-moist food in the oven until it both softens and develops external color. In this case, the parts of the food that are exposed to dry air in the oven gain color, while the submerged parts soften. This method is showcased by the Whole Roasted Spiced Cauliflower (page 94).

Common Cooking Methods

DRY HEAT

- **Baking** Dry cooking in an oven for longer periods.
- **Grilling** Cooking directly over a flame from below (see page 80).
- **Roasting** Cooking in an oven, with food surrounded by dry heat. If not using oil, add moisture during cooking (see page 86).
- **Toasting** Dry cooking in a hot pan, to release the oils and enhance the flavors of nuts, seeds, or spices.

MOIST HEAT

- **Blanching** Briefly submerging food in boiling water, followed by an ice-bath to stop the cooking process and retain color and crispness.
- **Poaching** Submerging food in a hot flavorful liquid until tender (see Poached Fruit recipes, page 276).
- **Pressure-cooking** Cooking with high-pressure steam, allows for an accelerated cooking process.
- **Steaming** Suspending food in a covered basket over simmering water. The healthiest of cooking methods.
- **Sautéing** Traditionally, oil is used to sauté, but you can use the Dry Sauté Method (page 78) with water or other flavorful liquid to soften onions, garlic, or other vegetables in a pan.

Whole Roasted Spiced Cauliflower

Serves 4

Gorgeous to look at and delicious to eat! The combination cooking method ensures the cauliflower is moist and tender inside, while the flavorful crust is crispy and browned.

½ cup pitted dates

¼ cup garlic cloves, or 3 tablespoons garlic paste (pages 69 and 70)

1 cup canned no-added-sodium crushed tomatoes

1 cup low-sodium vegetable broth

¼ cup roasted red peppers

1½ teaspoons onion granules

1 to 1½ teaspoons red pepper flakes

½ teaspoon smoked paprika

¼ teaspoon sea salt

½ cup lightly packed fresh cilantro leaves

1 large head cauliflower, trimmed

Preheat the oven to 375°F.

In a small saucepan, combine the dates and garlic and add water to cover. Bring to a simmer over medium heat and simmer until softened, about 15 minutes. Drain the dates and garlic and transfer to a food processor or a (preferably high-speed) blender.

Add the tomatoes, ½ cup of the broth, the roasted peppers, onion granules, red pepper flakes, paprika, and salt. Blend until smooth. Pulse in all but a few cilantro leaves (set those leaves aside for garnish).

Place the cauliflower cut-side down in a Dutch oven or deep roasting pan. Spoon half the sauce over the cauliflower, coating it completely. Pour the remaining ½ cup broth into the bottom of the pan. Cover with a lid or foil, making sure the foil does not touch the food. Roast for 25 minutes.

Remove the cauliflower from the oven and baste it with the drippings from the bottom of the pan. Spoon on the remaining sauce and roast, uncovered, until the cauliflower is easily pierced with a knife, 30 to 45 minutes more, depending on the size of your cauliflower. Remove from the oven and let cool.

Transfer the cauliflower to a cutting board and slice it into thick slabs. Serve with the pan juices drizzled over the top and garnish with the reserved cilantro leaves.

Per serving: 155 calories, 1 g total fat, 0 g saturated fat, 0 mg cholesterol, 280 mg sodium, 33 g total carbohydrate (8 g dietary fiber, 19 g sugar, 0 g added sugars), 6 g protein, 2 mg iron

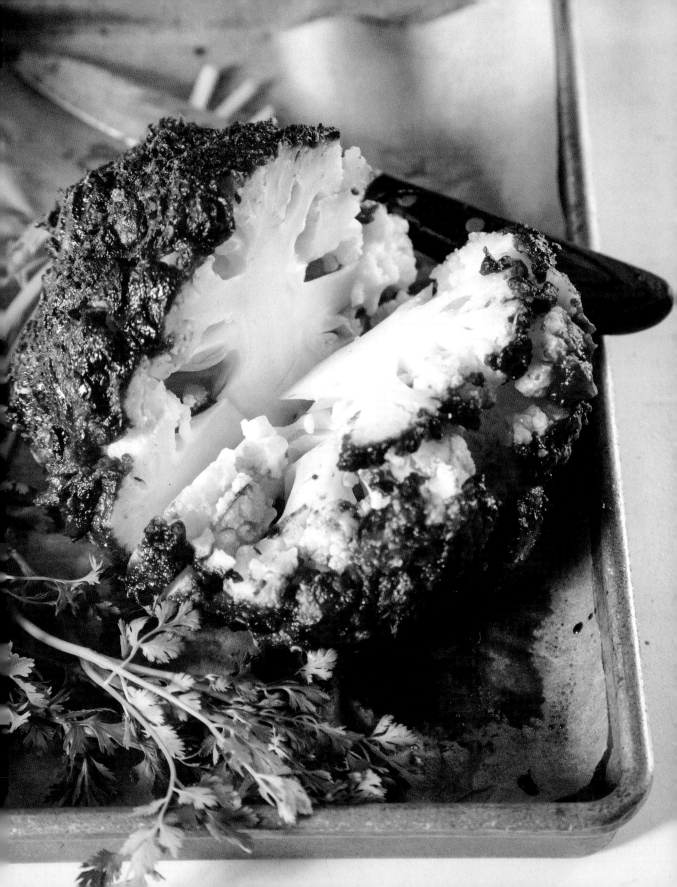

Low-and-Slow Cooking

Set it and forget it, as they say! If you have the time to cook slowly, your patience will be well rewarded. Cooking foods over low heat (175 to 200°F) for a longer time has a similar effect to reducing (see page 72): it caramelizes the natural sugars and intensifies the flavors in a food. This is a particularly good method to use for beans and stews, as it marries all the flavors over its long cooking time. As the moisture slowly evaporates, the other ingredients concentrate, creating rich layers of flavor. Many of the one-pot meals on pages 191 to 200 can be made using a slow cooker. Try this with the Wicked Good Pot of Cassoulet Beans (page 46) and the Veggie-Loaded Chili (page 193).

This page and opposite: Classic Celeriac Pot Roast, page 99

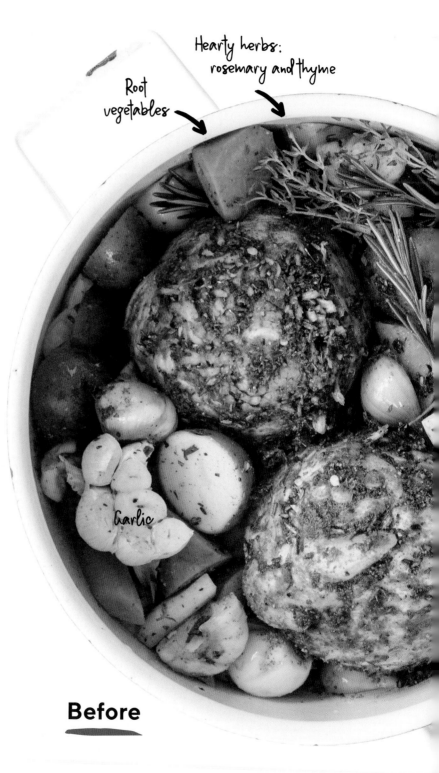

Root vegetables

Hearty herbs: rosemary and thyme

Garlic

Before

Slow cooking caramelizes
the vegetables

After

Celeriac is tender
and moist

Garlic and herbs
infuse flavor

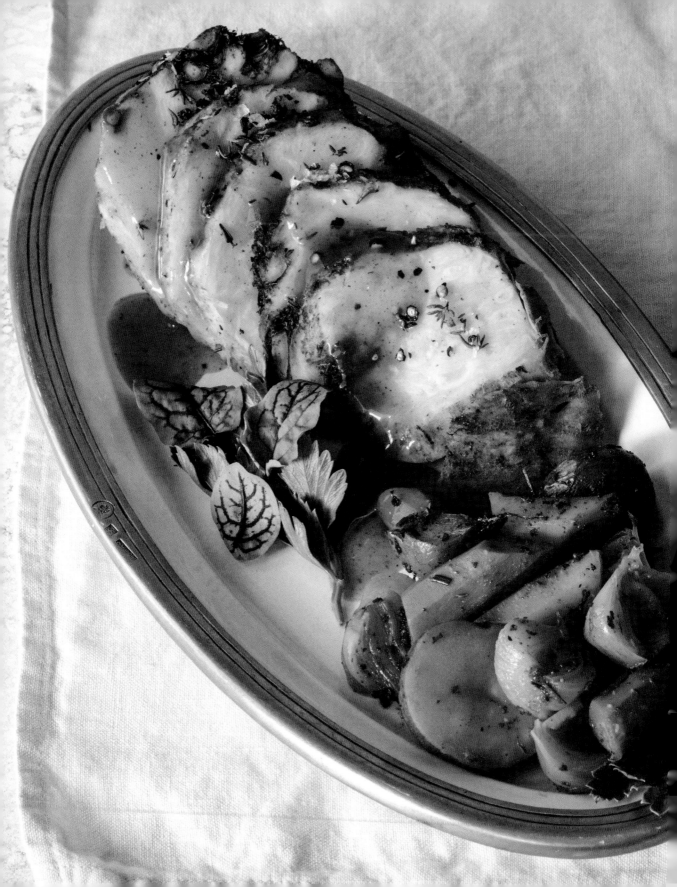

Classic Celeriac Pot Roast

Serves 8

A beautiful way to highlight plants at the center of the plate, this twist on a classic roast makes a low-calorie main dish or a side for any holiday meal. The long, slow cooking process caramelizes all the veggies to a festive sweetness, while leaving this roasted root juicy and tender. (See pages 86 and 87 for the roasting process.)

2 onions, quartered

2 large carrots, quartered

3 large russet potatoes, scrubbed and quartered

5 garlic cloves, smashed

½ cup low-sodium vegetable broth

½ teaspoon smoked paprika

½ teaspoon red pepper flakes

2 teaspoons freshly ground black pepper

½ teaspoon sea salt

1 large celeriac (celery root), trimmed and scrubbed

1 tablespoon onion granules

Juice of 1 lime

2 bay leaves

1 tablespoon chopped fresh thyme

1 tablespoon chopped fresh rosemary

½ cup lightly packed small fresh flat-leaf parsley leaves

If using the oven, preheat the oven to 400°F. If using a slow cooker, set the slow cooker to High.

In a Dutch oven or in the slow cooker, combine the onions, carrots, potatoes, garlic, ¼ cup of the broth, the paprika, red pepper flakes, 1 teaspoon of the black pepper, and the salt. Gently toss to completely coat the vegetables with the seasonings.

In a medium bowl, combine the whole celeriac, onion granules, lime juice, remaining ¼ cup broth, and 1 teaspoon black pepper. Gently toss to coat, then put the celeriac in the Dutch oven or slow cooker, nestling it into the other vegetables. Scrape the contents of the bowl into the Dutch oven or slow cooker. Add the bay leaves.

Cover, place the Dutch oven in the oven, and reduce the oven temperature to 300°F; if using a slow cooker, set it to Low. Cook until the celeriac is tender enough to be easily pierced with a knife, 3½ to 4 hours in the oven or 4 to 6 hours in the slow cooker, depending on size of celeriac.

Remove and discard the bay leaves. Carve the celeriac into slices and serve it with the vegetables and pan juices. Garnish with the thyme, rosemary, and parsley.

Note: If you have a substantial amount of natural juices from the vegetables remaining after the vegetables have been removed from the Dutch oven or slow cooker, you can thicken them into a gravy. Whisk together 1 teaspoon cornstarch and 2 tablespoons cold water to make a slurry, then whisk the slurry into the juices and cook over low heat or on Low until thickened, 2 to 3 minutes. If the gravy is too thick, stir in a little more vegetable broth.

Per serving: 183 calories, 1 g total fat, 0 g saturated fat, 0 mg cholesterol, 263 mg sodium, 41 g total carbohydrate (5 g dietary fiber, 4 g sugar, 0 g added sugars), 5 g protein, 3 mg iron

Baking in Salt

Salt baking is an ancient cooking method most commonly used for fish, but it works wonderfully for vegetables, too. Packing the vegetables in salt helps them retain their moisture and concentrates their natural sweetness, along with ensuring perfectly even cooking. The salt insulates the vegetables so they stay whole and yet become tender all the way through. Traditionally, egg whites are mixed with the salt before baking to help with moisture retention, but this is certainly not necessary. Be sure to keep the skin on the vegetables so they don't absorb the salt and you don't need to be concerned about excess sodium. Wipe off the salt well once the vegetables are done. Try our Carrot Lox recipe (opposite) or use the same baking method with beets, parsnips, and potatoes—salt-baked baby potatoes are highly addictive!

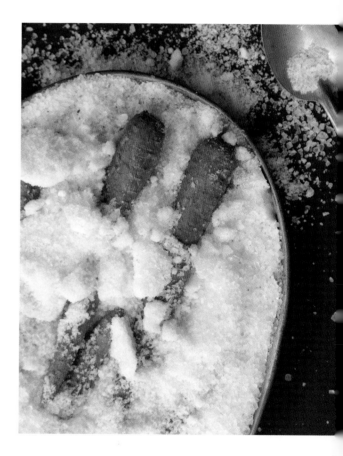

Carrot Lox

Makes 2 cups

These delicious sweet-and-smoky salt-baked carrots are reminiscent of traditional salmon lox in both color and flavor. You'll see them showcased on page 131 on a tartine that is sure to impress your brunch guests. You can also add this lox to the Penne Carbonara with Cauliflower (page 208). Don't worry about the large quantity of salt called for—this is not consumed, just used during the baking process to help lock in moisture and evenly bake the carrots.

3 cups coarse sea salt, plus more if needed

6 to 8 thick carrots, scrubbed but not peeled

½ teaspoon coriander seeds

½ teaspoon caraway seeds

2½ tablespoons unseasoned rice vinegar or coconut vinegar

1 tablespoon apricot paste (see page 56)

Juice of 1 orange

1 teaspoon smoked paprika

¼ teaspoon freshly ground black pepper

3 tablespoons minced fresh chives

Preheat the oven to 375°F. Line a rimmed baking sheet with parchment paper.

Sprinkle a layer of salt over the parchment. Place the carrots on salt, making sure they are not touching the sides of the pan to prevent burning. Pour the remaining salt over the carrots, rolling the carrots to coat them completely.

Roast for 60 to 75 minutes, until tender when pierced through one end with a knife. Remove from the oven and let cool on the pan.

When cool, wipe the salt from the carrots.

Use a mandoline or thin-bladed sharp knife to slice the carrots on an angle, making very wide, thin slices. Place the slices in a single layer on several baking sheets (these will take up quite a bit of space).

Combine the coriander and caraway seeds in a small sauté pan. Toast over medium heat, shaking the pan occasionally, until fragrant, 1 to 2 minutes. Transfer to a plate and let cool, then transfer to a spice grinder. Grind the coriander and caraway to a powder and transfer to a small bowl. Whisk in the vinegar, apricot paste, orange juice, smoked paprika, pepper, and chives. Pour the mixture over the carrots, turning gently to coat the slices. Let sit at room temperature until the mixture has been absorbed by the carrots, about 30 minutes. Serve cold, or keep in the fridge for up to five days.

Note: For a smokier flavor, you can smoke the carrots instead of using smoked paprika. After coating the slices with the vinegar mixture, cover the baking sheet with plastic wrap and use a smoking gun filled with dried rosemary to blow rosemary smoke under the plastic for 2 minutes. Seal the carrots under the plastic to trap the smoke. Let sit in the smoke for 3 to 5 minutes. Unwrap and use immediately. These smoked carrots make a great substitution for smoked salmon.

Per serving (¼ cup): 47 calories, 0 g total fat, 0 g saturated fat, 0 mg cholesterol, 38 mg sodium, 10 g total carbohydrate (2 g dietary fiber, 5 g sugar, 0 g added sugars), 1 g protein, 0 mg iron

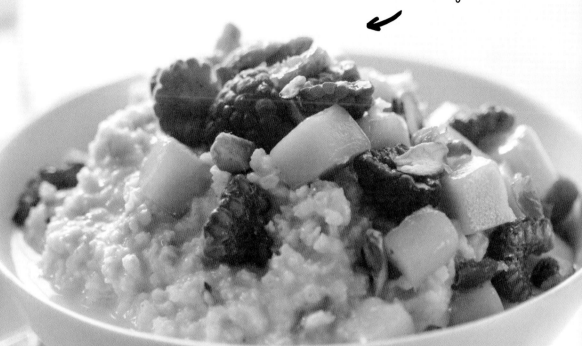

Mango Millet with Raspberries & Toasted Pistachios, page 116

CHAPTER 8

Starting Your Day Off Right

Some people swear by breakfast as the most important meal of the day. Others barely remember to grab a bite as they run out the door. Whether you like a hearty morning meal or a quick, light start to the day, we've got nourishing, whole foods, plant-based options for you in the pages ahead.

Making Your Own Nondairy Milks

If you choose to remove animal products from your diet, you'll want an alternative to dairy milk to use in cooking and for breakfast bowls. These days, you can find an amazing variety of unsweetened plant milks at your local grocery store, from soy milk to various nut milks to hemp milk, rice milk, oat milk, and more. But you might be surprised at how easy it is to make your own nondairy milk at home—and how fresh and delicious it tastes! All you need are a blender and a piece of cheesecloth (or a sprouting/nut milk bag or fine-mesh strainer). If you want to keep the healthy fiber, you don't even need to strain it--just stir it before use.

Keep in mind this basic formula: 1 cup nuts, seeds, or cooked oats to 4 cups filtered water. This will produce a silky nondairy milk. If you want it a bit thicker, more like a creamer, use 1 to 3 cups water. For a sweeter taste without adding dried fruit, use coconut water (with no sugar added) instead of filtered water.

Fresh Nut Milk or Seed Milk

Makes 4 cups

Use this creamy milk as a base for your smoothies, when cooking your oatmeal, or to pour over breakfast bowls.

1 cup raw nuts or seeds, such as blanched almonds or hulled hemp seeds

4 cups filtered water

3 tablespoons date paste (see page 56)

½ teaspoon vanilla bean paste, or ½ vanilla bean, split lengthwise and seeds scraped

Pinch of sea salt

Place all the ingredients in a high-speed blender and puree for 2 minutes.

Line a strainer with cheesecloth or a mesh sprouting or nut milk bag and set it over a large bowl. Pour the puree through the strainer and gently press on the solids to extract all the liquid.

Transfer the milk to a glass jar, seal, and refrigerate for up to 4 days.

Oat Milk: For a lower-fat milk made with oats, replace the nuts or seeds with 1¼ cups cooked plain oatmeal. If using old-fashioned rolled oats or coarser steel-cut oats, strain as directed. If using instant oats, skip the straining.

Per serving (1 cup): 206 calories, 15 g total fat, 1 g saturated fat, 0 mg cholesterol, 93 mg sodium, 13 g total carbohydrate (5 g dietary fiber, 7 g sugar, 0 g added sugars), 6 g protein, 2 mg iron

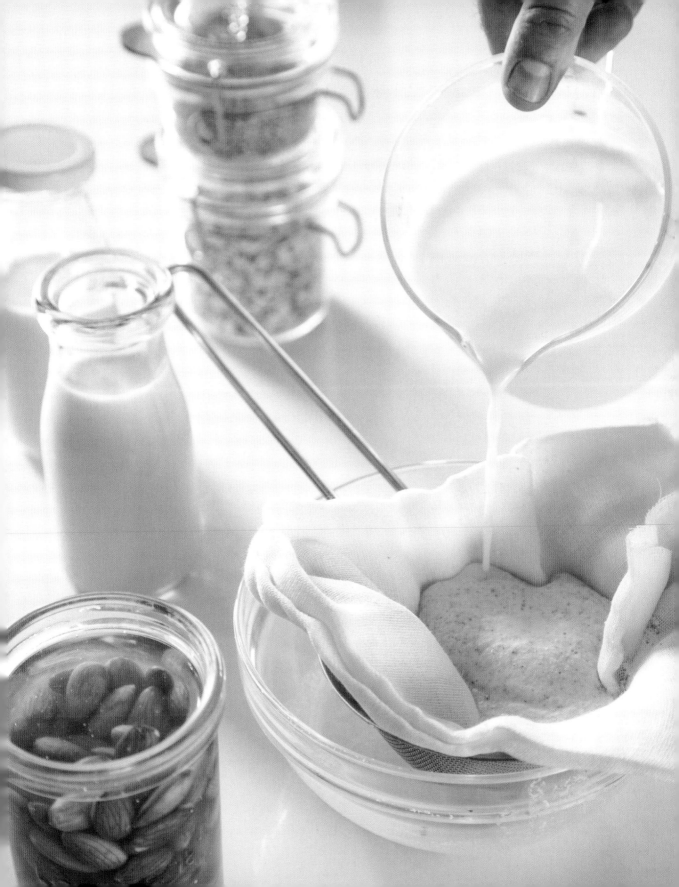

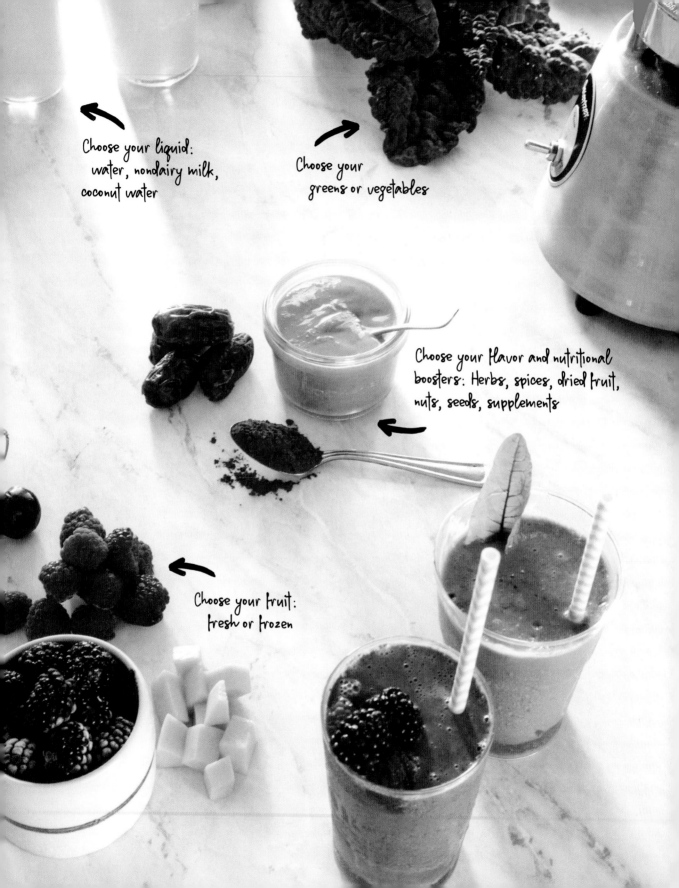

Choose your liquid:
water, nondairy milk,
coconut water

Choose your
greens or vegetables

Choose your flavor and nutritional
boosters: Herbs, spices, dried fruit,
nuts, seeds, supplements

Choose your fruit:
fresh or frozen

Building Smoothies

If you're in a hurry and need a quick breakfast, smoothies are a great opportunity to pack a lot of nutrients into something you can drink on the run. A tip for parents: If your kids (or spouse) won't drink a green smoothie due to the color, put it in a dark-colored sippy cup so they can't see it. With the right amount of fresh fruit, they won't taste all the greens you'll load in there.

Health Tip

If you're choosing to "drink your calories" in the form of a smoothie, sip it slowly to ensure you feel satisfied and don't overeat. Include lots of veggies and greens in addition to fruit to optimize health benefits. If you're trying to lose weight, consider reducing the calorie density of your smoothies by using water rather than soy or nut milk and using fewer nuts, seeds, and/or dried fruit.

Green Energy Smoothie

Makes two 12-ounce smoothies

This vegetable and fruit packed smoothie is a nutritious meal on the go. With the addition of matcha green tea powder (a very finely ground green tea, found in the tea section of most natural foods stores), this smoothie will give a kick of energy to start your day off right.

1 cup chopped peeled cucumber (about 1 medium)

1 cup unsweetened nondairy milk of your choice

2 or 3 green kale leaves, stemmed

1 cup baby spinach

1 cup frozen cubed mango

1 banana, peeled

3 tablespoons hemp hearts

1 teaspoon culinary-grade matcha

Combine all the ingredients in a (preferably high-speed) blender. Blend until smooth.

Per serving: 210 calories, 8 g total fat, 1 g saturated fat, 0 mg cholesterol, 120 mg sodium, 29 g total carbohydrate (3 g dietary fiber, 18 g sugar, 0 g added sugars), 8 g protein, 3 mg iron

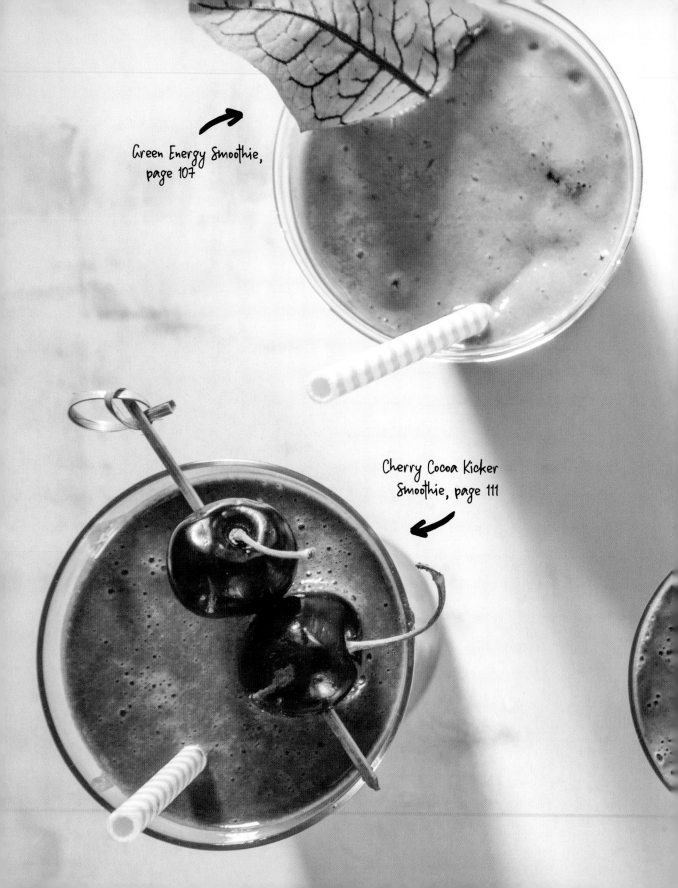

Green Energy Smoothie,
page 107

Cherry Cocoa Kicker
Smoothie, page 111

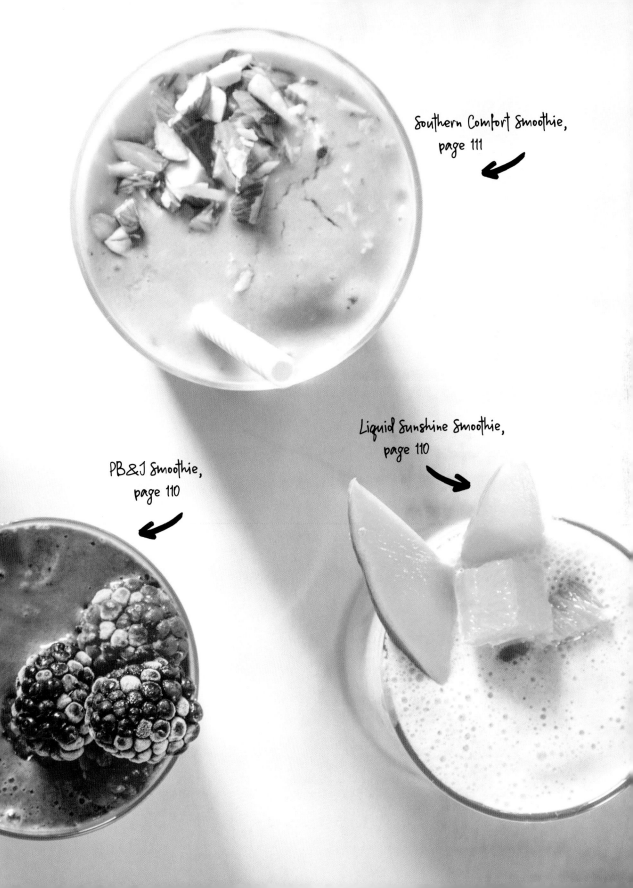

Southern Comfort Smoothie,
page 111

Liquid Sunshine Smoothie,
page 110

PB&J Smoothie,
page 110

PB&J Smoothie

Makes two 12-ounce smoothies

Familiar flavors in a new form. Garnish with fresh berries or crushed peanuts.

2 cups unsweetened soy milk or other nondairy milk

1½ cups fresh or frozen mixed berries

Juice of ½ lemon

3 tablespoons peanut butter or almond butter (no added oil, salt, or sugar)

3 dates, pitted, or 2 tablespoons date paste (see page 56)

Combine all the ingredients in a (preferably high-speed) blender. Blend until smooth.

Per serving: 306 calories, 17 g total fat, 2 g saturated fat, 0 mg cholesterol, 164 mg sodium, 31 g total carbohydrate (8 g dietary fiber, 16 g sugar, 0 g added sugars), 13 g protein, 3 mg iron

Liquid Sunshine Smoothie

Makes two 14-ounce smoothies

Summer in a glass! Garnish with a slice of fresh mango or orange.

2 cups unsweetened soy milk or other nondairy milk

½ cup fresh or frozen cubed mango

1 orange, peeled and seeded

½ yellow bell pepper, chopped

1 (1-inch) piece fresh turmeric, peeled

3 tablespoons hemp seeds

Ice, for serving (optional)

Combine all the ingredients except the ice (if using) in a (preferably high-speed) blender. Blend until smooth. Serve over ice or chilled.

Per serving: 230 calories, 12 g total fat, 1 g saturated fat, 0 mg cholesterol, 121 mg sodium, 24 g total carbohydrate (4 g dietary fiber, 13 g sugar, 0 g added sugars), 13 g protein, 3 mg iron

Cherry Cocoa Kicker Smoothie

Makes two 14-ounce smoothies

A decadent treat. Garnish with a dusting of unsweetened cocoa powder.

3 cups unsweetened soy milk or other nondairy milk

¾ cup fresh or frozen pitted cherries

1 banana, peeled

2 dates, pitted

5 kale leaves, stemmed

¼ cup unsweetened raw or toasted cocoa powder

½ teaspoon pure vanilla extract

Ice, for serving (optional)

Combine all the ingredients except the ice (if using) in a (preferably high-speed) blender. Blend until smooth. Serve over ice or chilled.

Per serving: 262 calories, 8 g total fat, 1 g saturated fat, 0 mg cholesterol, 174 mg sodium, 44 g total carbohydrate (8 g dietary fiber, 18 g sugar, 0 g added sugars), 14 g protein, 4 mg iron

Southern Comfort Smoothie

Makes two 10-ounce smoothies

The fall flavors of steamed sweet potato and warming nutmeg make this a soothing and filling meal-in-a-glass. Garnish with a drizzle of thinned-out date paste.

½ cup 1-inch cubes peeled sweet potato

2 cups unsweetened soy milk or other nondairy milk

3 dates, pitted, or 2 tablespoons date paste (see page 56)

¼ teaspoon pure almond extract

¼ teaspoon freshly grated nutmeg

Ice, for serving (optional)

Steam the sweet potato in a covered steamer basket over gently simmering water until tender, 10 to 15 minutes.

Transfer the sweet potato to a (preferably high-speed) blender. Add the remaining ingredients except the ice (if using) and blend until smooth. Serve over ice or chilled.

Per serving: 142 calories, 4 g total fat, 0 g saturated fat, 0 mg cholesterol, 128 mg sodium, 21 g total carbohydrate (2 g dietary fiber, 8 g sugar, 0 g added sugars), 8 g protein, 2 mg iron

Building Breakfast Bowls

Grains, fruits, nuts, and nondairy milk—these four categories offer endless variations for creating sweet, warming, satisfying breakfast bowls that will set you up for the day ahead. Some grains can be cooked the day before; oats can be simply soaked overnight (see Overnight Oatmeal, page 116); and others can be cooked in a slow cooker overnight so they're waiting for you, perfectly creamy and delicious, when you wake up in the morning (or they can just be simmered on the stovetop while you get ready for your day). Top with your favorite combo of fruits and nuts/seeds, add a splash of nondairy milk, and breakfast is served!

Coconut Brown Rice Pudding

Serves 6

Whenever you're cooking grains, it's worth making a double or triple batch. The leftovers can be used in so many ways, both savory and sweet, as this brown rice pudding demonstrates. This makes a great breakfast, topped with tropical fruit, or a satisfying dessert to follow a lighter meal.

2¾ cups cooked brown rice (see page 36)

1 (14-ounce) can coconut milk

1 cup unsweetened soy milk or other nondairy milk

3 tablespoons date or other dried fruit paste (see page 56)

1 vanilla bean, split lengthwise and seeds scraped, or 1 to 2 teaspoons pure vanilla extract

1 star anise pod

½ teaspoon sea salt

1 cup fresh berries or chopped (peeled, if necessary) fruit of your choice

Put the cooked rice in a medium saucepan if it isn't already in one. Add the coconut milk, soy milk, date paste, vanilla bean pod and seeds, star anise, and salt and bring to a simmer over medium heat. Cook, stirring continuously, until the rice begins to absorb the liquid and the mixture thickens to the consistency of a porridge, 10 to 15 minutes. If the rice sticks to the pan, reduce the heat.

Remove and discard the vanilla bean and star anise. Serve warm, topped with fresh berries or other fruit.

Per serving: 286 calories, 15 g total fat, 13 g saturated fat, 0 mg cholesterol, 222 mg sodium, 36 g total carbohydrate (4 g dietary fiber, 4 g sugar, 0 g added sugars), 5 g protein, 3 mg iron

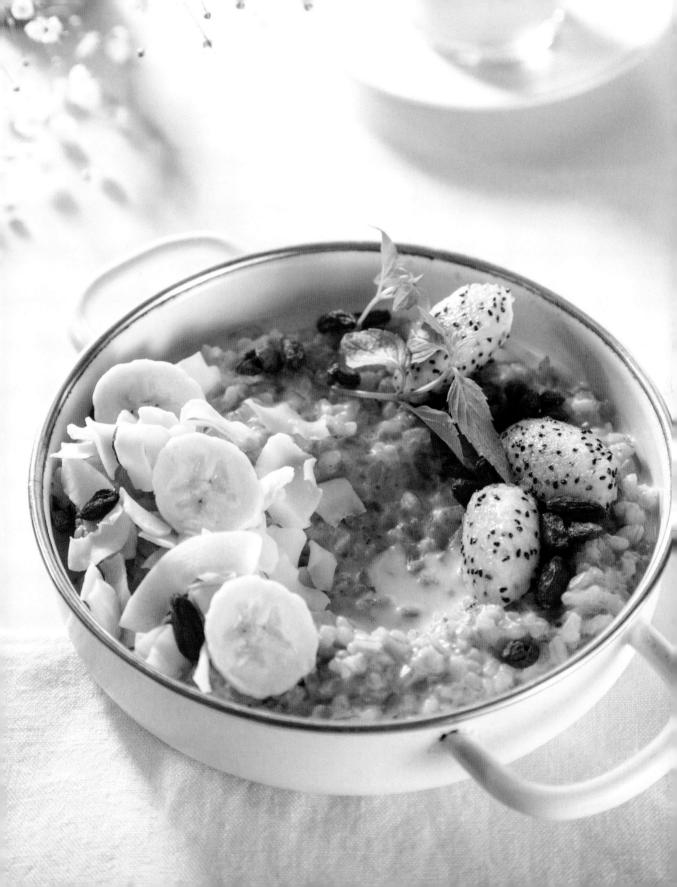

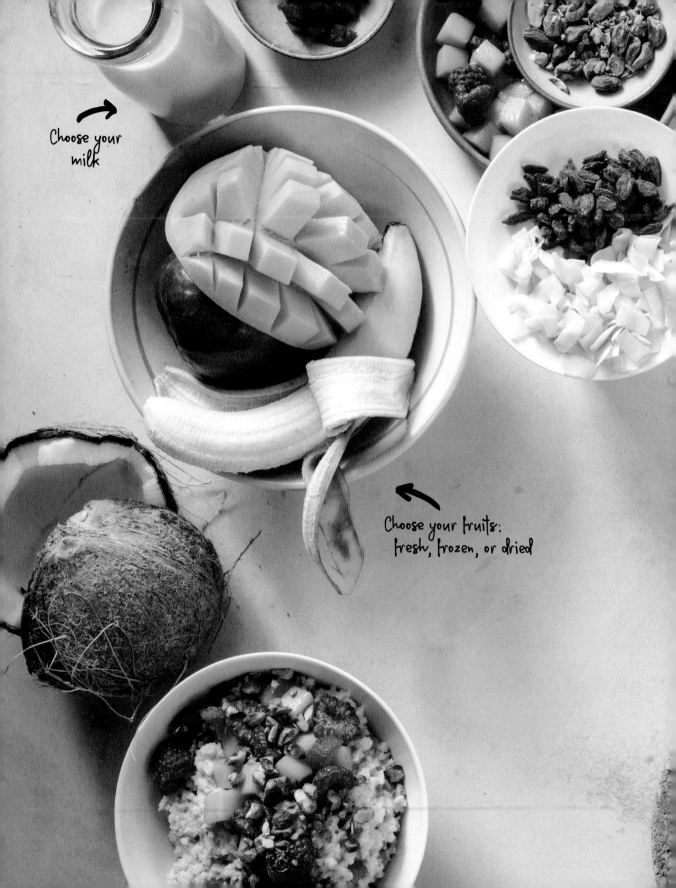

Choose your milk

Choose your fruits:
fresh, frozen, or dried

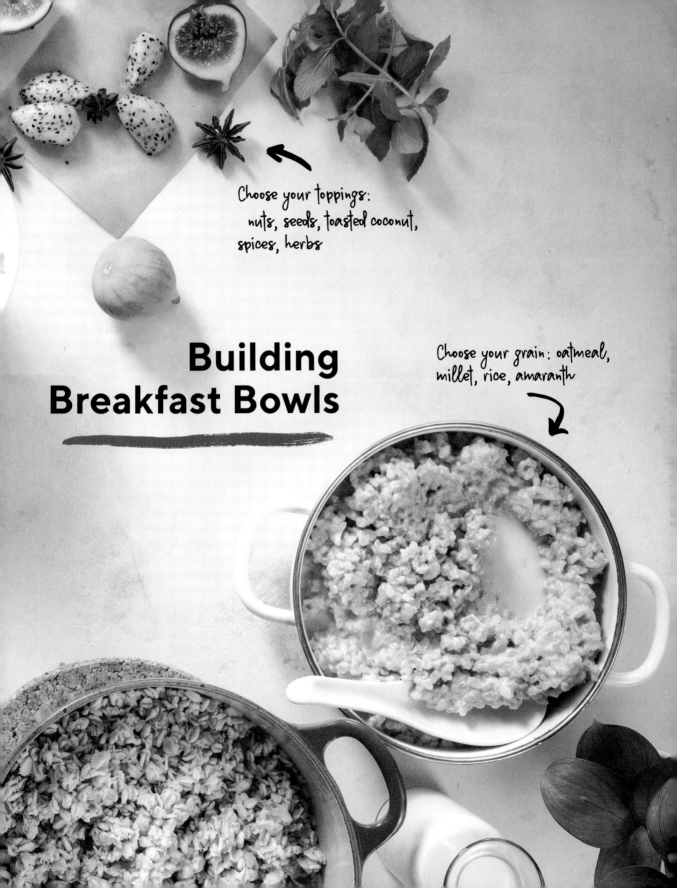

Choose your toppings:
nuts, seeds, toasted coconut,
spices, herbs

Building Breakfast Bowls

Choose your grain: oatmeal,
millet, rice, amaranth

Overnight Oatmeal

Serves 2

This low-cost, quick, and healthy breakfast is a great way to kick off the day. Simply mix the ingredients together and refrigerate overnight to soften the oats. The next morning, enjoy it cold or gently warmed in a small pot, topped with your favorite nuts and fruit.

1½ cups old-fashioned rolled oats

1½ cups unsweetened soy milk or other nondairy milk

½ teaspoon pure vanilla extract

Pinch of sea salt

¼ cup pecans or other nut or seed of your choice, toasted and chopped

1 cup fresh fruit (peaches, mango, berries, banana, etc., peeled, pitted and chopped as needed)

3 tablespoons dried fruit (dates, raisins, currants, apricots, etc.; optional)

In a medium bowl, combine the oats, milk, vanilla, and salt and stir well. Cover and refrigerate overnight.

In the morning, stir in half the nuts, seeds, and fresh and dried fruits. Divide the oatmeal between two bowls and top evenly with the remaining nuts, seeds, and fresh and dried fruits.

Per serving: 519 calories, 18 g total fat, 2 g saturated fat, 0 mg cholesterol, 271 mg sodium, 76 g total carbohydrate (11 g dietary fiber, 17 g sugar, 0 g added sugars), 17 g protein, 5 mg iron

Mango Millet with Raspberries & Toasted Pistachios

Serves 6

Mix up your morning bowl by using light and fluffy millet instead of oatmeal. You can substitute your favorite fruits and nuts to experiment with different toppings (pictured on page 102).

2½ cups unsweetened soy milk or other nondairy milk, plus more if needed

1 cup unsweetened coconut milk

1 cup dry millet

3 tablespoons minced dried apricots

½ teaspoon pure vanilla extract

¼ cup unsalted pistachios, toasted

1½ cups fresh or frozen cubed mango

¼ cup fresh or frozen raspberries

In a medium saucepan, combine the soy milk and the coconut milk. Bring to a boil over medium heat. Stir in the millet with a wooden spoon. Reduce the heat to medium-low and simmer, stirring occasionally, until the millet is creamy and tender, 20 to 25 minutes.

Add the apricots, vanilla, half the pistachios, and half the mango, reduce the heat to low, and cook for 2 to 3 minutes more. Add a splash of soy milk if needed to keep the millet creamy. Remove from the heat.

Serve the millet topped with the raspberries, remaining pistachios, and remaining mango.

Per serving: 286 calories, 12 g total fat, 8 g saturated fat, 0 mg cholesterol, 66 mg sodium, 38 g total carbohydrate (4 g dietary fiber, 8 g sugar, 0 g added sugars), 8 g protein, 3 mg iron

Plantastic Granola

Makes about 8 cups

Want the sweet, satisfying crunch of granola in the morning, without all the oil and refined sugar that comes in traditional varieties? Try this delicious homemade granola sprinkled over a bowl of fresh fruit for your breakfast or fruit parfaits for dessert (page 271). This recipe uses date sugar and date syrup, which add to its calorie density, so eat this sweet treat as a topping rather than by the bowlful.

Recipe by Lisa Rice

4 cups old-fashioned rolled oats	1 cup date syrup (see Notes)
1 cup sliced almonds	½ cup unsweetened applesauce
1 cup raw sunflower seeds	1 tablespoon pure vanilla extract
1 cup raw pumpkin seeds	⅓ cup dried cranberries
¼ cup date sugar (see Notes)	⅓ cup golden raisins
	⅓ cup dried Bing or tart cherries

Preheat the oven to 325°F. Line a rimmed baking sheet with parchment paper.

In a large bowl, combine the oats, almonds, sunflower seeds, pumpkin seeds, and date sugar.

In a small bowl, whisk together the date syrup, applesauce, vanilla, and ⅓ cup water. Pour the wet ingredients into the bowl with the oat mixture and stir with a large spoon or combine with your hands until well coated.

Spread the mixture in an even layer over the prepared pan.

Bake for 10 minutes, then stir with a metal spatula and bake for 10 minutes more, and stir. Repeat this baking and stirring until the granola is dry and golden, 25 to 30 minutes total. Remove from the oven and let cool completely on the pan.

Once cool, break up any big chunks of granola and mix in the cranberries, raisins, and cherries. Use immediately, or transfer to an airtight container such as a large mason jar. Store at room temperature away from heat and light for up to 3 weeks. Humidity will soften the granola. You can also store the jars in the freezer to keep the granola crisp longer.

Notes: Date sugar is made from dates that have been dried and ground. Look for it in the baking section of your market. You can find date syrup, such as Date Lady Pure Date Syrup, in the baking aisle as well, or order it online.

Make nut-free granola by omitting the almonds and adding an additional 1 cup oats. You can also replace the pumpkin seeds with unsweetened coconut flakes, if you like.

Choose any combinations of dried fruits you love, such as currants, raisins, chopped dried apricots, goji berries, mulberries, chopped dried figs, etc.

For flavor variations, try adding ¼ teaspoon pure almond extract or ¼ teaspoon ground cinnamon and/or cardamom.

Per serving (½ cup): 329 calories, 13 g total fat, 2 g saturated fat, 0 mg cholesterol, 13 mg sodium, 45 g total carbohydrate (5 g dietary fiber, 22 g sugar, 0 g added sugars), 10 g protein, 4 mg iron

Savory Scrambles

If your palate craves savory fare in the morning, you may find yourself seeking alternatives to eggs. Well, grab a skillet and start scrambling! Use these recipes as templates for endless combinations of vegetables, tofu, tempeh, beans, and even coconut meat that will add comfort to your morning menu. Here are a few ideas for scrambles and hash to get you started.

Pacific Northwest Mushroom Hash

Serves 4

A hearty taste of the northwest with local foraged mushrooms, dark greens, and potatoes, this makes a great standalone breakfast, or roll it up in a wrap with some greens and take it to go. If you can't get the mushrooms specified, any variety of wild mushroom will work. **Recipe by Whole Foods Market**

1 large yam or sweet potato, scrubbed and cut into bite-size pieces

2 large Yukon Gold potatoes, scrubbed and cut into bite-size pieces

¼ cup Marsala wine

½ cup finely chopped leeks (see Note, page 37)

8 ounces golden chanterelle mushrooms, chopped if large

8 ounces oyster or maitake mushrooms, chopped if large

3 garlic cloves, minced

Leaves from 2 sprigs rosemary

Pinch of sea salt

1½ teaspoons cracked black pepper

¼ cup low-sodium vegetable broth

2 tablespoons smoked paprika

4 large eggs, poached, for serving (optional)

Preheat the oven to 350°F. Line a baking sheet with parchment paper.

Arrange the yams and potatoes in a single layer on the prepared pan. Roast until the potatoes are barely tender but not completely soft, 8 to 10 minutes. Remove from the oven, drizzle with the wine, and shake the pan to coat the potatoes. Return the pan to the oven and roast until the potatoes are fork-tender, 4 to 6 minutes more.

Heat a large sauté pan over medium-high heat. When hot, add the leeks and dry sauté, stirring often, until they begin to stick to the pan and lightly brown, 1 to 2 minutes. Stir in the chanterelles, oyster mushrooms, garlic, rosemary, salt, and pepper and cook, stirring often, until the mushrooms begin to stick, 3 to 4 minutes. Add the broth and stir to deglaze the pan. Cook until the liquid has evaporated and the mushrooms are very tender. Stir in the yams, potatoes, and paprika.

If you eat eggs, serve each portion of hash topped with a poached egg.

Per serving (without egg): 250 calories, 1 g total fat, 0 g saturated fat, 0 mg cholesterol, 289 mg sodium, 52 g total carbohydrate (6 g dietary fiber, 8 g sugar, 0 g added sugars), 8 g protein, 3 mg iron

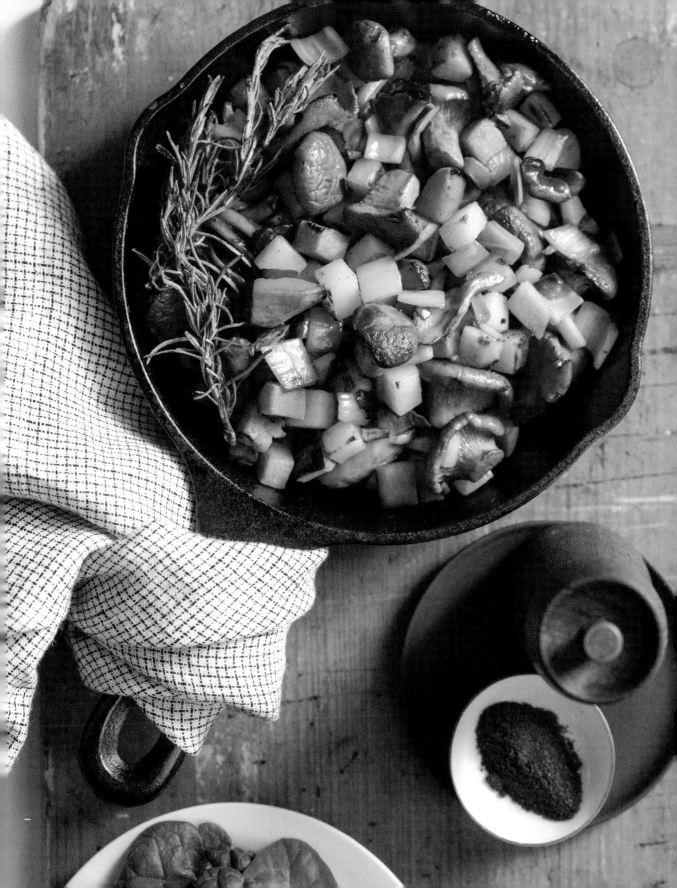

Tofu Scramble with Spinach, Peppers, & Basil

Serves 4

This savory breakfast dish gets its particular character from *kala namak*, or Indian black salt, which is high in sulfur and gives the tofu a flavor reminiscent of scrambled eggs. Serve with your favorite salsa or hot sauce, or try it in a breakfast burrito with black beans.

1½ (14-ounce) blocks extra-firm tofu, drained

2½ tablespoons low-sodium tamari

2 tablespoons nutritional yeast

½ teaspoon ground turmeric

½ teaspoon Indian black salt (kala namak) or sea salt (optional)

1 cup chopped white onion

3 garlic cloves, minced

¼ cup low-sodium vegetable broth

1 cup baby spinach

¼ cup chopped roasted red peppers

¼ cup chopped fresh basil

Freshly ground black pepper

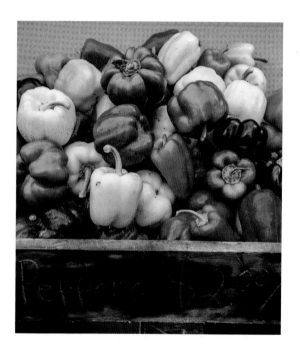

Crumble the tofu into a large bowl. Stir in the tamari, nutritional yeast, turmeric, and salt.

Heat a large sauté pan over medium-high heat. When hot, add the onion and cook until it begins to stick to the pan. Add the garlic and cook, stirring frequently to prevent burning, for 1 minute. Add the broth and stir to deglaze the pan.

Reduce the heat to medium and stir in the spinach, roasted peppers, and the tofu mixture. Cook, stirring to prevent sticking, until the tofu mixture is heated through and the spinach wilts, about 4 minutes. Remove from the heat.

Stir in the basil, season with black pepper, and serve.

Per serving: 205 calories, 9 g total fat, 1 g saturated fat, 0 mg cholesterol, 465 mg sodium, 10 g total carbohydrate (2 g dietary fiber, 2 g sugar, 0 g added sugars), 21 g protein, 4 mg iron

Coconut & Potato Spelt Wraps with Mango-Habanero Puree

Serves 2

A tasty and unusual scramble in a wrap, perfect for breakfast on the run. The use of a small amount of *kala namak* (Indian black salt) gives this a subtle egg-like flavor. **Recipe by Hiram Camillo**

POTATOES AND COCONUT

1 large russet potato, scrubbed and cut into ½-inch cubes

2 cups 1-inch pieces fresh or thawed frozen young Thai coconut meat

2 tablespoons nutritional yeast

2 teaspoons onion powder

2 teaspoons garlic powder

½ teaspoon hot mustard powder

¼ teaspoon Indian black salt (kala namak)

⅛ teaspoon sea salt

Spray oil

MANGO-HABANERO PUREE

2 ripe mangoes, pitted and peeled

1 habanero chile, seeded if less heat is desired

Juice of 1 lime

TO ASSEMBLE

2 large (8-inch) spelt or whole wheat wraps

½ cup thinly sliced red onion

For the potatoes and coconut, place the potatoes in a medium saucepan and add water to cover. Bring to a boil over high heat. Reduce the heat to medium and simmer until the potatoes are tender, about 10 minutes.

While the potatoes cook, heat a large skillet over medium heat. When hot, add the coconut meat, nutritional yeast, onion powder, garlic powder, mustard powder, and black salt. Dry sauté, stirring often, until the ingredients begin to stick to the pan and lightly brown, 8 to 10 minutes. Splash in a tablespoon or two of water to loosen anything stuck to the pan. Remove the pan from the heat and transfer the mixture to a plate to cool.

Wipe out the skillet and return it to medium heat. Lightly coat the skillet with spray oil. Drain the potatoes and add them to the hot pan. Cook, stirring often, until the potatoes are browned and crisp all over, 10 to 12 minutes. Season with the sea salt, remove the skillet from the heat, and set aside.

Transfer the cooled coconut mixture to a food processor and pulse to a coarse puree. Set aside.

For the mango-habanero puree, combine the mango, habanero, and lime juice in a high-speed blender and puree until smooth.

To assemble, in the center of each wrap, layer half the coconut mixture, then half the potatoes, half the onions, and finally a generous spoonful of the mango-habanero puree. Fold in the sides of the wrap and roll up to enclose. Serve. Save any leftover mango-habanero puree in the fridge for up to five days and use as a condiment.

Per serving: 643 calories, 7 g total fat, 2 g saturated fat, 0 mg cholesterol, 877 mg sodium, 136 g total carbohydrate (11 g dietary fiber, 60 g sugar, 0 g added sugars), 17 g protein, 4 mg iron

Building the Brunch Menu

Nothing says "weekend" like brunch: a mash-up of sweet and savory breakfast and lunch favorites. As its name makes clear, this leisurely meal is intended to keep you going till dinnertime, so be sure to make enough for even the hungriest guests. Include sweet and savory options, add a baked good, make sure you have a salad option and a few lighter choices, and you'll be set for a morning feast.

Whole Foodie Pancakes

Serves 2

These fluffy whole-grain pancakes are the perfect brunch food. Be sure to double or triple the batch—you'll be glad you did. If you have leftovers, it's easy to reheat them for the kids' breakfast. Top with fresh or stewed fruits, date paste, or chopped nuts.

1 cup whole wheat flour

⅓ cup unsweetened applesauce

2 tablespoons date paste (see page 56)

1 cup unsweetened almond milk or other nondairy milk

1 teaspoon baking powder

½ teaspoon baking soda

¼ teaspoon ground cinnamon

Pinch of sea salt (optional)

Fresh or poached berries, for serving (optional)

Vanilla Coconut Cream (page 271), for serving (optional)

In a medium bowl, combine the flour, applesauce, date paste, and almond milk. Mix thoroughly. Stir in the baking powder, baking soda, cinnamon, and salt (if using).

Heat a large nonstick pan over medium heat. When hot, pour in about ⅓ cup of the batter and cook until you see tiny bubbles forming on top and the bottom is browned, 2 to 3 minutes. Flip and cook until the other side is browned, about 2 minutes more. Transfer to a warm plate. Repeat with the remaining batter.

Serve with your favorite fresh or poached berries and vanilla coconut cream.

Banana-Nut Pancakes: Add half a mashed banana and ¼ cup chopped walnuts to the batter before cooking the pancakes.

Per serving: 277 calories, 3 g total fat, 0 g saturated fat, 0 mg cholesterol, 681 mg sodium, 58 g total carbohydrate (8 g dietary fiber, 11 g sugar, 0 g added sugars), 9 g protein, 3 mg iron

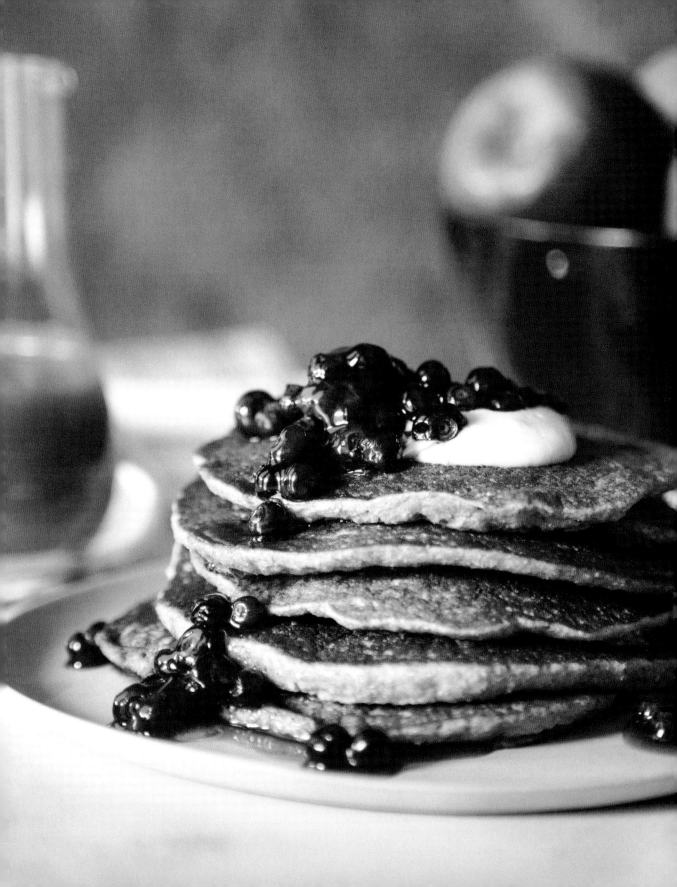

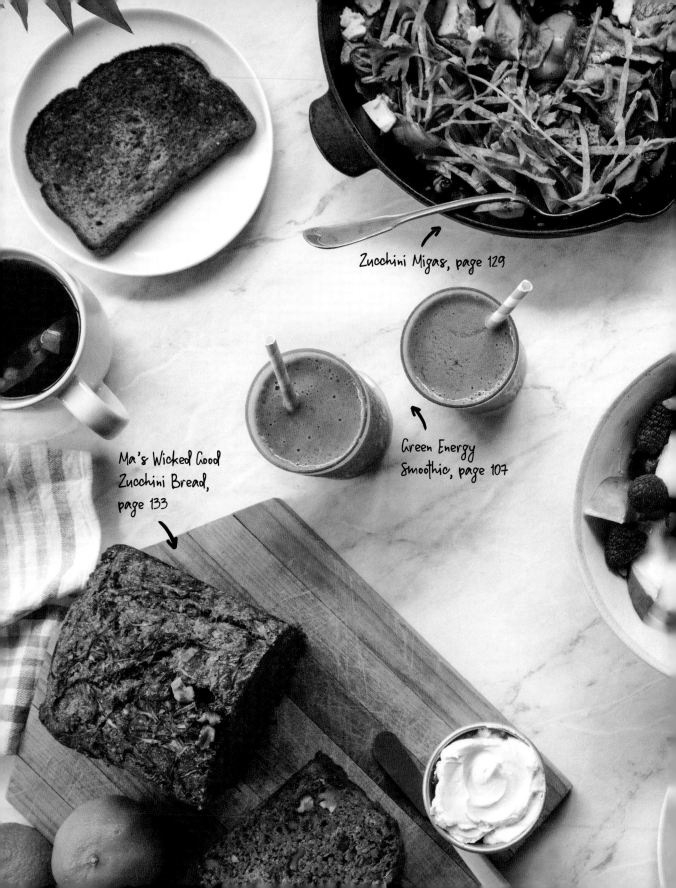

Zucchini Migas, page 129

Green Energy
Smoothie, page 107

Ma's Wicked Good
Zucchini Bread,
page 133

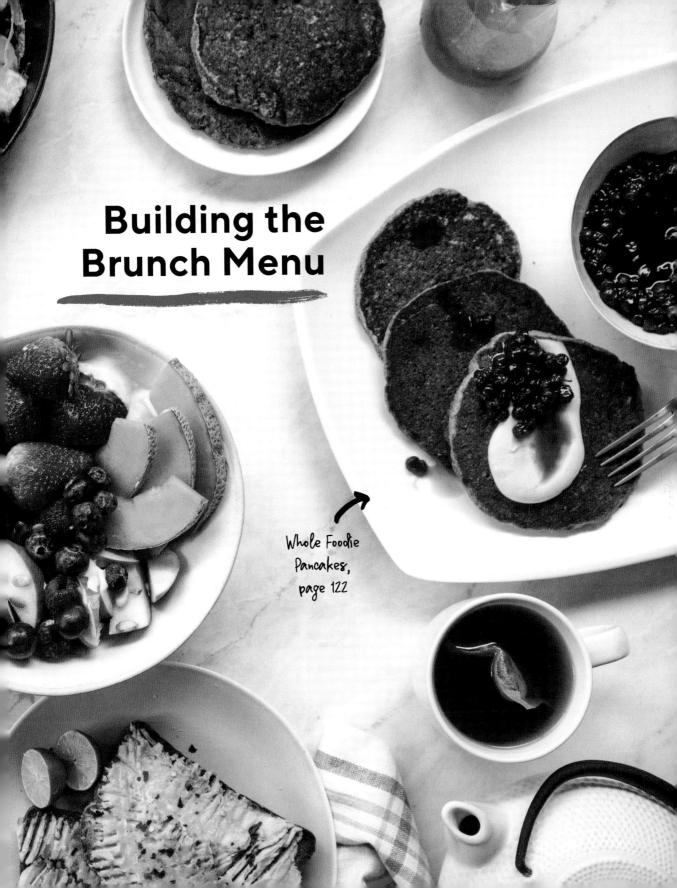

Building the
Brunch Menu

Whole Foodie
Pancakes,
page 122

Morning Dosas

Serves 6

Dosas—thin, crepe-like pancakes with a crispy texture and a tangy flavor from the fermented batter used to make them—are a South Indian specialty. Serve them with your favorite chutney, such as mango or coconut. You could also add a dollop of plain cashew sour cream (page 160) for richness. Note that this dish requires some advance planning because the batter needs to ferment overnight before cooking. **Recipe by Jess Kolko**

DOSA BATTER

2 cups dry short-grain brown rice

½ cup dry split hulled black lentils (urad dal)

2 teaspoons fenugreek seeds

Pinch of sea salt

FILLING

1 teaspoon cumin seeds

1 teaspoon black mustard seeds

2 small dried red chiles

1 onion, finely chopped

1 serrano chile, seeded, if less heat is desired, and finely chopped

1 (1-inch) piece fresh ginger, peeled and minced

2 to 4 garlic cloves, minced

1 teaspoon ground turmeric

½ teaspoon sea salt

1 pound Red Bliss or yellow new potatoes, cut into 1-inch cubes

1 cup fresh or frozen green peas

½ cup chopped fresh cilantro

Spray oil (for pan)

For the dosa batter, place the rice, lentils, and fenugreek in a medium bowl. Add water to cover and soak overnight.

The next morning, drain the mixture in a fine-mesh sieve and transfer to a food processor. Add 1 cup water and process until smooth, 2 to 3 minutes. Be patient and scrape down the sides of the processor as needed to make sure the batter is smooth. Add water as necessary to create a consistency like that of thin pancake batter. Scrape the batter into a medium bowl, cover it loosely with plastic wrap, and let it ferment at room temperature for 8 hours or up to overnight. As it ferments, the batter will develop air bubbles, which are important for leavening the dosas as they cook.

After fermenting, gently stir the salt into the batter. At this point, the batter can be stored in the refrigerator, covered, for up to 1 week. Before using it, add water, if necessary, to create a thin, runny consistency like crepe batter.

For the filling, heat a large nonstick skillet over medium heat. Add the cumin seeds and mustard seeds and toast, shaking the pan often, until fragrant and popping, 1 to 2 minutes. Stir in the dried chiles and onion and cook, stirring often, until the onion begins to stick to the pan and lightly brown, 3 to 4 minutes. Add 1 to 2 tablespoons water and stir to deglaze the pan and loosen the onion. Stir in the serrano, ginger, garlic, turmeric, and salt and cook for 1 minute.

Stir in the potatoes and ¾ cup water. Cover and simmer until the potatoes are tender, 15 to 20 minutes. Stir in the peas and simmer, uncovered, until all the liquid in the pan has evaporated. Remove from the heat. Stir in the cilantro and mash the potato mixture, leaving some small chunks. Set aside.

To cook the dosas, heat an 8-inch nonstick skillet or crepe pan over medium heat. When hot, coat it lightly with spray oil. Use a rounded ladle to spoon ¼ cup of the batter into the hot pan, then use the bottom of the ladle to quickly spread the batter into a thin, even layer over the pan. Cook, without flipping, until the edges look dry, 1 to 2 minutes. Transfer the dosa to a plate and repeat with the remaining batter.

Spoon ½ cup of the potato filling on one side of each cooked dosa and fold over the other side to enclose it. Serve hot.

Per serving: 360 calories, 3 g total fat, 0 g saturated fat, 0 mg cholesterol, 288 mg sodium, 78 g total carbohydrate (11 g dietary fiber, 3 g sugar, 0 g added sugars), 12 g protein, 4 mg iron

Brunch Inspiration from Around the World

It's natural that on a busy weekday morning, we reach for easy and familiar foods. But a weekend brunch is a great opportunity for creativity. To break out of the breakfast box, take your inspiration from other cultures that may choose dishes you've never considered to start the day. Here are a few examples:

- **Spice it up!** Try the Morning Dosa recipe (left), inspired by a South Indian specialty, or the Coconut & Potato Spelt Wraps with Mango-Habanero Puree (page 121), and pair with some hot chutneys and fresh tropical fruit salad. Mix up a smoothie featuring coconut water and banana (see our simple formula, page 106) or brew up a pot of fragrant Chai tea.

- **Morning Miso.** Take your cues from Japanese culture, and make a miso soup bar for brunch, featuring fresh chopped veggies, radishes, sea vegetables, brown rice, rice or buckwheat noodles, tofu, edamame, pickled ginger, and some Furikake seasoning. Your guests will have fun assembling their own bowls and may discover a new morning favorite. Serve with our Green Energy Smoothie featuring Matcha green tea powder (page 107).

- **Mediterranean Magic.** On a hot summer weekend, make a big fresh salad the center of your brunch table, adding beans, olives, juicy tomatoes, crunchy cucumbers, and other Mediterranean favorites. Some classic spreads like Dill Hummus (page 262), Harissa Vinaigrette (page 150) and Baba Ghanoush (page 262) will round out the meal, served with whole grain pita breads. Serve with a pitcher of fresh iced tea.

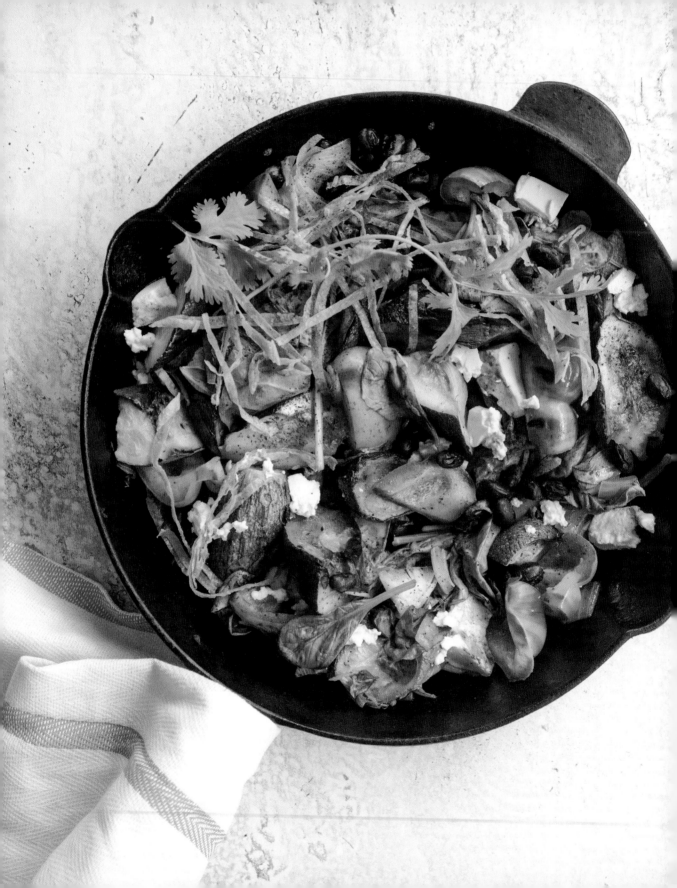

Zucchini Migas

Serves 3

Migas is a traditional Spanish, Mexican, and Tex-Mex dish that uses up leftover tortillas. Be sure to use chili powder (a mix of powdered mild red chiles and other spices) rather than crushed chiles or cayenne pepper, unless, of course, you want it extra hot!

2 zucchini

3 corn tortillas, cut into ¼- to ½-inch-wide strips

½ onion, finely chopped

2 garlic cloves, minced

¼ cup low-sodium vegetable broth

1 teaspoon chili powder

½ red bell pepper, cubed

½ cup cubed silken tofu

½ cup lightly packed baby spinach

¼ cup cooked black beans (see page 42) or canned no-added-sodium black beans, drained and rinsed

½ teaspoon minced jalapeño

1½ teaspoons nutritional yeast

½ teaspoon sea salt

¼ cup lightly packed fresh cilantro leaves

2 avocados, pitted, peeled, and sliced

Hot sauce (optional)

Preheat the oven to 350°F. Line two baking sheets with parchment.

Put the zucchini on one baking sheet and prick them with a fork. Spread the tortilla strips in a single layer over the other baking sheet. Bake the tortilla strips for 5 to 7 minutes, until they are crisp, flipping the strips halfway through. Bake the zucchini until it is fork-tender, 12 to 15 minutes, depending on size. (If you only have one sheet, bake the zucchini, then let the baking sheet cool slightly before baking the tortilla strips.) Remove from the oven as they are done and set aside to cool.

When the zucchini are cool enough to handle, cut them into bite-size cubes.

Meanwhile, heat a large sauté pan over medium-high heat. Add the onion and dry sauté, stirring often, until it begins to stick to the pan, 3 to 4 minutes. Add the garlic and cook for 1 minute. Add the broth and stir to deglaze the pan. Gently stir in the chili powder, bell peppers, zucchini, and tofu. Cook until the peppers are slightly softened, 3 to 4 minutes.

Stir in the spinach, black beans, jalapeño, and nutritional yeast and cook until the spinach wilts, 1 to 2 minutes.

Stir in the salt and cilantro and cook for 1 minute. Remove from the heat.

Divide the migas among three plates and scatter the toasted tortilla strips over each. Serve with the sliced avocado and your favorite hot sauce.

Per serving: 296 calories, 16 g total fat, 2 g saturated fat, 0 mg cholesterol, 451 mg sodium, 33 g total carbohydrate (10 g dietary fiber, 5 g sugar, 0 g added sugars), 9 g protein, 2 mg iron

Carrot Lox Tartine with Cashew Cream Cheese, Capers, & Shallot

Serves 6

The salt-baking method used for these carrots creates a flavor very similar to traditional salmon lox, making them a perfect accompaniment to nondairy cream cheese and capers. An elegant addition to any brunch menu, this dish was inspired by our dear friend Tal Ronnen, chef of Crossroads Kitchen in Los Angeles. Look for garlic flowers at the farmers' market—they add a pretty finish to the dish.

½ cup Kite Hill almond cream cheese or Cashew Cream Cheese (page 264)

6 slices seeded low-sodium whole-grain bread

1 cup Carrot Lox (page 101)

3 tablespoons drained and rinsed capers

2 small shallots, sliced into thin rings

6 dill sprigs

Garlic flowers (optional)

Divide the cream cheese among the slices of bread and spread evenly. Cut each slice in half diagonally. Top with the carrot lox, capers, shallot, dill sprigs, and garlic flowers (if using).

Per serving: 177 calories, 6 g total fat, 0 g saturated fat, 0 mg cholesterol, 344 mg sodium, 24 g total carbohydrate (2 g dietary fiber, 6 g sugar, 0 g added sugars), 7 g protein, 1 mg iron

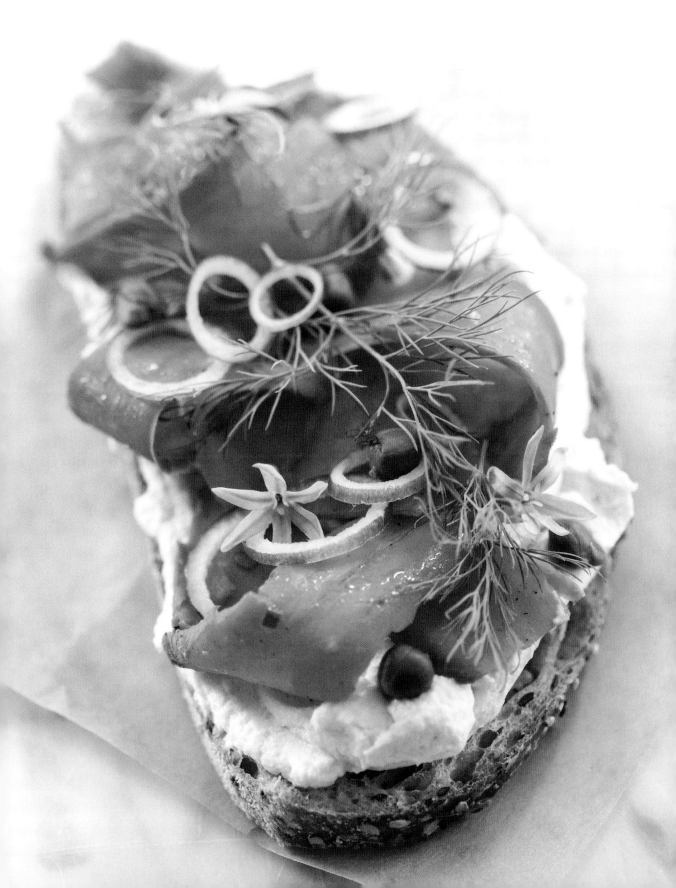

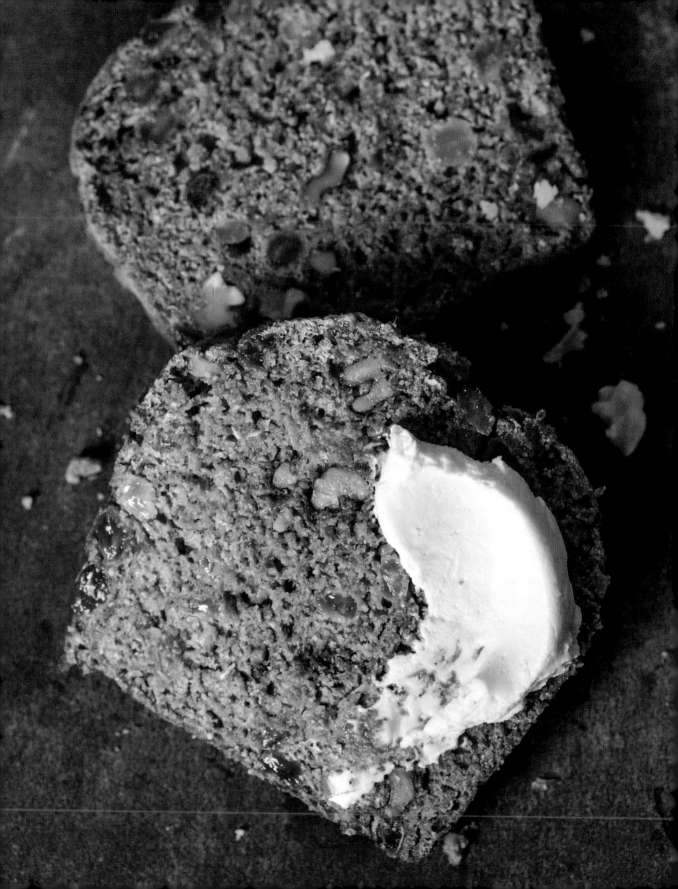

Ma's Wicked Good Zucchini Bread

Makes one 8 by 4-inch loaf (about 10 slices)

Zucchini is one of the most versatile vegetables. It works well in sweet and savory dishes due to its water content and pliability once cooked. This is not your traditional sweet zucchini bread—it's a little more savory. This bread is moist and filling and makes a great addition to the brunch menu. Use a serrated knife to cut the finished loaf into ¾-inch-wide pieces, and if you have any left over, freeze individual slices wrapped in plastic. **Recipe by Beverly Burl, supermom extraordinaire**

Spray oil (for pan)

1 or 2 small zucchini

1 cup raisins

3 cups whole wheat flour

1 teaspoon baking soda

1 teaspoon baking powder

1 teaspoon ground cinnamon

Pinch of sea salt

1 cup unsweetened almond milk

¾ cup unsweetened applesauce

½ cup date paste (see page 56)

½ cup walnuts, toasted and chopped

Nondairy cream cheese, such as Kite Hill brand or Cashew Cream Cheese (page 264) (for serving, optional)

Preheat the oven to 325°F. Lightly coat the bottom and sides of an 8 by 4-inch loaf pan with spray oil.

Grate the zucchini on the large holes of a box grater into a large bowl (you should have about 3 cups). Reserve a few tablespoons of the shredded zucchini in a small bowl to top the bread before baking. Stir the raisins into the remaining zucchini in the large bowl and set aside.

In a medium bowl, whisk together the flour, baking soda, baking powder, cinnamon, and salt. In a small bowl, whisk together the almond milk, applesauce, date paste, and walnuts. Add the milk mixture to the zucchini mixture and stir to combine, then stir in the flour mixture. The batter will be thick.

Scrape the batter into the prepared loaf pan and sprinkle the reserved shredded zucchini on top. Bake until golden brown and a knife inserted into the center comes out clean, about 1 hour. Remove from the oven and let cool in the pan for 10 minutes. Remove from the pan and set on a wire rack to cool completely.

Cut the loaf into ten slices and serve with your favorite nondairy cream cheese, if desired.

Note: For sweeter zucchini bread, increase the date paste to 1 cup and add a few minutes to the baking time.

Per serving (1 slice): 250 calories, 5 g total fat, 1 g saturated fat, 0 mg cholesterol, 237 mg sodium, 48 g total carbohydrate (6 g dietary fiber, 19 g sugar, 0 g added sugars), 7 g protein, 2 mg iron

Baked Tofu, Chimichurri, & Roasted Vegetable Club

Serves 4

This satisfying sandwich is a great brunch addition, highlighting roasted vegetables paired with the wonderful flavors of Argentina's chimichurri sauce. You'll probably have extra sauce left over, so try using it tossed over portobello caps before grilling for a meaty side dish. Make extra tofu, too—it's great to have on hand for snacks, bowls, and salads.

TOFU AND VEGETABLES

1 (14-ounce) package extra-firm tofu, drained

1½ tablespoons low-sodium tamari

1 sweet potato, scrubbed but not peeled

1 zucchini, cut into ¼-inch-thick planks

1 small eggplant, cut into ¼-inch-thick planks

1 red bell pepper, quartered lengthwise

¼ teaspoon sea salt

½ teaspoon freshly ground black pepper

CILANTRO CHIMICHURRI

½ avocado, pitted and peeled

1 cup loosely packed chopped fresh cilantro

1½ cups loosely packed chopped fresh parsley

2 tablespoons chopped shallot

2 tablespoons apricot paste (see page 56)

3 tablespoons white wine vinegar

Juice of ½ lime

¼ teaspoon sea salt

½ teaspoon fresh ground black pepper

½ serrano chile, seeded, if less heat is desired, and chopped

TO ASSEMBLE

¾ cup Kite Hill cream cheese or Cashew Cream Cheese (page 264)

8 slices low-sodium whole-grain bread

1 cup baby spinach

For tofu and vegetables, preheat the oven to 350°F. Line two baking sheets with parchment paper.

Wrap the drained tofu in a few layers of paper towels, then sandwich it between two plates and weight down the top plate with a heavy book. Press for at least 10 minutes and up to 1 hour. Cut the pressed tofu block crosswise into 8 rectangular planks, each about the size of a domino.

Place the tofu planks in a single layer on one of the prepared baking sheets. Drizzle with the tamari, turning the tofu to coat evenly (handle the planks gently to avoid breaking). Bake until the tofu is golden brown and slightly firm, about 30 minutes, using a spatula to carefully turn the tofu halfway through the cooking time. Lift the tofu on the parchment paper off the baking sheet and set it aside. Increase the oven temperature to 400°F.

Pierce the sweet potato several times with a fork and set it on the oven rack. Roast until fork-tender, 30 to 45 minutes, depending on the size of the sweet potato. Set aside to cool.

Meanwhile, spread the zucchini, eggplant, and bell pepper in a single layer on the second prepared baking sheet and sprinkle them all over with the salt and black pepper. Roast the vegetables with the sweet potato until slightly softened, about 10 minutes. Carefully flip the vegetables with a spatula and roast until tender and lightly browned, 8 to 10 minutes more. Set aside to cool.

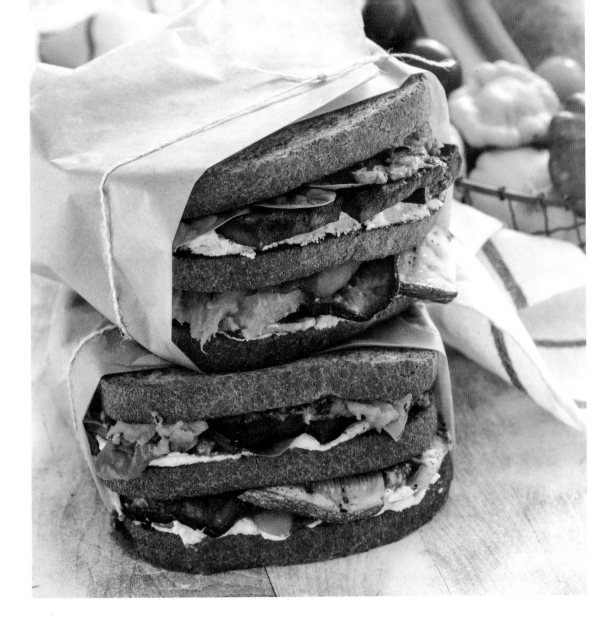

For the chimichurri, combine all the chimichurri ingredients in a food processor or high-speed blender and process or blend to a coarse puree, about 30 seconds. Set aside.

To assemble, divide the cream cheese between 4 slices of the bread and spread evenly. Cut the sweet potato in half lengthwise and scoop out the flesh; spread one-quarter of the sweet potato flesh over the cream cheese on each of those slices. Layer on the baked tofu, roasted vegetables, and spinach, dividing them evenly. Spread a layer of the chimichurri over each of the remaining 4 bread slices and set them chimichurri-side down over the tofu and vegetables to close the sandwiches.

Slice each sandwich in half diagonally and serve. Any leftover chimichurri sauce can be stored in the fridge for up to a week.

Per serving: 535 calories, 19 g total fat, 1 g saturated fat, 0 mg cholesterol, 859 mg sodium, 65 g total carbohydrate (8 g dietary fiber, 11 g sugar, 0 g added sugars), 29 g protein, 7 mg iron

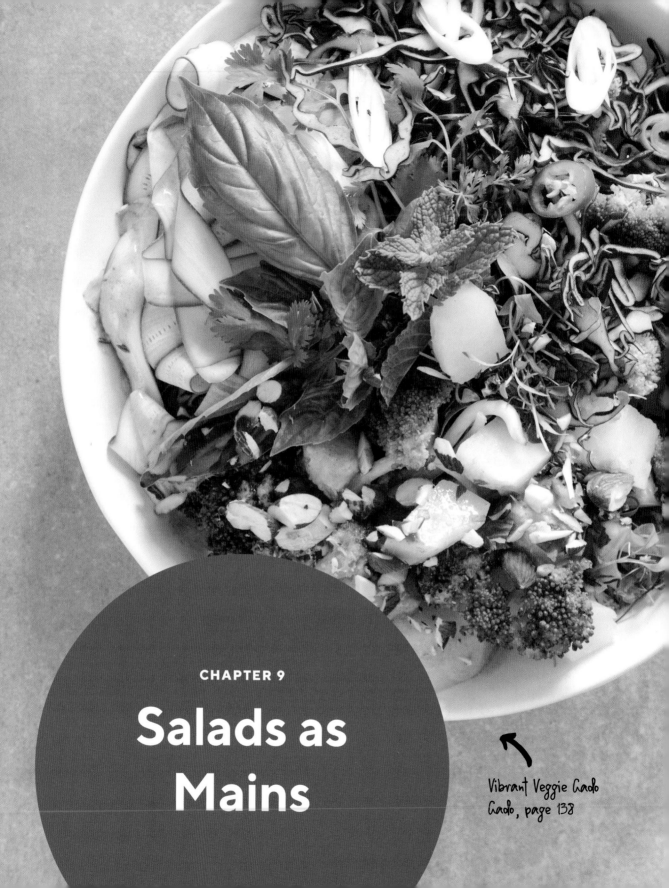

CHAPTER 9

Salads as Mains

Vibrant Veggie Gado
Gado, page 138

"Side salads," step aside! Salads can make satisfying and delicious main dishes; with the addition of raw vegetables, nuts and seeds, whole grains, or beans, they become the centerpiece of a meal. Toss with a delicious oil-free dressing (see page 153 for a simple formula and some of our favorite dressings), and you've got a fresh, vibrant lunch or dinner.

Leafy greens form the base of many salads, and these nutrient-dense foods are some of the healthiest options on the menu. Don't stop at the familiar varieties (put down that iceberg!)—try mixing it up with bitter greens like watercress, dandelion, chicory, or arugula, or leaves that aren't green at all, like radicchio, red oak-leaf lettuce, or red cabbage. Sprouts and microgreens also add a fresh, spicy kick to your salad. If you're not used to eating a lot of greens and find some of the flavors too intense, start with milder varieties like baby spinach, butter lettuces, and romaine.

Want the best possible greens for a fraction of the price? Grow your own! Depending on your kitchen and outdoor space, growing your own food is one of the most rewarding gifts for yourself and family, and a great way to get kids invested in healthy eating. For pennies on the dollar, you can grow your own sprouts in jars to use as a vibrant, fresh addition to any meal. You can also grow microgreens and sprouts in trays and, if you have outdoor space, use planter boxes for lettuces and herbs. Those with a garden can plant rows of green abundance!

Chef's Tip

"Nothing can compare to growing your own greens and vegetables from seed, then harvesting and incorporating them into your family meals to share with the ones you love. I have been growing all my sprouts and microgreens in an Urban Cultivator, one of my newest favorite kitchen tools. The size of a wine fridge, it gives you the ability to grow fresh greens and sprouts year-round in your kitchen. I highly recommend checking it out!"—**Chad Sarno**

Building Green and Vegetable Salads

These colorful and crunchy combinations of greens and raw veggies are perfect when you want a lighter meal or to serve in smaller portions as side dishes or appetizers. As you build your salad, consider flavor profiles and textures. Add a little crunch, throw in some fresh herbs to elevate your salad, and fill it out with steamed, blanched, or roasted veggies.

Vibrant Veggie Gado Gado

Serves 4

This Indonesian-inspired dish, packed with nutrients, features a combination of raw and lightly cooked vegetables, including zucchini noodles. Spicy Almond-Chile Sauce makes it especially memorable. It makes a delicious side salad or, when served in larger portions with the optional protein, a satisfying main meal. (Pictured on page 136.) **Recipe by Whole Foods Market**

2 cups cubed red potatoes

1½ cups small broccoli florets

4 cups zucchini noodles (zoodles; see Note)

1 cup finely shredded red cabbage

1 cup finely shredded green cabbage

¾ cup bean sprouts

¾ cup chopped mixed fresh mint, basil, and cilantro leaves

3 green onions, cut into 2-inch matchsticks

1 cup Almond-Chile Sauce (page 158)

2 limes, cut into wedges

Ninja Squirrel Sriracha sauce or other hot sauce

Grilled tofu, poached fish, or poached chicken, for serving (optional)

Steam the potatoes and broccoli in a covered steamer basket over gently simmering water until tender, about 6 minutes for the potatoes and 3 minutes for the broccoli. Remove from the heat.

Divide the zucchini noodles among four bowls, placing them in the center of each bowl. Evenly divide the potatoes, broccoli, shredded red and green cabbage, bean sprouts, and the green onions among the bowls. Scatter with the chopped herbs. Pour ¼ cup of the almond-chile sauce over each bowl.

Serve each bowl with 2 lime wedges for squeezing and plenty of sriracha.

Note: You can buy precut zucchini noodles at Whole Foods Market. To make them yourself, use a spiralizer, julienne slicer, or mandoline to slice 3 or 4 medium zucchini into long, thin strips. If using a spiralizer, use one of the smaller blades; if using a julienne slicer or mandoline, slice the zucchini lengthwise into strips.

Per serving: 243 calories, 11 g total fat, 1 g saturated fat, 0 mg cholesterol, 295 mg sodium, 32 g total carbohydrate (8 g dietary fiber, 9 g sugar, 0 g added sugars), 10 g protein, 3 mg iron

Grilled Romaine Hearts & Vegetable Salad

Serves 4

Ever tried grilling your greens? If not, you're missing out. Grilling adds a nice charred flavor and texture to your summer salads. If you grow your own veggies, they can go straight from the garden to the grill. (Pictured on next page.)

Leaves and thin stems from 1 bunch cilantro

Leaves and thin stems from 1 bunch parsley

½ cup white wine vinegar

4 garlic cloves

3 tablespoons pine nuts

½ teaspoon red pepper flakes

½ teaspoon sea salt

½ teaspoon freshly ground black pepper

4 romaine hearts, halved lengthwise

2 ears corn, shucked

2 poblano chiles

1 bunch green onions or baby leeks

2 avocados, pitted, peeled, and cubed

2 ripe tomatoes, cored and cut into small wedges

Heat a grill to medium-high.

In a food processor, combine the cilantro, parsley, vinegar, garlic, pine nuts, red pepper flakes, salt, and black pepper. Process to a thick, coarse puree.

Use a pastry brush to brush half the herb puree over the romaine hearts, corn, poblanos, and green onions.

Grill the vegetables directly over the heat until just tender but still crisp, turning them for even cooking. The green onions will cook fastest (2 to 4 minutes), then the romaine hearts and poblanos (5 to 7 minutes), and finally the corn (8 to 10 minutes). As the vegetables are done, transfer them to a cutting board.

Serve these beautiful grilled vegetables family-style on a platter with the avocados and tomatoes. Alternatively, for a composed salad, cut the vegetables into bite-size pieces, cut the corn kernels from the cobs, transfer all the vegetables to a bowl, and add the avocado and tomato. Toss gently until combined. Serve warm, with the remaining herb puree alongside.

Per serving: 375 calories, 17 g total fat, 2 g saturated fat, 0 mg cholesterol, 383 mg sodium, 53 g total carbohydrate (23 g dietary fiber, 13 g sugar, 0 g added sugars), 15 g protein, 9 mg iron

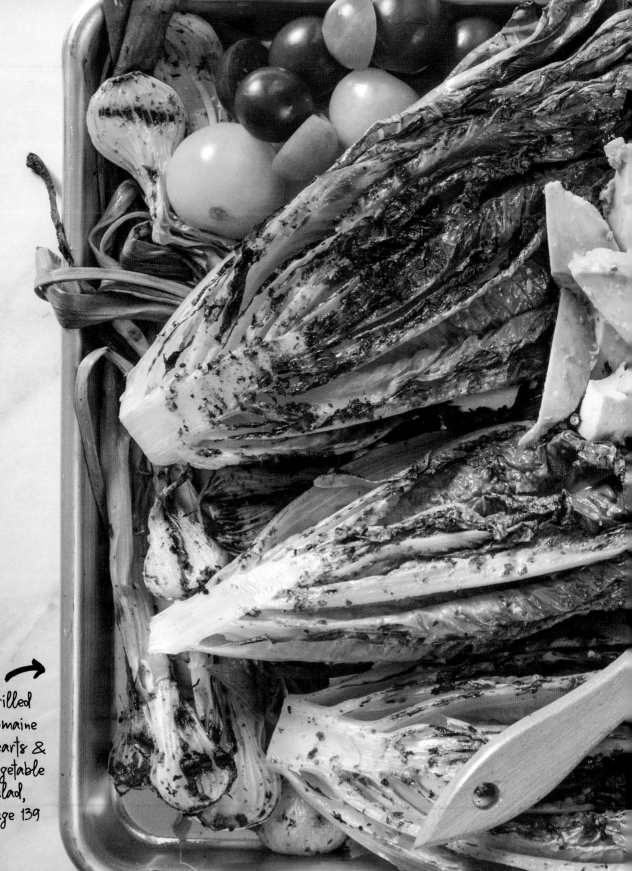

Grilled
Romaine
Hearts &
Vegetable
Salad,
page 139

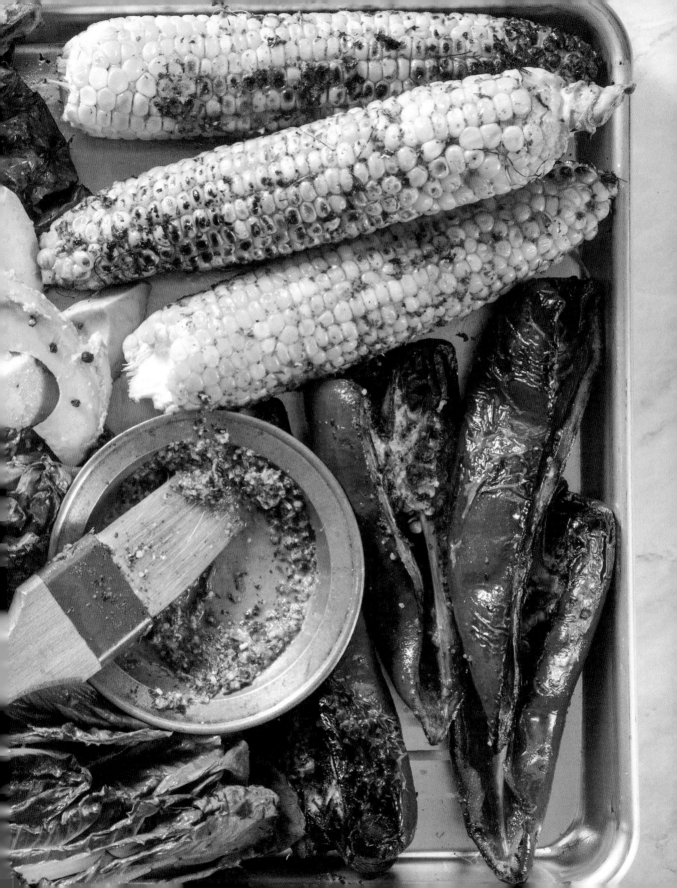

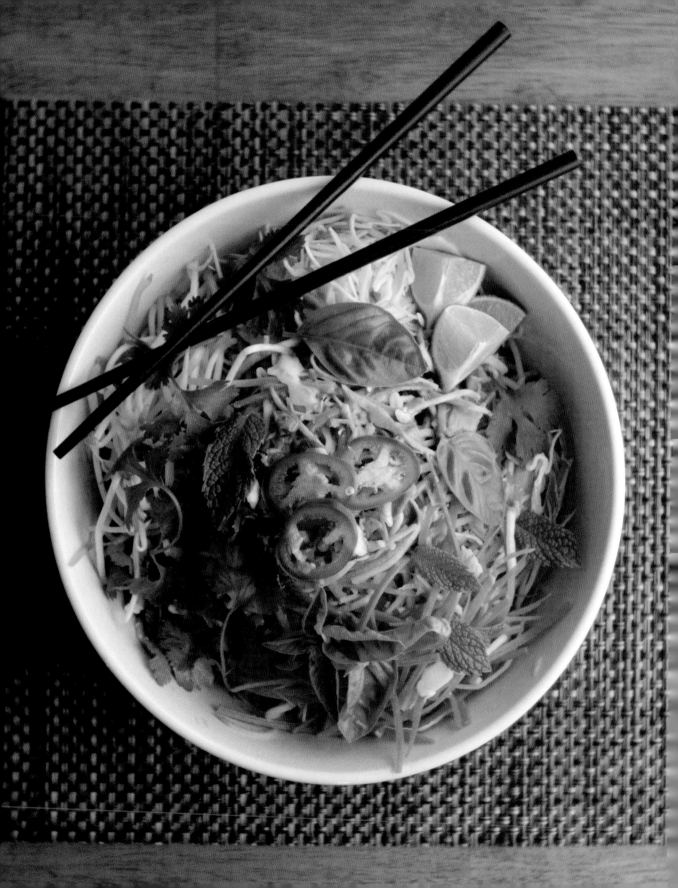

Roots & Fruits Pad Thai Salad

Serves 6

This colorful, flavorful salad is a raw twist on a classic Thai dish. Garden and root veggies complement the natural sweetness of green apples and pears, and the fresh herbs tie it all together with their distinctive flavors. Use various colors of carrots and cabbage to bring even more beauty, taste, and texture to this nutrient-packed salad.

½ head green cabbage, shredded

2 green apples, cored and cut into matchsticks

2 large carrots, cut into matchsticks

1 small kohlrabi, peeled and cut into matchsticks

1 pear, cored and cut into matchsticks

1 small celeriac root, peeled and cut into matchsticks

2 cups fresh bean sprouts

1½ cups Almond-Chile Sauce (page 158)

½ cup packed fresh cilantro leaves

½ cup packed fresh basil leaves, cut into thin strips

½ cup torn fresh mint leaves

2 jalapeños, seeded and cut into paper thin slices (optional)

½ cup crushed raw almonds (optional)

1 lime, cut into wedges (optional)

There are two ways to serve this: You can prep each vegetable one at a time, rinse each with cold water, drain, and serve them in separate bowls or serving dishes with the dressing, sprouts, herbs, and optional items on the side. This will give each diner the option to create an individual bowl with bits of color and flavor as they see fit. Or you can combine the vegetables in a big bowl for everyone to dig into. If that's your preference, prep each vegetable, rinse each with cold water, drain, then add everything to a large bowl, including the sprouts and optional items. Mix together the dressing and herbs, pour over the top, and serve the entire bowl family-style, with lime wedges alongside for squeezing, if desired.

Notes: It's fun to serve this salad in a large mason jar. Place the dressing in the bottom of the jar, then layer the fruits and vegetables in true rainbow fashion. To serve, turn the jar upside down to let the dressing coat the veggies, shake, and serve. Perfect for an office lunch.

Substitute or try adding different shaved raw veggies and fruits like rutabaga, golden beets, and/or green papaya.

Per serving: 251 calories, 12 g total fat, 1 g saturated fat, 0 mg cholesterol, 361 mg sodium, 30 g total carbohydrate (9 g dietary fiber, 16 g sugar, 0 g added sugars), 9 g protein, 3 mg iron

Potato Salad with Grilled Onion & White Bean Aioli

Serves 4

This low-fat and nutritious twist on potato salad uses blended white beans to create the creaminess usually achieved with mayonnaise. Grilled onions add a nice touch of sweetness. Serve on a bed of butter lettuce.

Spray oil (for grill)

1 Vidalia onion, sliced crosswise into ¼- to ½-inch-thick rounds

1 pound small new potatoes, halved or quartered if large

2 celery stalks, finely chopped

¼ cup chopped fresh parsley

3 tablespoons chopped fresh dill

3 tablespoons drained and rinsed small capers

1 cup cooked white beans (see page 42) or canned no-added-sodium white beans, drained and rinsed

2 tablespoons Dijon mustard

1½ tablespoons sherry vinegar (see Note)

2½ tablespoons grated fresh horseradish, or 1½ tablespoons prepared horseradish (see Note)

½ teaspoon freshly ground black pepper

Heat a grill to medium-high or heat a grill pan over medium-high heat. Lightly coat the grill grates or pan with spray oil. Add the onion and grill until browned all over, 2 to 3 minutes per side, rotating the onion once or twice for even browning. Transfer to a cutting board and finely chop.

Meanwhile, steam the potatoes in a steamer basket set over gently simmering water until tender, 8 to 10 minutes. Remove from the heat and let cool.

When the potatoes have cooled, transfer them to a medium bowl and stir in the celery, grilled onion, parsley, dill, and capers. Set aside.

In a high-speed blender, combine the beans, mustard, vinegar, horseradish, pepper, and 3 tablespoons water. Blend until smooth, 1 to 2 minutes.

Pour the bean mixture over the potatoes and toss to coat. Serve at room temperature, or cover and refrigerate for up to 3 days. Return to room temperature before serving.

Note: Prepared horseradish is made with vinegar. If you use prepared horseradish instead of fresh, cut back the amount of sherry vinegar to 2½ teaspoons.

Per serving: 193 calories, 1 g total fat, 0 g saturated fat, 0 mg cholesterol, 309 mg sodium, 39 g total carbohydrate (10 g dietary fiber, 4 g sugar, 0 g added sugars), 8 g protein, 3 mg iron

Moroccan Kale & Hemp Seed Salad

Serves 6

Lemony, garlicky, and aromatic, this kale salad makes a substantial and satisfying meal. The dressing is creamy yet retains some texture from the seeds. If you can't find the ras el hanout spice blend, you can substitute za'atar or ground cumin. **Recipe by Chef Pete Cervoni**

DRESSING

1¼ cups raw unhulled sesame seeds

½ cucumber, thinly sliced into half-moons, unpeeled

1 tablespoon grated lemon zest

¼ cup fresh lemon juice

1 tablespoon chopped garlic

2 to 4 teaspoons ras el hanout spice blend

¾ teaspoon fine pink Himalayan salt

¼ cup filtered water

SALAD

7 cups packed finely shredded lacinato or Tuscan kale leaves

2½ cups packed finely shredded red cabbage

½ cucumber thinly sliced into half-moons, unpeeled

1 cup thinly sliced green onions

1 cup halved grape tomatoes

½ cup chopped Kalamata olives

½ cup hulled hemp seeds

¼ cup dried currants

For the dressing, combine all the dressing ingredients in a high-speed blender and blend until the dressing is as smooth as possible (the sesame seeds will not completely break down), stopping to scrape down the sides of the blender jar once or twice.

To make the salad, combine the kale and cabbage in a large bowl. Pour on the dressing and firmly massage the dressing into the greens with your hands to break down the tough fibers of the greens, soften them, and fully flavor them, about 1 minute. The greens should feel softer and almost wilted when fully massaged.

Add the cucumber, green onions, tomatoes, olives, and ¼ cup of the hemp seeds. Toss gently to combine. Garnish with the remaining ¼ cup hemp seeds and the currants.

Per serving: 362 calories, 25 g total fat, 4 g saturated fat, 0 mg cholesterol, 244 mg sodium, 26 g total carbohydrate (9 g dietary fiber, 7 g sugar, 0 g added sugars), 16 g protein, 7 mg iron

Grain and Bean Based Salads

Cooked whole grains and beans can be easily tossed into any greens-based salad to turn it into a well-rounded meal. But sometimes you crave a heartier salad, where grains or beans form the base and are complemented by crunchy veggies, fragrant herbs, and a fresh or creamy dressing. These recipes are sure to satisfy, served as they are or atop a bed of fresh greens.

Brown Rice Salad with Mandarin, Mint, & Jalapeño

Serves 4

This rice dish is perfect to wrap in lettuce and top with avocado and your favorite hot sauce. It makes a great accompaniment to Greek Vegetable Kabobs with Tzatziki (page 81).

2 cups cooked brown rice (see page 36), cooled

2 tablespoons minced shallot

1 garlic clove, minced

¼ cup chopped red bell pepper

2 seedless mandarin oranges, peeled and chopped

3 tablespoons sunflower seeds or shelled pistachios, toasted

Grated zest and juice of ½ lemon

2 tablespoons finely chopped fresh mint

2 tablespoons chopped fresh parsley leaves

1 jalapeño (see Note), seeded, if less heat is desired, and minced

½ teaspoon sea salt

¼ teaspoon freshly ground black pepper

Combine all the ingredients in a large bowl and mix gently.

Note: If you'd like even less heat, don't use the full jalapeño.

Per serving: 184 calories, 4 g total fat, 0 g saturated fat, 0 mg cholesterol, 293 mg sodium, 37 g total carbohydrate (4 g dietary fiber, 5 g sugar, 0 g added sugars), 4 g protein, 1 mg iron

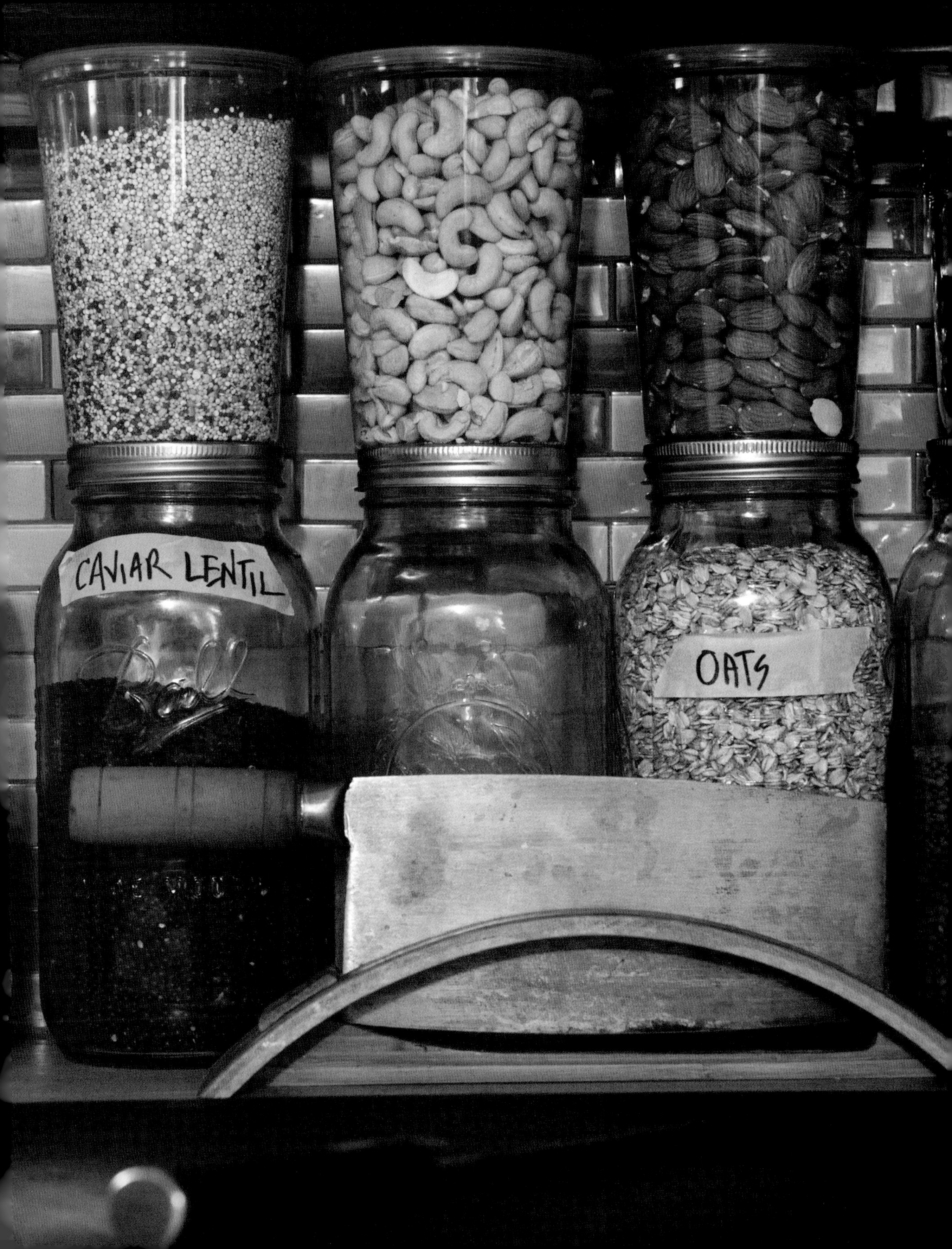
CAVIAR LENTIL
OATS

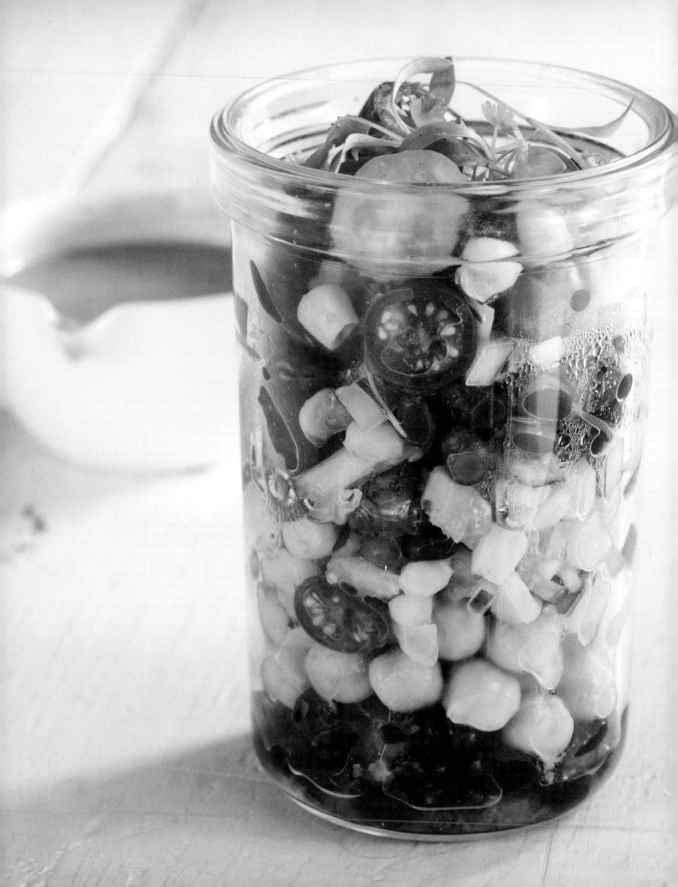

Layered Hearty Bean Salad with Dijon Vinaigrette

Serves 6

This bean salad gives new meaning to the term *hearty*. Once you get the hang of the formula, you can experiment with multiple variations on this satisfying and nutritious dish. Try adding different beans, including fresh green beans or fava beans. Throw in some multicolored bell peppers, carrots, jicama, or avocado. This salad is a meal in itself, or serve it atop some shredded lettuce.

DRESSING

2½ tablespoons apple cider vinegar

3 tablespoons unseasoned rice vinegar

3 tablespoons date paste (see page 56)

2 tablespoons Dijon mustard

1 garlic clove, minced

1½ teaspoons Mum's Spice Blend (page 67) or your favorite spice blend

¼ teaspoon freshly ground black pepper

1 teaspoon Sriracha, or to taste

SALAD

1 pint small cherry tomatoes, halved lengthwise

½ cup thawed frozen corn kernels

½ red onion, finely chopped

1 celery stalk, finely chopped

3 tablespoons drained and rinsed capers

1 (15-ounce) can no-added-sodium black beans, drained and rinsed

1 (15-ounce) can no-added-sodium chickpeas, drained and rinsed

1 (15-ounce) can no-added-sodium red beans, drained and rinsed

For the dressing, combine all the dressing ingredients in a jar or small bowl and shake or whisk until blended.

For the salad, in a large bowl, combine the tomatoes, corn, onion, celery, and capers. Line up six 1-pint mason jars (or small salad bowls if you don't have jars) and layer the ingredients as follows, making roughly 1-inch layers of each: black beans, corn mixture, chickpeas, corn mixture, red beans, corn mixture. Continue layering until the jars are filled. Pour on dressing shortly before serving.

Per serving: 210 calories, 1 g total fat, 0 g saturated fat, 0 mg cholesterol, 300 mg sodium, 40 g total carbohydrate (9 g dietary fiber, 6 g sugar, 0 g added sugars), 11 g protein, 2 mg iron

Moroccan Barley & Cauliflower Salad with Harissa Vinaigrette

Serves 6

The blend of earthy barley and crunchy cauliflower is nicely set off by the rich pine nut cream, and elevated by the signature North African harissa spice blend. This no-oil harissa vinaigrette retains all the flavor of traditional harissa paste. Try rubbing it on vegetables before grilling, or using it as a sauce for steamed greens. If you want more of these delicious flavors, double the vinaigrette recipe!

PINE NUT PUREE

½ cup pine nuts

3 tablespoons garlic paste (pages 69 and 70)

1 teaspoon grated lemon zest

¼ teaspoon sea salt

BARLEY SALAD

2 cups cooked barley (see page 36), cooled

3 tablespoons dried currants

2 tablespoons pine nuts, toasted

1 tablespoon minced fresh chives

2 tablespoons fresh lemon juice

HARISSA VINAIGRETTE

½ teaspoon caraway seeds

½ teaspoon cumin seeds

½ teaspoon coriander seeds

¼ cup minced roasted red pepper

2 small mandarin oranges, peeled, seeded, and minced

2 tablespoons minced fresh chives

1 garlic clove, minced

¼ teaspoon sea salt

3 cups small cauliflower florets

4 baby cucumbers, sliced lengthwise into ribbons

For pine nut puree, soak the pine nuts in hot water to cover for 15 minutes. Drain and transfer to a food processor or high-speed blender. Add the garlic paste, lemon zest, and salt and blend until smooth, about 30 seconds, adding a tablespoon or two of water if necessary to reach the desired consistency. Set aside.

For the barley salad, in a medium bowl, mix together the barley, currants, pine nuts, chives, and lemon juice. Set aside.

For the harissa vinaigrette, heat a small sauté pan over medium heat. Add the caraway, cumin, and coriander seeds and toast, shaking the pan often, until fragrant, 1 to 2 minutes. Remove from the heat and transfer to a plate to cool, then transfer to a spice grinder. Grind the spices to a powder and transfer to a small bowl. Stir in the roasted pepper, oranges, chives, garlic, and salt, mixing well.

Steam the cauliflower in a covered steamer basket over gently simmering water until just tender, about 5 minutes. Remove from the steamer and set aside.

To assemble, spoon some pine nut puree on each plate, followed by a spoonful of barley salad, a row of blanched cauliflower florets, and a row of sliced cucumber. Finish with a drizzle of vinaigrette.

Note: You could also present this dish on a platter instead of on individual plates. Toss the barley with the pine nut puree and spread the mixture over a platter. Toss the cauliflower and cucumbers with the vinaigrette and place on the barley before serving.

Per serving: 202 calories, 9 g total fat, 1 g saturated fat, 0 mg cholesterol, 220 mg sodium, 29 g total carbohydrate (5 g dietary fiber, 9 g sugar, 0 g added sugars), 5 g protein, 2 mg iron

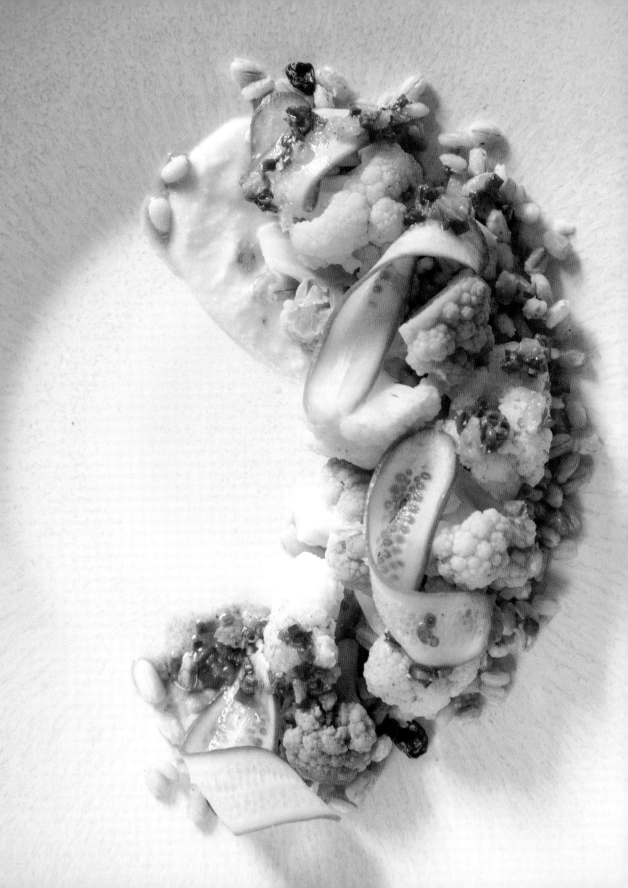

CHAPTER 10

Sauce It Up!

It's all about the sauce! If the sauce is good, you'll enjoy it on anything. Sauces, dressings, and marinades are essential elements of whole foods, plant-based cooking. A great sauce will offer the opportunity to build flavor into your dishes, turning them from average to amazing.

Dressings

Conventional salad dressings tend to involve large quantities of oil and sugar. But prepare to be surprised, because it's easy to make delicious dressings using whole-food ingredients. There are two types of dressing: creamy dressings, which are blended, and vinaigrettes, which are shaken or whisked. Here's a simple formula for each.

Creamy Dressing Formula (blended until smooth)

Whole-food fat + Acid + Spices + Natural sweeteners (optional) + Salt (optional)

Vinaigrette Formula (shaken or whisked)

Acids + Spices + Natural sweeteners + Salt (optional)

BUILD YOUR DRESSINGS FROM A BASE

Make a big batch of a simple base dressing, such as a creamy cashew dressing or an oil-free vinaigrette, and then add different herbs, spices, and seasonings to create variations when you are ready to use it. You'll see an example of how this works with the Cashew Ranch Dressing on page 156, which can be adapted to make a Green Goddess Dressing or a Thousand Island Dressing.

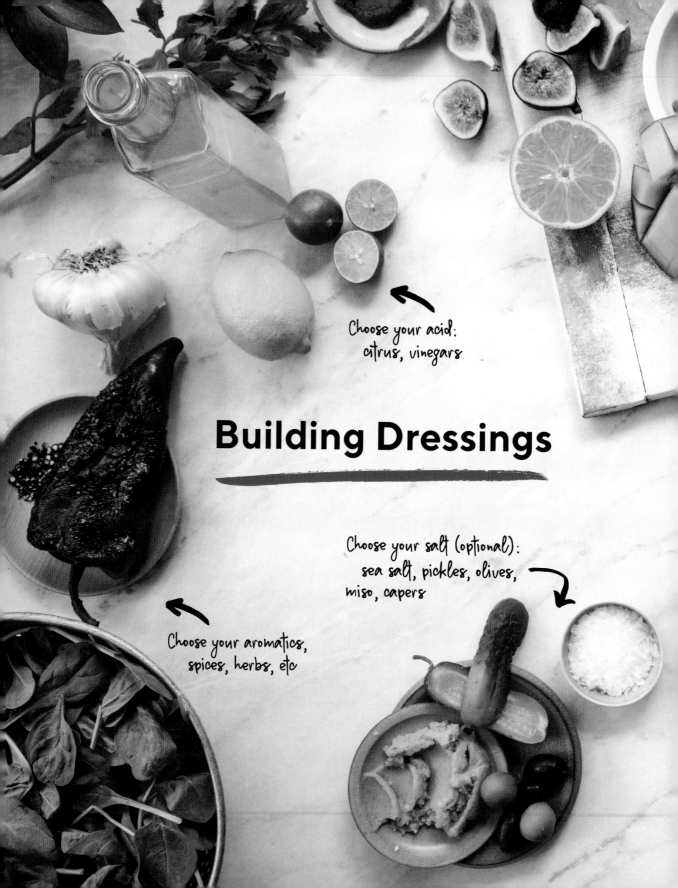

Choose your acid:
citrus, vinegars

Building Dressings

Choose your salt (optional):
sea salt, pickles, olives,
miso, capers

Choose your aromatics,
spices, herbs, etc

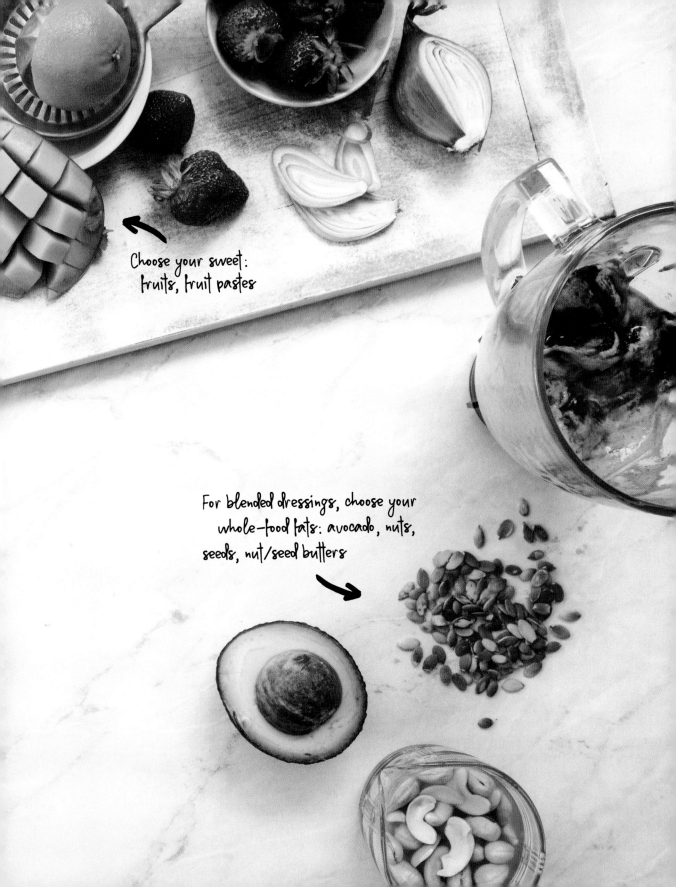

Choose your sweet:
fruits, fruit pastes

For blended dressings, choose your
whole-food fats: avocado, nuts,
seeds, nut/seed butters

Cashew Ranch Dressing

Makes 2½ cups

Serve this as a salad dressing or as a dip for Tofu Bites (page 250), or drizzle it on Sweet Potato BBQ Pizza (page 238). Get a head start by soaking the cashews the night before.

1 cup raw cashews

¾ cup unsweetened soy milk or other nondairy milk

1 tablespoon distilled white vinegar

Juice of ½ lemon

1 garlic clove

2 teaspoons onion powder

1 teaspoon cracked black pepper

Pinch of dry mustard

1½ teaspoons chopped fresh chives

1 tablespoon chopped fresh dill

Soak cashews in water to cover at room temperature for at least 3 hours or up to overnight. Drain and rinse the cashews, then transfer them to a (preferably high-speed) blender. Add the nondairy milk, vinegar, lemon juice, garlic, onion powder, pepper, and mustard. Process until very smooth, 1 to 2 minutes.

Add the fresh herbs and briefly pulse until just incorporated. Use immediately or refrigerate in an airtight container for up to 2 days.

Green Goddess Dressing: Replace the soaked cashews with 2 pitted, peeled, and chopped avocados.

Thousand Island Dressing: Omit the chives. Blend 1½ tablespoons tomato paste, 1 teaspoon Dijon mustard, and a pinch of chipotle powder (adjust for desired heat) into the dressing, transfer to a small bowl, and fold in ¼ cup minced dill pickle and 1½ tablespoons minced fresh parsley.

Per serving (¼ cup): 74 calories, 5 g total fat, 1 g saturated fat, 0 mg cholesterol, 11 mg sodium, 5 g total carbohydrate (1 g dietary fiber, 1 g sugar, 0 g added sugars), 3 g protein, 1 mg iron

Citrus-Miso Dressing

Makes about 1½ cups

A light, simple dressing that pairs great with grilled or raw vegetables. Use this as a base recipe and pulse in your favorite spice and herb combinations: For an Italian dressing, pulse in minced sun-dried tomatoes and basil. For Thai style, pulse in ginger, chile, and cilantro. The sky's the limit.

2 oranges, preferably mandarins or tangerines, peeled

½ cup white miso paste

1 tablespoon tahini

1 tablespoon unseasoned rice vinegar

1 tablespoon chopped fresh ginger

1 teaspoon low-sodium tamari

Combine all the ingredients in a high-speed blender and blend until smooth, 1 to 2 minutes. Use immediately or refrigerate in an airtight container for up to 1 day.

Per serving (2 tablespoons): 38 calories, 1 g total fat, 0 g saturated fat, 0 mg cholesterol, 380 mg sodium, 7 g total carbohydrate (0 g dietary fiber, 4 g sugar, 0 g added sugars), 2 g protein, 1 mg iron

Strawberry-Chile Vinaigrette

Makes 1¼ cups

Sweet fresh strawberries and spicy chiles make a wonderful summer vinaigrette. **Recipe by Brian Stafford**

1 poblano chile

1 jalapeño

2 cups ripe fresh strawberries, stemmed

½ apple, peeled, cored, and chopped

3 tablespoons unseasoned rice vinegar

8 large fresh mint leaves

Leaves from ½ bunch cilantro

Preheat the broiler. Line a baking sheet with parchment paper.

Put the poblano and jalapeño on the prepared baking sheet and broil until their skins are charred all over, 8 to 10 minutes, turning them to blacken all sides. Transfer them to a bowl, cover with plastic wrap, and set aside to steam for 15 minutes. When cool enough to handle, use a clean dishtowel or paper towel to wipe off the charred skin; discard the skin. Use a paring knife to remove and discard the stems, cores, and seeds and place the flesh of both chiles in a high-speed blender.

Add the strawberries, apple, and vinegar and blend until smooth, 30 to 40 seconds. Add the mint and cilantro and pulse just until finely chopped, to give you those bursts of flavor.

Use immediately or refrigerate in an airtight container for up to 1 day.

Per serving (2½ tablespoons): 25 calories, 0 g total fat, 0 g saturated fat, 0 mg cholesterol, 2 mg sodium, 5 g total carbohydrate (1 g dietary fiber, 3 g sugar, 0 g added sugars), 1 g protein, 1 mg iron

Fig-Balsamic Dressing

Makes about 2 cups

Use this as a punchy salad dressing or a glaze for grilled vegetables.

¾ cup balsamic vinegar

¼ cup fig paste (see page 56)

¼ cup low-sodium tamari

1 tablespoon minced shallot

1½ teaspoons minced fresh parsley

2 teaspoons minced fresh rosemary

¼ teaspoon freshly ground black pepper

Combine all the ingredients and ¼ cup water in a bowl or glass jar. Whisk or cover and shake well until combined. Use immediately or refrigerate for up to 4 days.

Per serving (2 tablespoons): 18 calories, 0 g total fat, 0 g saturated fat, 0 mg cholesterol, 178 mg sodium, 3 g total carbohydrate (0 g dietary fiber, 2 g sugar, 0 g added sugars), 1 g protein, 0 mg iron

Marinades and Sauces

The terms *sauce*, *marinade*, and *dressing* are often used interchangeably, as are the foods they refer to. We like to make marinades a bit punchier than dressings, because they're designed to be absorbed by the food and to caramelize during the cooking process. That means higher acidity, more sweetness, and an extra boost of spices and aromatics. Some of the recipes in this section—for example, the Asian BBQ Sauce (page 161)—can be used as either a marinade or a sauce.

Almond-Chile Sauce

Makes 1½ cups

The smooth creaminess of almonds carries the heat of the chiles over your palate. This sauce is featured in Vibrant Veggie Gado Gado (page 138) and Roots & Fruits Pad Thai Salad (page 143).

½ cup smooth almond butter (no added oil, salt, or sugar)

¾ cup warm water

2½ tablespoons fresh lime juice

2½ tablespoons low-sodium tamari or soy sauce

1 tablespoon minced fresh ginger

½ teaspoon minced fresh garlic

¼ to ½ teaspoon red pepper flakes

Combine all the ingredients in a high-speed blender and blend until smooth, 1 to 2 minutes. Use immediately or store in an airtight container in the refrigerator for up to 2 weeks.

Per serving (2 tablespoons): 69 calories, 6 g total fat, 1 g saturated fat, 0 mg cholesterol, 144 mg sodium, 2 g total carbohydrate (1 g dietary fiber, 1 g sugar, 0 g added sugars), 3 g protein, 0 mg iron

Spicy BBQ Tahini Sauce

Makes 1½ cups

Simple and flavor-packed, this creamy sauce brings any bowl of veggies alive.

½ cup tahini

⅓ cup hot pepper sauce, such as Tabasco

1 tablespoon no-added-sodium tomato paste

1 tablespoon nutritional yeast

1 teaspoon ground cumin

1 teaspoon chili powder

½ teaspoon smoked paprika

½ teaspoon coarse sea salt

½ teaspoon freshly ground black pepper

Combine all the ingredients and ⅓ cup water in a blender or bowl and blend or mix until smooth. Use immediately or refrigerate in an airtight container for up to 3 days.

Per serving (2 tablespoons): 63 calories, 5 g total fat, 1 g saturated fat, 0 mg cholesterol, 158 mg sodium, 3 g total carbohydrate (1 g dietary fiber, 0 g sugar, 0 g added sugars), 2 g protein, 1 mg iron

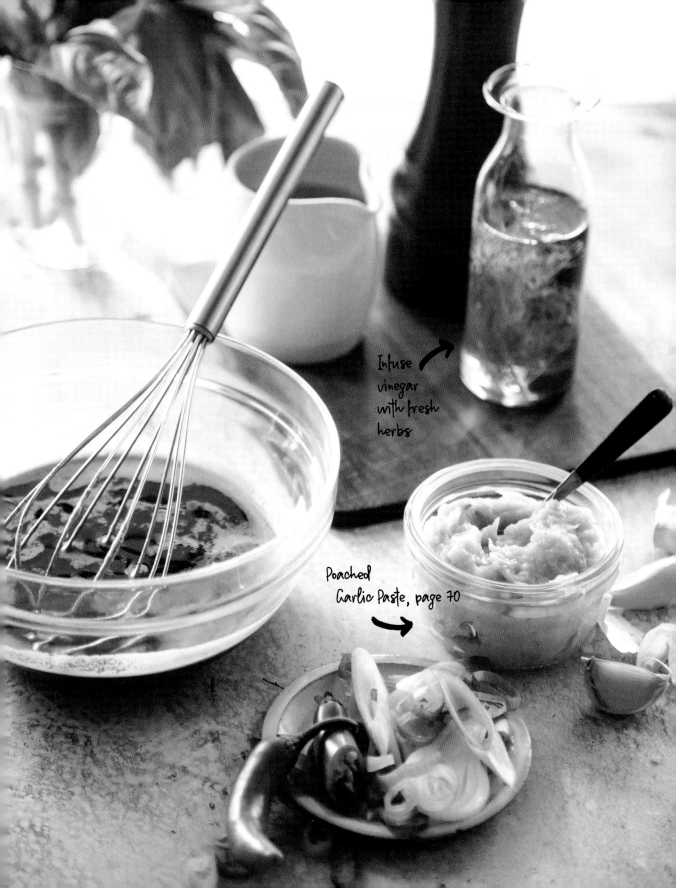

Infuse vinegar with fresh herbs

Poached Garlic Paste, page 70

Jalapeño Cashew Sour Cream

Makes about 2 cups

This plant-based alternative to sour cream is incredibly versatile, and you'll see it show up in multiple recipes in this book; it's especially delicious on Sweet Potato Enchiladas (page 242). You can omit the jalapeños and replace the cilantro with different herbs to create variations that fit the flavor profile of whatever dish you're making.

1 cup raw cashews

2 tablespoons fresh lime juice

2 tablespoons nutritional yeast

2 jalapeños, halved

¼ cup fresh cilantro leaves

½ teaspoon sea salt

½ teaspoon freshly ground black pepper

½ cup warm water, or as needed

Soak the raw cashews in warm water to cover for at least 3 hours or overnight. Drain and rinse the cashews, then transfer to a high-speed blender.

Add the lime juice, nutritional yeast, jalapeños, cilantro, salt, and pepper and blend until silky smooth, 4 to 5 minutes. As you blend, add just enough of the warm water to get the mixture moving and make a creamy, pourable sauce. Use immediately or refrigerate in an airtight container for up to 3 days.

Plain Cashew Cream: For a plain sour cream, omit the jalapeños and cilantro in the recipe above. If a more neutral, less sour flavor is desired, omit the lime juice as well. If using in sweet dishes, use only cashews and water.

Per serving (2 tablespoons): 43 calories, 3 g total fat, 1 g saturated fat, 0 mg cholesterol, 75 mg sodium, 2 g total carbohydrate (0 g dietary fiber, 1 g sugar, 0 g added sugars), 2 g protein, 0 mg iron

Asian BBQ Sauce

Makes about 3 cups

This sweet, spiced sauce is excellent paired with mushrooms, in a stir-fry, or as a glaze for grilled vegetables. You'll see it in a number of recipes in this book, including Roasted Mushroom Tacos (page 245) and Sweet Potato BBQ Pizza (page 238).

1 cup diced onion

1 cup canned no-added-sodium crushed tomatoes

⅓ cup apple cider vinegar

3 tablespoons low-sodium tamari or soy sauce

¼ cup no-added-sodium tomato paste

¼ cup date paste (see page 56)

2 tablespoons minced fresh ginger

2 garlic cloves

¾ teaspoon freshly ground black pepper

½ teaspoon smoked paprika

½ teaspoon ground cinnamon

1 bay leaf

½ serrano chile, minced (optional)

Heat a medium saucepan over medium-high heat. When hot, add the onion and dry sauté, stirring often, until it begins to stick to the pan and lightly brown, 3 to 4 minutes. Add the remaining ingredients, reduce the heat to medium-low, and bring to a slow simmer. Cook for 10 minutes, until reduced in volume and slightly thickened.

Remove from the heat and remove the bay leaf. Carefully transfer the sauce to a high-speed blender or food processor and blend until smooth. Use immediately as a stir-fry sauce or dipping sauce, or refrigerate in an airtight container for up to 1 week.

Sweet BBQ Sauce: For a more traditional sweet-and-spicy BBQ sauce, omit the ginger and cinnamon.

Per serving (¼ cup): 39 calories, 0 g total fat, 0 g saturated fat, 0 mg cholesterol, 162 mg sodium, 9 g total carbohydrate (1 g dietary fiber, 5 g sugar, 0 g added sugars), 1 g protein, 1 mg iron

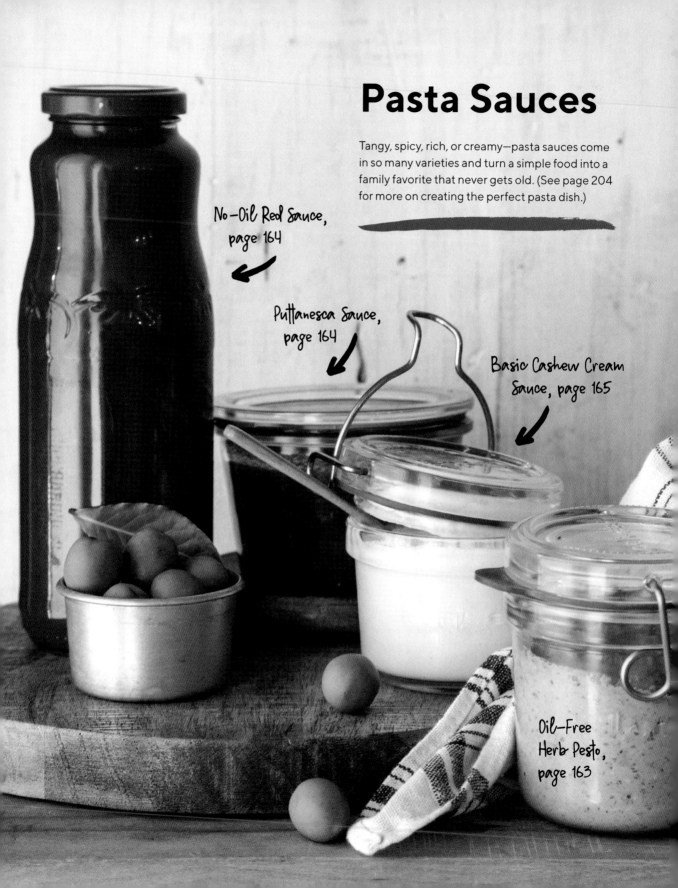

Pasta Sauces

Tangy, spicy, rich, or creamy—pasta sauces come in so many varieties and turn a simple food into a family favorite that never gets old. (See page 204 for more on creating the perfect pasta dish.)

No-Oil Red Sauce, page 164

Puttanesca Sauce, page 164

Basic Cashew Cream Sauce, page 165

Oil-Free Herb Pesto, page 163

Oil-Free Herb Pesto

Makes about 2 cups

Use as a sauce for pasta or pizza or as a spread for sandwiches and wraps. For pasta sauce, dilute the pesto a bit more with a splash of vegetable broth, soy milk, or water to thin it out.

2 cups lightly packed chopped fresh basil leaves

¼ cup chopped fresh parsley leaves

¼ cup chopped leeks (see Note on cleaning leeks, page 37)

2 garlic cloves

½ cup toasted pine nuts

2 tablespoons nutritional yeast

½ avocado, pitted and peeled

½ teaspoon sea salt

Combine all the ingredients in a food processor and pulse until finely chopped. Pulse in just enough water, 1 tablespoon at a time, to get things moving and break the mixture down to a coarse and chunky puree—it should not be completely smooth. You should only need a tablespoon or two of water. Refrigerate for up to 5 days.

Per serving (2 tablespoons): 38 calories, 3 g total fat, 0 g saturated fat, 0 mg cholesterol, 75 mg sodium, 2 g total carbohydrate (1 g dietary fiber, 0 g sugar, 0 g added sugars), 1 g protein, 1 mg iron

CHEF'S Tip

EXTEND YOUR PESTO

Traditionally, pesto is made with fresh herbs. However, you can make pesto go a lot further by adding other greens, such as spinach or kale, creating a mellower flavor and a delicious source of all the nutrients found in leafy greens.

Pesto Combinations

You don't have to make pesto with basil! Try the following delicious herb and nut combinations:

- **Thyme and almond**
- **Rosemary and hazelnut**
- **Cilantro and cashew**
- **Parsley and walnut**

No-Oil Red Sauce

Makes 10 cups

A great red sauce is the cornerstone of many Italian dishes. The secrets to success are quality ingredients and cooking time. Your choice of tomatoes will determine whether the sauce is sweet or acidic, so be sure to choose good-quality tomatoes (San Marzano tomatoes are a good choice because they are always picked ripe and are therefore sweeter). And don't skimp on the cooking time—your patience will be rewarded if you give this sauce the time it needs for the flavors to concentrate. Double the recipe, since you'll enjoy using this for days to come or you can freeze it for another meal!

2 onions, finely chopped

2 carrots, finely grated or chopped

½ cup low-sodium vegetable broth

1 (15-ounce) jar roasted red peppers, drained

2 (28-ounce) cans no-added-sodium whole plum tomatoes, with their juices

¼ cup no-added-sodium tomato paste

¼ cup garlic cloves, smashed

1½ teaspoons freshly ground black pepper

½ teaspoon sea salt

3 bay leaves

½ cup fresh basil leaves, torn by hand (optional)

Heat a large saucepan over medium-high heat. Add onions and carrots and dry sauté, stirring often, until the onions begin to stick to the pan and lightly brown, 3 to 4 minutes. Add the broth and stir to deglaze the pan. Cook, stirring now and then, until the onions are translucent, 2 to 3 minutes.

Stir in the roasted peppers, whole tomatoes with their juices, tomato paste, garlic, black pepper, and salt. Bring to a simmer, then reduce the heat to low and simmer for 1 to 2 hours. (The longer the sauce simmers, the more concentrated the flavors become.)

Remove from the heat and let cool slightly. Blend directly in the pot with an immersion blender until smooth (or carefully transfer to an upright blender and blend until smooth, then return the sauce to the pot). Add the bay leaves. Bring to a simmer over medium heat and simmer gently for 20 minutes.

Remove the pot from the heat, remove the bay leaves, and stir in the basil (if using). Use immediately or transfer to airtight containers and refrigerate for up to 5 days or freeze for up to 2 months.

Puttanesca Sauce: After blending the sauce, stir in ¼ cup chopped Kalamata olives, 3 tablespoons drained and rinsed capers, 1 teaspoon red pepper flakes, and 3 tablespoons dulse leaves torn into small pieces (optional—this seaweed adds a flavor reminiscent of the anchovies in a traditional puttanesca). Simmer 15 to 20 minutes. Just before using, stir in 2 tablespoons chopped fresh parsley.

Per serving (1 cup): 79 calories, 0 g total fat, 0 g saturated fat, 0 mg cholesterol, 242 mg sodium, 17 g total carbohydrate (5 g dietary fiber, 6 g sugar, 0 g added sugars), 2 g protein, 1 mg iron

Basic Cashew Cream Sauce

Makes about 4 cups

This rich, creamy sauce is a base recipe that you'll see in numerous applications throughout this book. Try it on pasta, or stir it into risotto (pages 37 and 40) to create an authentic creamy texture. Like a traditional cream sauce, it will reduce in volume and thicken when cooked or baked. See the notes following the recipe for more variations on this versatile sauce.

1½ cups raw cashews

3 cups low-sodium vegetable broth

1 cup chopped onion

¼ cup garlic cloves

2 tablespoons nutritional yeast (optional)

1 teaspoon sea salt (optional)

Soak the cashews in warm water to cover for at least 3 hours or up to overnight. Drain and rinse the cashews, then transfer to a (preferably high-speed) blender.

In a small saucepan, combine the broth, onion, and garlic. Bring to a simmer over medium-high heat and simmer until the garlic and onion are very soft, 5 to 8 minutes. Remove from the heat and let cool slightly, then transfer the contents (liquid and vegetables) of the pan to the blender with the cashews. Add the nutritional yeast and sea salt, if desired. Blend until very smooth, a few minutes in a high-speed blender like a Vitamix or slightly longer in a standard blender.

Use immediately or transfer to an airtight container and refrigerate for up to 1 week or freeze for up to 3 months.

Notes: For a lower-fat alternative, use only ¼ cup cashews and add 2½ cups chopped cauliflower. Simmer the cauliflower with the garlic and onion until very soft, then proceed with the recipe.

For a delicious pasta sauce, sauté some chopped onion in a large skillet until translucent, then add your choice of vegetables such as fresh peas, asparagus, and/or mushrooms. Deglaze the pan with a little white wine, then add the finished sauce and bring to a gentle simmer. Add pasta (cooked al dente) and toss well with the warm cream sauce. Garnish with chopped fresh parsley, oregano, or other herbs.

Rich Cheeze Sauce: Add ½ cup roasted yellow peppers or ½ cup steamed carrots or butternut squash to the blender.

Per serving (¼ cup): 70 calories, 5 g total fat, 1 g saturated fat, 0 mg cholesterol, 29 mg sodium, 5 g total carbohydrate (1 g dietary fiber, 2 g sugar, 0 g added sugars), 2 g protein, 1 mg iron

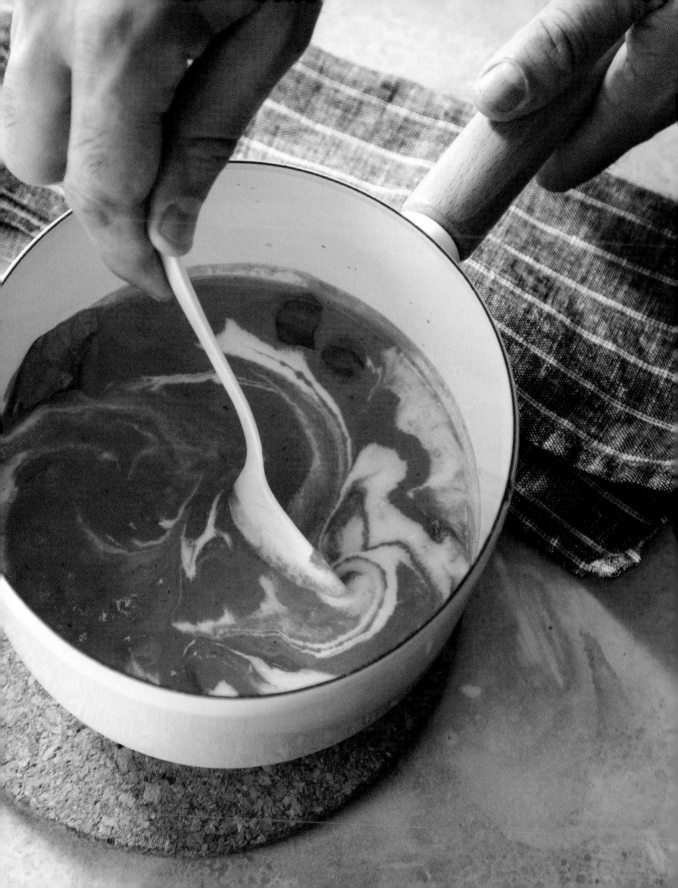

Roasted Red Pepper Sauce

Makes 3 cups

This versatile sauce can be tossed with pasta, used as a pizza sauce, or thinned out with some added vegetables and beans to make a sweet and aromatic soup. You can buy roasted red peppers in a jar (no added sodium or oil), or roast your own. The cashew cream adds richness and helps carry the flavors of the sweet peppers and fragrant basil.

3 cups chopped roasted red bell peppers

3 tablespoons pine nuts, toasted

⅔ cup chopped onion

½ teaspoon red pepper flakes

3 garlic cloves, minced

¼ cup low-sodium vegetable broth

½ cup unsweetened soy milk or Basic Cashew Cream Sauce (page 165)

¼ cup chopped fresh basil

¼ teaspoon sea salt

¼ teaspoon freshly ground black pepper

Combine the roasted peppers and pine nuts in a high-speed blender and blend until smooth, 1 to 2 minutes.

Heat a large skillet over medium heat. When hot, add the onion and red pepper flakes and dry sauté, stirring often, until the onion begins to stick to the pan and lightly brown, 3 to 4 minutes, stirring often. Stir in the garlic and cook for 1 minute. Add the broth and cook until the liquid evaporates, 2 to 3 minutes.

Whisk in the red pepper puree and soy milk until thoroughly combined. Simmer, stirring a few times to prevent burning, until the mixture is heated through and bubbling, 3 to 4 minutes. Remove from the heat and stir in basil, salt, and black pepper. Refrigerate for up to 5 days.

Per serving (½ cup): 61 calories, 3 g total fat, 0 g saturated fat, 0 mg cholesterol, 115 mg sodium, 7 g total carbohydrate (2 g dietary fiber, 3 g sugar, 0 g added sugars), 2 g protein, 1 mg iron

Autumn Veggie Bowl,
page 172

Autumn Veggie Bowl,
page 172

CHAPTER 11

Bowl Meals

Dinner doesn't need to be plated! There's something wonderfully comforting about getting your hands around a warm bowl filled with healthy goodness. From carefully assembled Wellness Bowls to hearty soups to satisfying one-pot meals, the recipes in this chapter are designed to be served in the round. Make sure you have a set of big bowls on hand—wooden, glass, from a local potter—everyone needs a favorite bowl for these dishes.

Constructing Wellness Bowls

Wellness Bowls include all the elements of a balanced meal, using toppings and sauces to tie them together with distinctive flavors. Featuring grains, beans, greens, veggies, and more, they're a great way to get four or more of the Essential Eight foods (see chapter 2) in one meal.

Chef's Tip

THINK TEXTURE!

When putting together a bowl meal, don't just think about the flavors you want to include—consider the textures, too. From the crunch of croutons or toasted nuts and seeds to the silkiness of avocado or silken tofu to the pleasing chewiness of whole grains, a variety of contrasting textures will activate your palate.

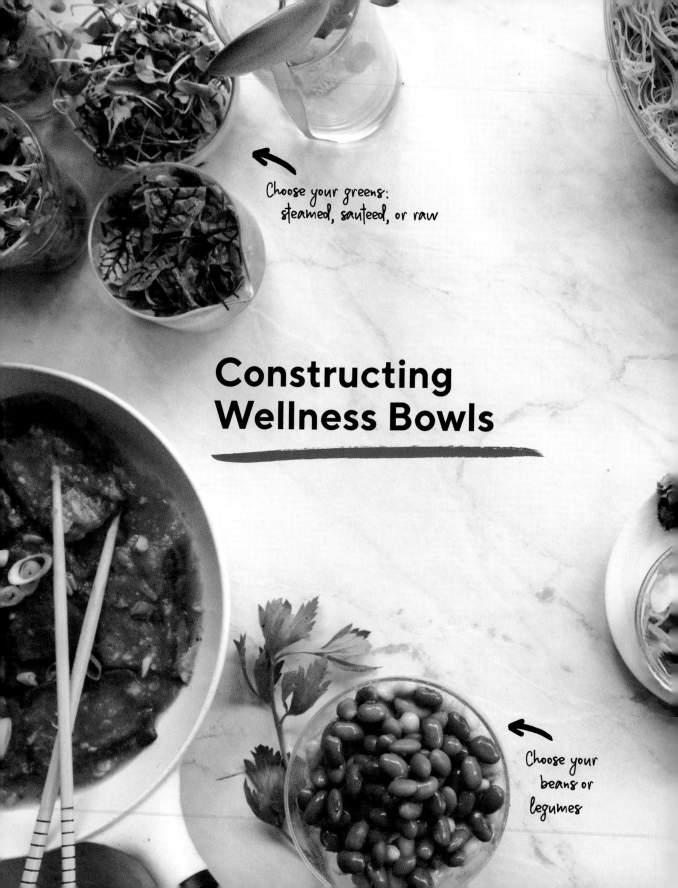

Choose your greens:
steamed, sauteed, or raw

Constructing
Wellness Bowls

Choose your
beans or
legumes

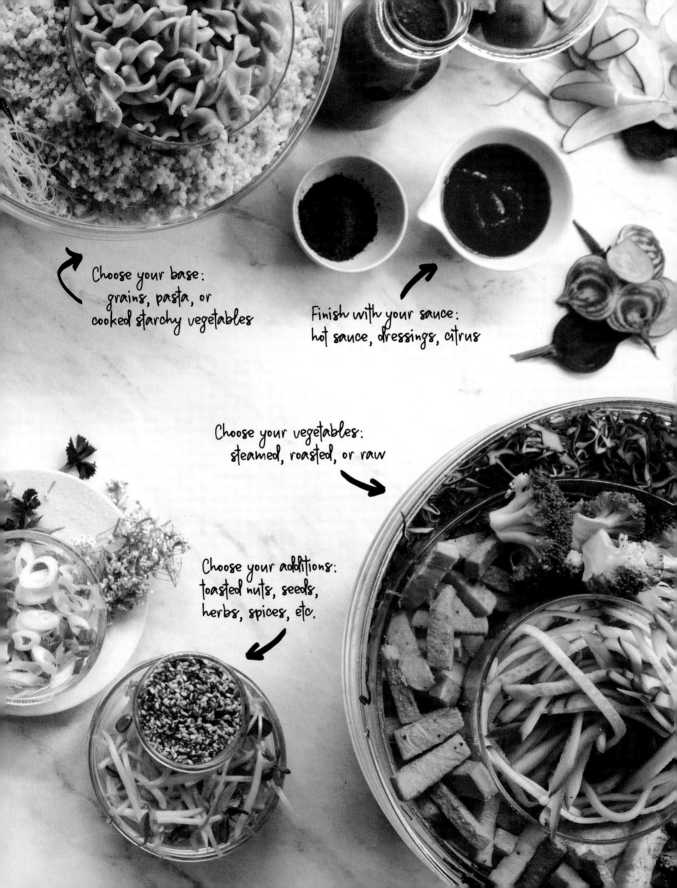

Choose your base:
grains, pasta, or
cooked starchy vegetables

Finish with your sauce:
hot sauce, dressings, citrus

Choose your vegetables:
steamed, roasted, or raw

Choose your additions:
toasted nuts, seeds,
herbs, spices, etc.

Autumn Veggie Bowl

Serves 4

Celebrate fall with this hearty and comforting bowl of roasted roots and greens, complemented by the tart sweetness of balsamic syrup. If you want to kick up the heat, add fresh chiles. (Pictured on page 168.) **Recipe by Whole Foods Market**

2 cups bite-size cubes peeled sweet potato

2 cups bite-size cubes peeled rutabaga

2 cups halved Brussels sprouts

3 tablespoons white balsamic vinegar

1 tablespoon garlic granules

1 teaspoon freshly ground black pepper

¼ teaspoon cayenne pepper

¼ cup low-sodium vegetable broth

1 head curly kale, stemmed, leaves torn or chopped into bite-size pieces

4 cups cooked quinoa (see page 36)

2 tablespoons fresh lemon juice (from about 1 lemon)

3 tablespoons small fresh parsley leaves

½ cup halved pitted cherries

½ cup pecans, toasted and chopped

½ teaspoon sea salt

White Balsamic Syrup (page 72)

Nondairy ricotta such as Kite Hill or feta cheese, crumbled, (optional)

Preheat the oven to 400°F. Line a rimmed baking sheet with parchment paper.

In a bowl, toss together the sweet potato, rutabaga, Brussels sprouts, vinegar, garlic granules, black pepper, and cayenne. Spread the vegetables in a single layer on the prepared baking sheet and roast for 20 minutes, stirring halfway through to brown the vegetables on more than one side. When the vegetables are fork-tender, remove from the oven and sprinkle evenly with the broth. Let cool.

Steam the kale leaves in a covered steamer basket over gently simmering water until just tender, 2 to 3 minutes.

Place the cooked quinoa in a large bowl and toss with the lemon juice, parsley, cherries, pecans, and salt.

To assemble, place a generous amount of the quinoa salad in the center of each bowl, followed by the roasted vegetables and steamed kale. Finish with a drizzle of white balsamic syrup and some crumbled cheese (if using).

Per serving (without cheese): 490 calories, 15 g total fat, 1 g saturated fat, 0 mg cholesterol, 425 mg sodium, 74 g total carbohydrate (13 g dietary fiber, 17 g sugar, 0 g added sugars), 15 g protein, 6 mg iron

"Fried" Farro with Caramelized Fennel & Tofu

Serves 6

This unique take on classic fried rice lets you create that sticky, savory favorite without reaching for the oils. The farro adds a pleasing chewy bite to the dish. You'll want to cook it in advance (see page 36). If you're gluten-free, you can substitute brown rice. This recipe calls for a lot of chopped vegetables, but using a mandoline or food processor attachment will save on prep time. Be sure to have them all prepped before you start cooking.

1 cup thinly sliced fennel, rinsed

1 onion, finely chopped

¼ cup low-sodium vegetable broth, plus more as needed

2 cups sliced shiitake mushrooms

1 cup thinly sliced red or green cabbage

1 red bell pepper, cut into thin 1-inch-long strips

1 (16-ounce) block firm tofu, cut into 1-inch cubes

1 tablespoon minced fresh ginger

1 tablespoon minced fresh garlic

¼ cup low-sodium tamari or soy sauce

4 cups cooked farro (see page 36)

1 teaspoon granulated onion

1 teaspoon freshly ground black pepper

½ teaspoon red pepper flakes

¾ cup packed mixed fresh cilantro and flat-leaf parsley leaves

2 teaspoons toasted mixed white and black sesame seeds

1 lime, cut into wedges

Heat a large sauté pan or wok over medium-high heat. When the pan is hot, add the fennel and onion and dry sauté, stirring frequently, until they begin to stick and turn slightly translucent and you see some browning on the bottom of the pan. Add 2 to 3 tablespoons broth and stir to deglaze the pan. Cook, stirring frequently and adding 2 to 3 tablespoons of broth when vegetables begin to stick, until the vegetables turn golden brown, 4 to 5 minutes.

Add the mushrooms, cabbage, bell pepper, tofu, ginger, and garlic and cook, stirring frequently, until the mushrooms are wilted, 2 minutes more.

Add the tamari and cook for 1 minute. Add the farro and stir to keep it from sticking to the pan. Stir in the granulated onion, black pepper, red pepper flakes, and herbs (save a pinch of the herbs for garnish). Heat well until very hot, a couple of minutes more. Remove the skillet from the heat.

Plate the "fried" farro and garnish with the reserved fresh cilantro and parsley and the sesame seeds. Serve with the lime wedges for squeezing.

Notes: Try substituting button, oyster, or maitake mushrooms for the shiitakes.

Replace one of the vegetables with 1 cup broccoli or cauliflower florets.

If you like spicy food, add some chopped fresh Thai chiles or red jalapeños.

Per serving: 295 calories, 6 g total fat, 0 g saturated fat, 0 mg cholesterol, 424 mg sodium, 45 g total carbohydrate (8 g dietary fiber, 3 g sugar, 0 g added sugars), 19 g protein, 5 mg iron

Citrus-Sesame-Glazed Tofu Bun Cha

Serves 6

This variation on the traditional Vietnamese favorite is the perfect one-bowl meal. The freshness of the raw vegetables and the light vermicelli balance the flavor of the citrusy, spicy-sweet glazed tofu. Swap in your favorite vegetables for the tofu if you prefer—the glaze is terrific on eggplant as well.

TOFU

2 (14-ounce) blocks extra-firm tofu, drained

3 tablespoons low-sodium tamari or soy sauce

CITRUS-SESAME GLAZE

2 small oranges or mandarins, peeled

1 cup chopped pineapple

3 tablespoons unseasoned rice vinegar

3 tablespoons apricot paste (see page 56)

2 garlic cloves, minced

2 tablespoons finely minced lemongrass

½ teaspoon minced fresh Thai chile (optional)

2 tablespoons arrowroot powder

TO ASSEMBLE

3 tablespoons sesame seeds, toasted (see page 61)

1 (0.8-ounce/227-g) package brown rice vermicelli noodles

¼ cup unseasoned rice vinegar

3 tablespoons low-sodium tamari or soy sauce

¼ cup low-sodium vegetable broth

1 cup cucumber matchsticks (about 2 inches long)

2 cups shredded romaine lettuce

8 radishes, sliced paper-thin

¼ cup thinly sliced green onion

¼ cup torn or chopped fresh mint

¼ cup unsalted dry-roasted peanuts (optional)

2 fresh red Thai chiles, thinly sliced (optional)

2 limes, cut into wedges

For the tofu, preheat the oven to 350°F. Line a baking sheet with parchment paper.

Wrap the drained tofu in a few layers of paper towels, then sandwich it between two plates and weight down the top plate with a heavy book. Press for at least 10 minutes and up to 1 hour. Cut each pressed tofu block lengthwise into 3 slabs, for a total of 6 slabs.

Cover the tofu slabs with the tamari; handle the slabs gently to avoid breaking them. Arrange the slabs in a single layer on the prepared baking sheet, then bake until the tofu is golden and slightly firm, about 30 minutes, turning the tofu halfway through the cooking time. Remove and let rest while making the glaze.

For the citrus-sesame glaze, combine the oranges, pineapple, vinegar, and apricot paste in a high-speed blender and blend until smooth. Pour the mixture into a small saucepan and stir in the garlic, lemongrass, and chile (if using). Bring to a low boil over medium-high heat, then reduce the heat to medium-low and simmer until reduced by one-third, 10 to 12 minutes.

Continues

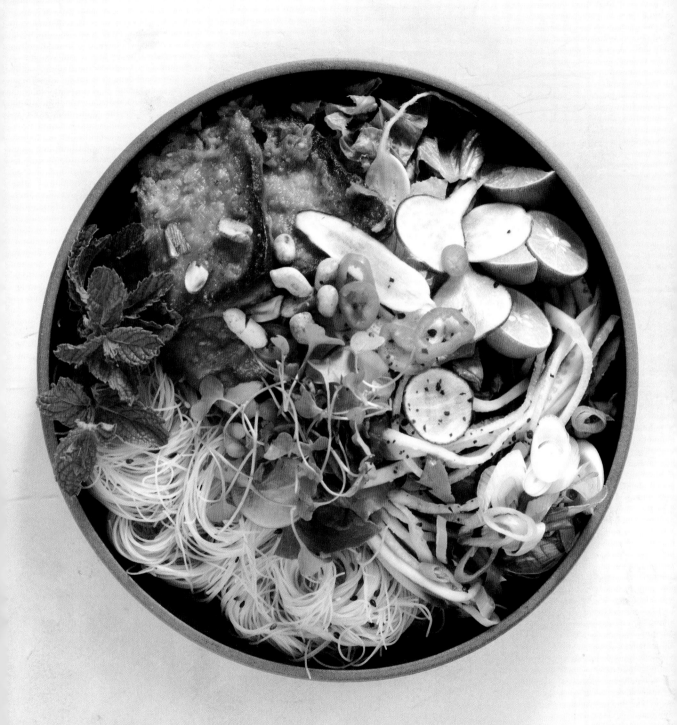

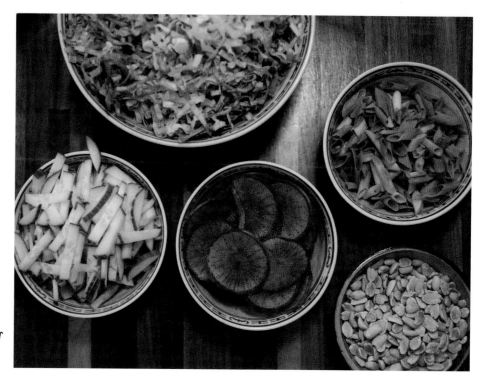

When serving this dish at a dinner party, let guests assemble their own bowls

In a cup, whisk together the arrowroot powder and ¼ cup cold water. While whisking, slowly pour the arrowroot slurry into the glaze. Simmer until thickened, another minute or two; the glaze should coat the back of a spoon and not run off quickly. Remove from the heat.

To assemble, place two large sauté pans over medium-high heat. Add enough citrus glaze to coat the bottom of each pan. Position the tofu slabs in the pans so they are not touching and cook for 2 minutes. Flip gently using a wide spatula and add more glaze to the top of the tofu. (This glaze thickens quickly, so it will only need an additional minute or two on the heat.)

Remove from the heat and transfer the tofu to a large platter. Sprinkle with 2 tablespoons of the sesame seeds.

Bring a large pot of water to a boil. Turn off the heat, add the vermicelli, and soak for 3 minutes, stirring once or twice. Drain and rinse under cold water. Place the rice noodles in a large bowl.

In small bowl, mix the vinegar, tamari, and remaining 1 tablespoon sesame seeds. Pour half the sauce over the rice noodles and toss gently to coat; set aside. Stir the broth into the remaining sauce and set aside.

Place a generous amount of seasoned noodles in the center of each of six bowls. Place piles of the cucumber, lettuce, radishes, green onion, and mint around the noodles in each bowl. Top each bowl of noodles with 2 slabs of glazed tofu, the peanuts, and the chiles (if using), and serve with lime wedges for squeezing.

Per serving: 338 calories, 7 g total fat, 1 g saturated fat, 0 mg cholesterol, 623 mg sodium, 57 g total carbohydrate (2 g dietary fiber, 12 g sugar, 0 g added sugars), 15 g protein, 3 mg iron

Chickpea-Nut & Broccoli Satay

Serves 8

Here's a fantastic chickpea satay that satisfies on all fronts! Serve it to a crowd with cooked brown rice and spicy cabbage slaw. The sauce can be made the day before and will keep in the refrigerator for a couple of weeks. Make extra so you can try it on salads and other veggie and grain bowls; it's even great on oatmeal!

PEANUT SAUCE

1 cup smooth peanut butter (no added oil, salt, or sugar)

⅓ cup low-sodium tamari or soy sauce

2 tablespoons minced fresh ginger

1 teaspoon minced fresh garlic

Juice of 3 limes

½ teaspoon smoked paprika

½ teaspoon freshly ground black pepper

SATAY

3 (14-ounce) cans chickpeas, drained and rinsed

1 small red onion, chopped

1 (16-ounce) block tofu, cubed

3 cups small broccoli florets

3 celery stalks, sliced into thin half-moons

1 red bell pepper, chopped

½ bunch kale, stemmed, leaves torn into small pieces

2 tablespoons white and/or black sesame seeds

¾ cup chopped mixed fresh cilantro and mint, plus a few sprigs for garnish

½ teaspoon coarse sea salt (optional)

½ to 1 teaspoon red pepper flakes (optional)

Preheat the oven to 350°F. Line a large (13 by 9-inch or 3-quart) baking dish with parchment paper.

For the peanut sauce, combine all the peanut sauce ingredients in a high-speed blender. Blend on low to start, then increase the speed, adding warm water as needed to get the mixture moving (you may need as much as 1 cup warm water, but use as little as possible, as the sauce should be thick). The sauce is done when it mixes easily at high speed. Set aside while you make the satay.

For the satay, toss the chickpeas and onion in the prepared baking dish and roast until chickpeas are beginning to dry and crisp up, 15 to 20 minutes.

Remove the baking dish from the oven and add the tofu, broccoli, celery, and bell pepper. Add the peanut sauce and stir until everything is coated. Return the baking dish to the oven and bake, uncovered, for 20 minutes more, stirring occasionally. Remove from the oven, stir in the kale, and bake for 5 minutes more.

Remove the dish from the oven and stir in the sesame seeds and the cilantro and mint. Sprinkle with the salt and red pepper flakes (use more or less to your liking), and garnish with the herb sprigs.

Per serving: 507 calories, 24 g total fat, 4 g saturated fat, 0 mg cholesterol, 795 mg sodium, 43 g total carbohydrate (13 g dietary fiber, 9 g sugar, 0 g added sugars), 29 g protein, 5 mg iron

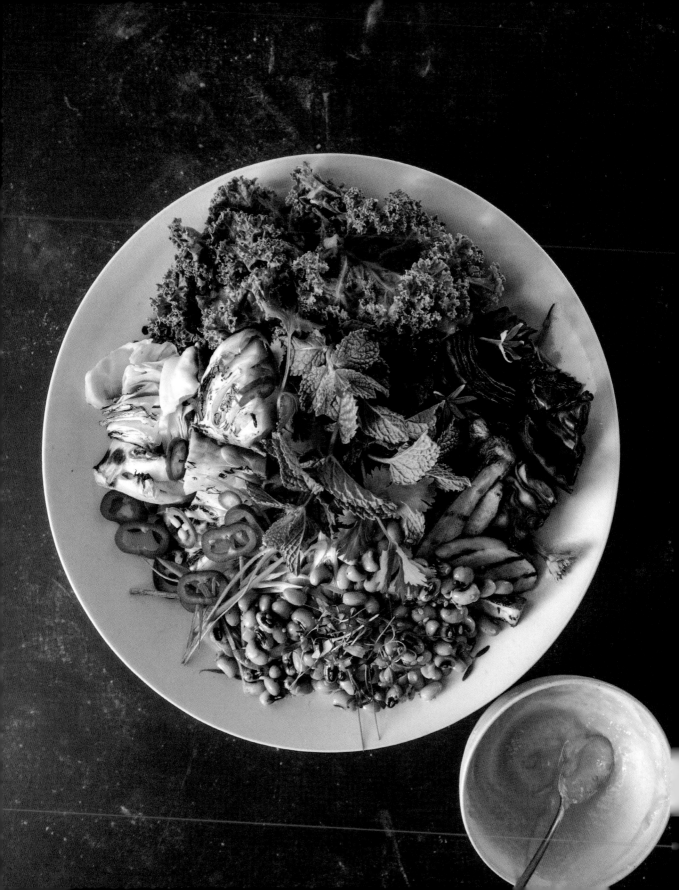

Summer Chopped Bowl

Serves 4

Grillin' is not just for burgers! This hearty veggie bowl makes a satisfying standalone meal, pairing the fresh crispness of kale with the sweet char of grilled onions and cabbage. Aromatic herbs make it pop, and beans round out the nutritional benefits. You can use chickpeas, white beans, black beans, or any other variety you like.

½ head green or red cabbage, cut into 3 wedges

1 zucchini, sliced lengthwise into ¼- to ½-inch-thick planks, or 6 baby zucchini, halved

1 sweet white onion, sliced crosswise into ¼- to ½-inch-thick rounds

½ teaspoon sea salt

¼ teaspoon freshly ground black pepper

Spray oil (for grill)

3 tablespoons sesame seeds

1 cup cooked beans of your choice (see page 42) or no-added-sodium canned beans, drained and rinsed

2 tablespoons low-sodium vegetable broth

6 green curly kale leaves, stemmed, leaves chopped

½ cup Citrus-Miso Dressing (page 156)

3 cups cooked quinoa (see page 36)

3 green onions, thinly sliced

Juice of ½ lemon

1 Thai chile, sliced into thin rounds

¼ cup chopped fresh cilantro

¼ cup chopped fresh mint

Heat a grill to high or heat a grill pan over high heat.

Season the cabbage, zucchini, and onion with ¼ teaspoon of the salt and the pepper.

Lightly coat the grill or pan with spray oil. Place the vegetables on the grill and cook until browned, 3 to 4 minutes per side. Remove from the grill, keeping the vegetables separate. Coarsely chop the cabbage and onion, and cut the zucchini into bite-size cubes. Set each aside separately.

In a medium sauté pan, toast the sesame seeds over medium heat until they begin to pop and smell fragrant, 1 to 2 minutes. Stir in the beans, broth, and remaining ¼ teaspoon salt and cook just until the beans are heated through, 3 to 4 minutes. Remove from the heat.

In a medium bowl, toss the kale with half the dressing to lightly coat. Set aside the remaining dressing.

In a medium bowl, toss the quinoa with the green onions and lemon juice. Place the quinoa mixture in the center of a serving bowl and arrange the grilled cabbage, onion, zucchini, beans, chile, and kale in separate piles around the quinoa. Combine the cilantro and mint and add them as the last pile on the salad.

Serve warm, with the remaining dressing on the side.

Per serving: 387 calories, 8 g total fat, 0 g saturated fat, 0 mg cholesterol, 709 mg sodium, 61 g total carbohydrate (12 g dietary fiber, 13 g sugar, 0 g added sugars), 18 g protein, 6 mg iron

Spicy Hoppin' John

Serves 6

This comforting Southern-inspired meal of black-eyed peas, rice, and greens gets an extra kick from the spicy tahini sauce. Southerners traditionally eat this dish on New Year's Day to bring prosperity, but we think it tastes good any day of the year, and your body will benefit from its nutritional riches.

BLACK-EYED PEAS

2 cups dry black-eyed peas, soaked in water to cover overnight

3 garlic cloves, smashed

1 teaspoon apple cider vinegar

¾ teaspoon granulated onion

½ teaspoon smoked paprika

½ teaspoon freshly ground black pepper

½ teaspoon coarse sea salt

2 large bay leaves

TO SERVE

1 pound lacinato (Tuscan) kale or red Russian kale, rinsed and stemmed

1 cup chopped fresh flat-leaf parsley

6 cups cooked brown rice or other whole grain (see page 36)

1½ cups Spicy BBQ Tahini Sauce (page 158)

2 cups halved cherry tomatoes

1 lime, cut into wedges

Plate the beans, kale, and brown rice. Top the rice with tahini sauce and top the kale with the cherry tomatoes. Serve with lime wedges for squeezing.

Per serving: 609 calories, 13 g total fat, 2 g saturated fat, 0 mg cholesterol, 579 mg sodium, 110 g total carbohydrate (14 g dietary fiber, 5 g sugar, 0 g added sugars), 25 g protein, 8 mg iron

For the black-eyed peas, drain and rinse the peas, then transfer them to a medium saucepan. Add water to cover by about 2 inches. Add the garlic, vinegar, granulated onion, paprika, pepper, salt, and bay leaves. Cover and bring to a low boil over medium-high heat. Boil for 5 minutes, then reduce the heat to medium-low and simmer until the beans are tender but not mushy, 45 to 50 minutes.

To serve, shred the kale by hand into bite-size pieces. Steam the kale in a covered steamer basket over gently simmering water until bright green, 2 to 3 minutes.

Remove the bay leaves from the beans and stir in the parsley.

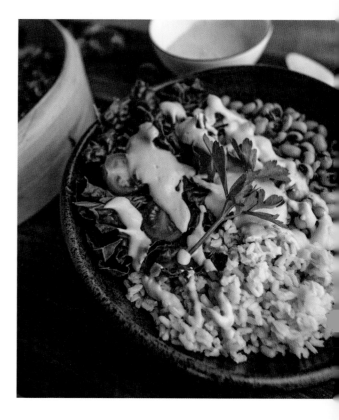

Soups

Soup is a simple term that contains a world of possibilities. From piquant broths to hearty beans, vegetables to creamy nondairy chowders to soft, earthy lentils—there's an endless variety of flavors, textures, and nutritional richness that all fit the category of "soup." The recipes that follow demonstrate just a few of the many variations you can create. We hope you'll be inspired to design your own!

Chef's Tip

YOU CAN MAKE CREAMY SOUPS WITHOUT CREAM!

Beans, well-cooked starchy vegetables, nondairy milk, or a few soaked nuts will all add a creamy texture to a soup when blended in a high-speed blender. For best results, carefully strain the liquids from the solids before you blend—that way, you can add the liquid a little at a time and ensure your soup doesn't get too thin.

Begin with Broth

The foundation of almost every good soup is a flavorful broth or stock. You can easily purchase low-sodium vegetable broth, but making your own will add an extra layer of delicious homemade flavor to your soups. When you make your own broth with whole-food ingredients, you can control the quality and the sodium levels, and you can tailor the combination of vegetables and aromatics to fit the dish you're making. Making broth is a great way to use any scraps and peels from your veggies (although whole vegetables make the best broth), as well as items that may be slightly blemished. Be sure to use quality ingredients, however, as they'll give your broth the best flavor.

Avoid using potato peelings or onion skins or ingredients that could discolor the broth, such as red cabbage or beets. Just combine everything, including your favorite herbs and spices, in a big pot, simmer for 1 to 2 hours, then strain the broth and discard the solids.

Vegetable broth is a key ingredient in a whole foods, plant-based diet—besides soups, you'll find it useful for sautéing, roasting, and thinning out sauces. Water does not add flavor to your recipes, so be sure to always reach for a flavorful liquid like broth instead. If you do need to purchase a ready-made broth, choose an organic, low-sodium variety without added oil or MSG.

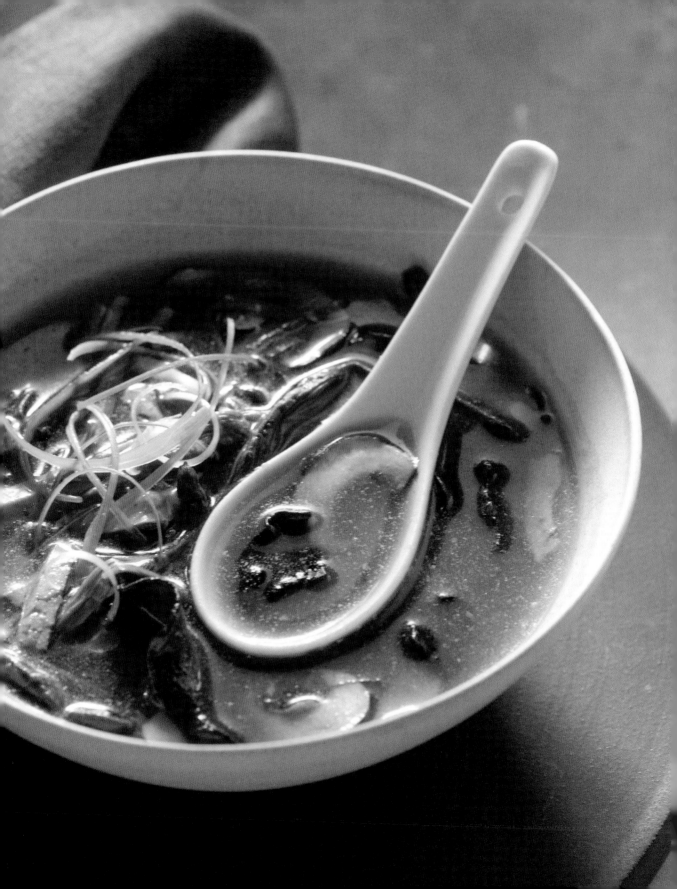

Hot-and-Sour Soup

Serves 6

Hot-and-sour soup brings together a variety of ingredients that create its distinctive, contrasting flavors. Feel free to use a variety of mushrooms. Dried tiger lily buds can be found in most Asian markets. To make this a heartier soup, just add cooked jasmine rice to the bowl prior to ladling in the soup. **Recipe by Beverly Burl, supermom extraordinaire**

⅓ cup dried tiger lily flower buds (see headnote)

¼ cup dried wood ear mushrooms

6½ cups low-sodium vegetable broth

3 tablespoons plus 1 teaspoon cornstarch

3 tablespoons low-sodium soy sauce

2½ tablespoons apple cider vinegar

4 ounces cremini (baby bella) or other mushrooms, thinly sliced

1 (14-ounce) block extra-firm tofu, drained and cut into matchsticks

1 teaspoon Ninja Squirrel Sriracha

Pinch of ground white pepper

1½ teaspoons Ener-G Egg Replacer

2 green onions, chopped

Soak the tiger lilies and wood ear mushrooms in warm water to cover until they are soft, about 15 minutes. Drain and cut into narrow strips.

In a small bowl, mix ½ cup of the broth with 3 tablespoons of the cornstarch until the cornstarch has dissolved. Set aside.

Pour 2 tablespoons of the broth into a small bowl and set aside.

Pour the remaining broth (a scant 6 cups) into a soup pot and bring to a simmer over medium heat. Stir in the shredded tiger lilies and wood ears, 2 tablespoons of the soy sauce, and the vinegar. Simmer for 5 minutes.

Pour the remaining 1 tablespoon soy sauce into a medium bowl and mix in the remaining 1 teaspoon cornstarch until the cornstarch has dissolved. Add the fresh mushrooms and toss to coat. Set aside.

Reduce the heat under the soup pot to low. Stir in the mushrooms, then the cornstarch-broth mixture and the tofu. Cook gently, stirring occasionally, until thickened, 3 to 5 minutes.

Stir in the Sriracha and white pepper, and remove from the heat.

Add the egg replacer to the bowl with the reserved 2 tablespoons broth and stir until dissolved. Gradually stir the egg replacer mixture into the warm soup, then let sit for 5 minutes.

Ladle into small bowls and garnish with the green onions.

Per serving: 122 calories, 4 g total fat, 0 g saturated fat, 0 mg cholesterol, 447 mg sodium, 12 g total carbohydrate (1 g dietary fiber, 3 g sugar, 0 g added sugars), 9 g protein, 2 mg iron

Dal with Toasted Spices & Coconut

Serves 4

This aromatic bowl of comfort is a great addition to any Indian-inspired meal. As the dal simmers, the lentils will begin to "melt," creating a creamy texture. To make it a main dish, serve it with a bowl of brown basmati rice. You can also try a topping of sliced avocado and sliced chiles to add extra kick.

1 tablespoon black mustard seeds

1 cup chopped onion

1½ teaspoons ground cumin

1½ teaspoons ground coriander

½ to 1 small red serrano pepper, depending on your heat tolerance

2 cups diced tomatoes (about 2 fresh tomatoes)

1½ cups uncooked split red or yellow lentils

4 cups low-sodium vegetable broth

1 (15-ounce) can light coconut milk

Juice of 1 lemon

2 cups chopped kale, rinsed and stemmed

Sea salt (optional)

Heat a soup pot over medium heat. When hot, add the mustard seeds and toast, shaking the pan now and then, until you smell the spice, about 1 minute. Add the onion and cook, stirring continuously until the onion is golden and begins to stick to the pot. Add the cumin and coriander and toss in the pan for 30 seconds to toast the spices.

Stir in the serrano and tomatoes and cook, stirring once or twice, for 2 minutes. Add the lentils, broth, coconut milk, and lemon juice and bring to a boil over high heat. Reduce the heat to low, cover, and simmer, stirring occasionally, until the lentils are tender, 30 to 35 minutes. Remove from the heat.

Just before serving, stir in the kale. Season with salt, if desired, and serve hot.

Per serving: 398 calories, 8 g total fat, 4 g saturated fat, 0 mg cholesterol, 539 mg sodium, 64 g total carbohydrate (10 g dietary fiber, 10 g sugar, 0 g added sugars), 20 g protein, 7 mg iron

Spring Minestrone Soup with Barley

Serves 6

This fresh and vibrant meal-in-a-bowl combines grains, beans, and veggies. If you have cooked barley on hand, this recipe comes together in less than twenty minutes. Substitute a gluten-free grain such as brown rice, if desired, and enjoy with your favorite whole-grain bread. **Recipe by Whole Foods Market**

½ cup chopped yellow onion

6 garlic cloves, minced

1 tablespoon minced fresh oregano

1 tablespoon minced fresh thyme

½ teaspoon red pepper flakes

½ teaspoon sea salt

¼ teaspoon freshly ground black pepper

4 cups low-sodium vegetable broth

1 (28-ounce) can no-added-sodium crushed tomatoes

1 (4-inch) Parmesan cheese rind (optional)

¾ cup chopped zucchini

2 cups chopped rainbow chard or other chard leaves

1 (15-ounce) can no-added-sodium white beans, drained and rinsed

1¼ cups cooked barley (see page 36)

¼ cup chopped fresh basil

3 tablespoons chopped fresh parsley

Grated Parmesan cheese, for serving (optional)

Heat a large soup pot over medium-high heat. When hot, add the onion and dry sauté, stirring often until it begins to stick to the pan and lightly brown, 3 to 4 minutes. Stir in the garlic, oregano, thyme, red pepper flakes, salt, and black pepper and cook until garlic begins to stick to the pan, 1 to 2 minutes.

Stir in the broth and crushed tomatoes. If using, add the Parmesan rind. Bring to a boil, then reduce the heat to medium-low and simmer, uncovered, 6 to 8 minutes.

Stir in the zucchini, chard, beans, and barley. Simmer until the zucchini is just tender, 8 to 10 minutes.

Stir in the basil and parsley. Serve hot, topped with grated Parmesan, if desired.

Per serving: 172 calories, 1 g total fat, 0 g saturated fat, 0 mg cholesterol, 342 mg sodium, 34 g total carbohydrate (8 g dietary fiber, 7 g sugar, 0 g added sugars), 8 g protein, 5 mg iron

Coconut Lemongrass Soup

Serves 4

This fragrant, golden soup nourishes all the senses. Aromatic turmeric and ginger are balanced by the creamy coconut milk. Be sure to add the herbs at the end to keep them fresh. If you prefer a lighter soup, use a mix of light and regular coconut milk, or thin it with water. You can swap out the sweet potatoes and tofu for your favorite vegetables.

½ cup finely chopped onion

½ stalk lemongrass (white part only)

1 tablespoon minced fresh ginger

1 tablespoon minced garlic

1 teaspoon minced fresh Thai or serrano chile

2 teaspoons no-added-sodium curry powder

2½ cups low-sodium vegetable broth

1½ cups finely chopped peeled sweet potatoes

2 (14-ounce) cans coconut milk

Juice of ½ lime

1 teaspoon grated fresh turmeric, or ½ teaspoon ground

½ teaspoon sea salt

1 cup cubed firm tofu

Leaves from ¼ bunch cilantro

Leaves from ¼ bunch Thai basil

Heat a medium soup pot over medium-high heat. When hot, add the onion and dry sauté, stirring often, until it begins to stick to the pan and lightly brown, 3 to 4 minutes. Smash the lemongrass with the back of a knife to "bruise" it and release its aromas. Add the lemongrass, ginger, garlic, chile, and curry powder to the pot with the onion and cook for 1 minute. Add about ¼ cup of the broth and stir to deglaze the pan.

Add the sweet potatoes and remaining 2¼ cups vegetable broth. Simmer for 5 minutes.

Add the coconut milk, lime juice, turmeric, and salt. Reduce the heat to medium-low and simmer, 10 to 12 minutes. Add the tofu and remove from the heat. Stir in the cilantro and basil, reserving a few sprigs for garnish. Let steep for 5 minutes before serving.

Serve hot, garnished with the reserved herbs.

Per serving: 574 calories, 48 g total fat, 38 g saturated fat, 0 mg cholesterol, 457 mg sodium, 24 g total carbohydrate (3 g dietary fiber, 5 g sugar, 0 g added sugars), 16 g protein, 10 mg iron

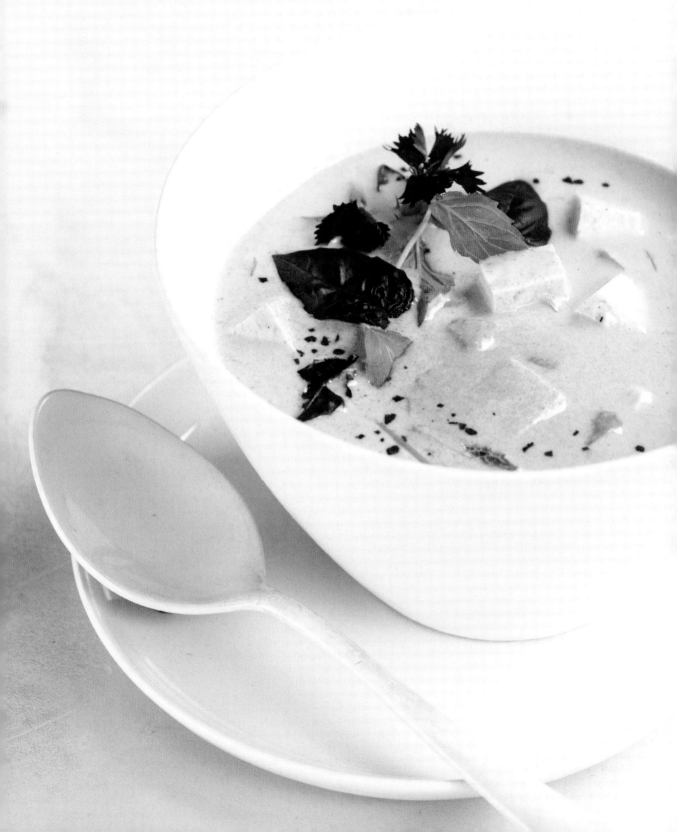

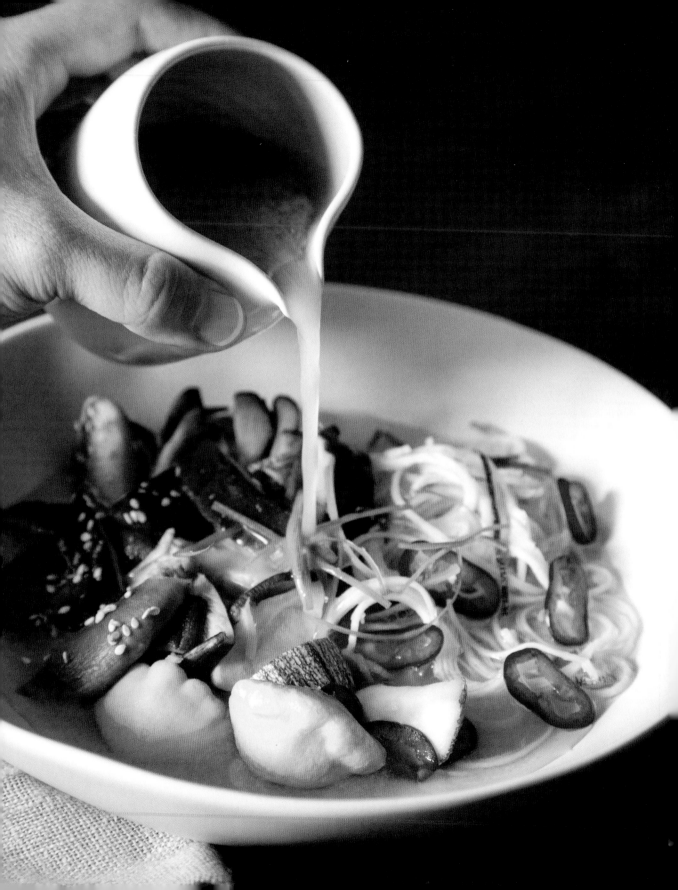

Zucchini Noodle Bowl with Green Onion & Miso

Serves 4 as a first course

This vibrant, fresh miso soup is best assembled at the table for optimum freshness and flavor. Be sure to have all your ingredients prepped and ready to go before you start cooking. Umeboshi vinegar, made from umeboshi plums, adds a distinctive sour and salty note; look for it in the Asian foods aisle at your local market. For a more robust meal, cooked jasmine rice or cellophane noodles can be added to the bowl before you ladle in the soup.

6 dried shiitake mushrooms

2 tablespoons minced fresh ginger

3 cups low-sodium vegetable broth

2 tablespoons white miso paste

1 tablespoon low-sodium soy sauce

2 teaspoons umeboshi vinegar

½ cup quartered small pattypan squash or cubed zucchini

1 zucchini, spiralized with the thin blade, noodles cut in half

3 green onions, chopped (about ½ cup)

2 tablespoons sesame seeds, toasted (see page 61)

1 small Thai red chile, thinly sliced (optional)

Soak the shiitake mushrooms in hot water to cover until softened, about 15 minutes. Drain and thinly slice.

Heat a medium saucepan over medium heat. Add the ginger and 1 tablespoon of the broth and simmer, stirring continuously, until fragrant, 30 to 60 seconds.

Stir in the remaining broth, the miso, soy sauce, and vinegar and raise the heat to medium-high. Bring to a simmer. Add the pattypans and simmer for 2 minutes more.

Divide the zucchini noodles and shiitakes among four small bowls. Pour the miso broth over the top and garnish with the green onions, sesame seeds, and sliced chile (if using).

Per serving: 85 calories, 2 g total fat, 0 g saturated fat, 0 mg cholesterol, 528 mg sodium, 14 g total carbohydrate (2 g dietary fiber, 5 g sugar, 0 g added sugars), 4 g protein, 2 mg iron

Mushroom Chowda with Herbes de Provence

Serves 6

This creamy corn-and-mushroom chowder is delicious served with crusty whole-grain bread or Garlic Bread (page 71). **Recipe by Lisa Rice**

½ cup raw cashews, soaked for 3 hours or up to overnight

1 large onion, diced

2 large celery stalks, diced

1 large carrot, diced

1 large garlic clove, minced

8 cups low-sodium vegetable broth

1½ tablespoons herbes de Provence

1 large Yukon Gold potato, diced

1 head cauliflower, cut into florets

1 cup fresh or thawed frozen corn kernels

3 cups oyster mushrooms (including stems), coarsely chopped

1½ teaspoons kelp granules or flaked nori

¼ cup chickpea miso paste

½ head kale, stemmed, leaves torn into bite-size pieces

Pinch of sea salt

½ teaspoon cracked black pepper

Drain and rinse the cashews.

Heat a large soup pot over medium-high heat. When hot, add the onion, celery, and carrot and dry sauté, stirring often, until the onion begins to stick to the pan, 4 to 6 minutes. Add the garlic and cook for 1 minute. Add ½ cup of the broth and stir to deglaze the pan.

Stir in herbes de Provence and cook for 1 minute more. Stir in the potato, cauliflower, and 7 cups of the broth and bring to a boil. Reduce the heat to medium-low and simmer until the potato and cauliflower are fork-tender, about 10 minutes. Stir in the corn and cook for 3 minutes more.

Meanwhile, heat a large skillet over medium heat. When hot, add the mushrooms and their stems and cook until they release their liquid and begin to stick to the pan, 3 to 4 minutes. Add the remaining ½ cup broth and stir to deglaze the pan. Stir in ½ teaspoon of the kelp or nori and cook until the mushrooms are very tender, 3 to 4 minutes more. Remove from the heat and set aside.

Transfer 2 cups of the soup to a (preferably high-speed) blender and add the drained cashews, miso, and remaining 1 teaspoon kelp or nori. Blend until smooth. Spoon the mixture into the soup and stir to combine.

Add the kale and mushrooms to the pot and cook until the kale turns bright green and wilts slightly, 2 to 3 minutes.

Ladle into bowls and season with the salt and pepper before serving.

Note: This recipe is great for using up the bits and bobs of vegetables in your refrigerator or freezer. Fresh or frozen peas, parsnips, green beans, snap peas, broccoli, asparagus, cabbage, sweet potatoes, partially used onions or green onions, mushrooms, spinach, chard, collards, etc. Just cook the harder vegetables first, add the softer vegetables later, and wilt the greens in at the end.

Per serving: 181 calories, 5 g total fat, 1 g saturated fat, 0 mg cholesterol, 787 mg sodium, 28 g total carbohydrate (5 g dietary fiber, 9 g sugar, 0 g added sugars), 8 g protein, 3 mg iron

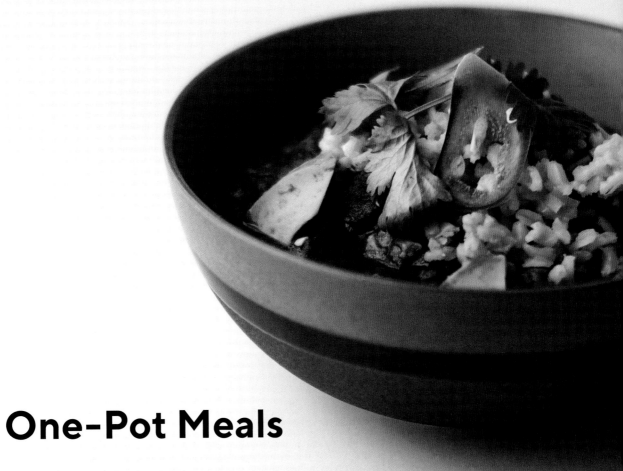

One-Pot Meals

Stews, chilies, curries, tagines, goulashes—one-pot meals are a busy whole foodie's friend. They ensure you get all the nutrition you need, while saving you time and energy washing dishes. With everything cooking at the same time in the same pot, you don't need to worry about following complex instructions. And you'll build flavor as the ingredients combine during cooking. Cultures around the world have developed their own distinct variations on this theme, taking advantage of the opportunity to build flavors as they work through the recipe.

Building Soups and Stews

Being empowered in the kitchen means opening up the fridge and working with the ingredients you have on hand. Soups and stews are a great way to use up those week-old veggies, or highlight some favorites for a comforting one-pot meal. Just use the Dry Sauté Method (see page 78) to start your soup with onions and garlic. Add your favorite vegetables, chopped, shredded, or diced and cook for a few minutes until you get some browning on the bottom of the pot. Add a liquid—vegetable broth, canned or pureed tomatoes, or nondairy milk. Add raw, frozen, or cooked grains and/or canned or frozen beans and allow to simmer. (Note: If using dried beans, remember to allocate much more time for soaking and cooking them; see page 42.) Season with your choice of acids, other aromatics, spices, or herbs, and enjoy with your favorite whole-grain bread for a one-pot meal of comfort.

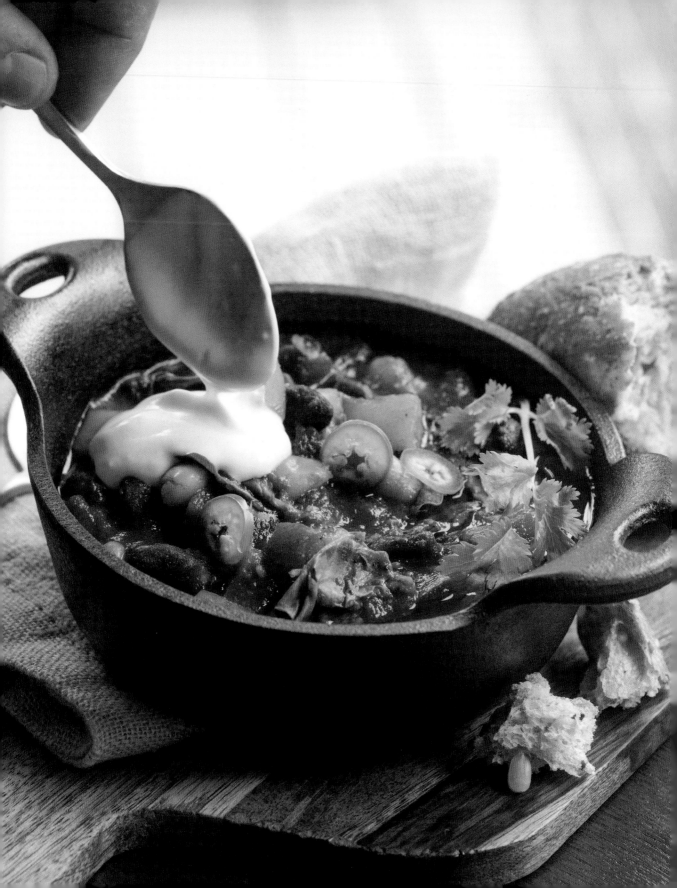

Veggie-Loaded Chili

Serves 6

Do you like your chili spicy? We sure do, and this recipe is no exception. If you're more cautious with the heat, you can eliminate the chipotle powder and pickled jalapeños. This will taste even better the next day, once all the flavors have married.

1 small onion, chopped

6 garlic cloves, minced

2¼ cups low-sodium vegetable broth

2 tablespoons ground cumin

1½ tablespoons chili powder

1 tablespoon chipotle powder

1 tablespoon paprika

1 cup cubed small new potatoes (skin-on)

1 (28-ounce) can no-added-sodium crushed tomatoes

1 (4-ounce) can no-added-sodium pickled jalapeños, drained and chopped

1 (4-ounce) can no-added-sodium chopped green chiles

1 cup diced zucchini

1 cup cooked black beans (see page 42) or canned no-added-sodium black beans, drained and rinsed

1 cup cooked pinto beans (see page 42) or canned no-added-sodium pinto beans, drained and rinsed

1 cup cooked kidney beans (see page 42) or canned no-added-sodium kidney beans, drained and rinsed

½ teaspoon sea salt

1 cup chopped or baby kale leaves

½ cup chopped fresh cilantro, plus some leaves for garnish

Heat a large soup pot over medium heat. When hot, add the onion and dry sauté, stirring often, until it begins to stick to the pan and lightly brown, 3 to 4 minutes. Stir in the garlic, then add ¼ cup of the broth and stir to deglaze the pan. Cook until most of the liquid has evaporated, 1 to 2 minutes.

Stir in the cumin, chili powder, chipotle, and paprika and cook, stirring often, until they smell fragrant, 1 to 2 minutes.

Add the potatoes and remaining 2 cups vegetable broth, and simmer until the potatoes are fork-tender, 5 to 8 minutes.

Reduce the heat to medium-low and add the tomatoes, jalapeños, green chiles, zucchini, all the beans, and the sea salt. Cover and simmer, 10 to 12 minutes.

Remove from the heat and stir in the kale and cilantro. Let sit until kale is wilted, 2 to 3 minutes.

Serve hot, garnished with cilantro.

Notes: For more flavor, top each serving with chopped avocado and a dollop of cashew sour cream (follow the recipe on page 160, omitting the jalapeño).

Serve with your favorite whole-grain seeded bread.

Per serving: 221 calories, 2 g total fat, 0 g saturated fat, 0 mg cholesterol, 415 mg sodium, 38 g total carbohydrate (11 g dietary fiber, 7 g sugar, 0 g added sugars), 11 g protein, 5 mg iron

Wild Mushroom & Kale Ragout over Soft Polenta

Serves 6

Cozy up to this belly-warming, heart-healthy bowl of life. We use cashew sour cream in both the polenta and the ragout to give it a smooth, creamy texture. For a complete meal, serve this dish with a large salad and roasted vegetables or another steamed green.

POLENTA

5 cups low-sodium vegetable broth, plus more as needed

1⅓ cups coarse polenta

¼ teaspoon sea salt

¼ cup nutritional yeast

½ teaspoon smoked paprika

½ teaspoon freshly ground black pepper

½ cup Cashew Sour Cream (page 160, made without the jalapeño and cilantro)

½ cup chopped fresh flat-leaf parsley

MUSHROOM AND KALE RAGOUT

1 large onion, finely chopped

3 garlic cloves, minced

2 shallots, cut into thin matchsticks

1 pound wild mushrooms, coarsely chopped

¼ cup dry sherry or Marsala wine

1 cup low-sodium mushroom broth or vegetable broth

1 (14-ounce) can no-added-sodium white beans, drained and rinsed

1 teaspoon dried thyme

½ teaspoon rubbed sage

1 teaspoon chopped fresh rosemary, plus a few sprigs for garnish

1 bunch kale, stemmed, leaves torn into bite-size pieces

1 cup Cashew Sour Cream (page 160, made without the jalapeño and cilantro)

¼ cup chopped fresh flat-leaf parsley

¼ teaspoon sea salt

½ teaspoon freshly ground black pepper

For the polenta, in a medium saucepan, bring the vegetable broth to a boil. While whisking, slowly stream in the polenta and continue whisking to avoid lumps. When fully incorporated, add the salt, nutritional yeast, paprika, and pepper.

Reduce the heat to very low and simmer, whisking almost continuously to prevent burning on the bottom, until the polenta pulls away from the sides of the pan when stirred, about 30 minutes. Add more broth if necessary to prevent sticking.

Remove from the heat. Whisk in the cashew sour cream and parsley and set aside.

For the ragout, heat a large skillet over medium-high heat. Add the onion, garlic, and shallots and dry sauté, stirring often, for 1 minute. Add the mushrooms and cook, stirring now and then, until they are soft, the liquid they release has evaporated, and they begin to brown, 3 to 4 minutes. Add the sherry and stir to deglaze the pan, then simmer until most of the liquid has evaporated.

Add the mushroom broth, beans, thyme, sage, and rosemary. Bring to a boil, then reduce the heat to low and simmer for 10 to 15 minutes.

Fold in the kale and cook until it is wilted and bright green, 3 minutes. Stir in the cashew sour cream, parsley, salt, and pepper. Cook for 3 minutes more, then remove from the heat.

To assemble, divide the polenta among six bowls, top with the ragout, and garnish with rosemary sprigs.

Notes: Try using all different kinds of mushrooms to vary the recipe.

Replace the kale with broccoli or green beans cut into ½-inch pieces.

Substitute your favorite dried or canned bean for the white beans.

Per serving: 487 calories, 11 g total fat, 2 g saturated fat, 0 mg cholesterol, 850 mg sodium, 75 g total carbohydrate (10 g dietary fiber, 8 g sugar, 0 g added sugars), 17 g protein, 6 mg iron

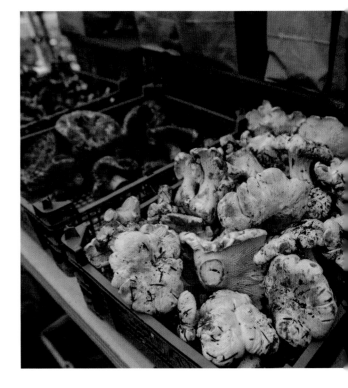

Thai Curry Chickpeas, Collards, & Rice

Serves 6

Curry, coconut, and chickpeas are an aromatic match made in heaven. The optional tofu will bulk up the dish if desired. This dish tastes even better on day two, when the flavors have married, so be sure to make extra.

3 (14-ounce) cans chickpeas, drained and rinsed

1 large onion, finely chopped

3 celery stalks, sliced on an angle into thin half-moons

2 carrots, finely chopped

1 teaspoon minced fresh ginger

1 teaspoon minced fresh garlic

Pinch of sea salt

Pinch of freshly ground black pepper

½ cup coconut milk

2 tablespoons red curry paste

1 (14-ounce) block of firm tofu, drained, cut into 1-inch cubes (optional)

1 bunch collards, stemmed, coarsely chopped and rinsed

½ cup chopped fresh cilantro

2 teaspoons white and/or black sesame seeds

6 cups cooked brown rice, preferably jasmine rice (see page 36)

2 limes, cut into wedges

Preheat the oven to 350°F.

Place chickpeas in a large (13 by 9-inch or 3-quart) baking dish. Bake, stirring now and then, until the chickpeas begin to crisp up, 15 to 20 minutes.

Heat a large saucepan over medium-high heat. Add the onion, celery, carrots, ginger, garlic, salt, and pepper. Cook, stirring frequently, for 3 minutes. Add the coconut milk, red curry paste, and 1 cup water and simmer for a few minutes. If using, add cubed tofu. Pour the mixture over the chickpeas and bake for 15 to 20 minutes.

Meanwhile, steam the chopped collards in a covered steamer basket over gently simmering water until wilted and bright green, 3 to 5 minutes.

Remove the baking dish from the oven and scatter on the cilantro and sesame seeds.

Serve the chickpeas with the rice, collards, and lime wedges for squeezing.

Per serving (without tofu): 554 calories, 7 g total fat, 1 g saturated fat, 0 mg cholesterol, 802 mg sodium, 108 g total carbohydrate (19 g dietary fiber, 11 g sugar, 0 g added sugars), 19 g protein, 4 mg iron

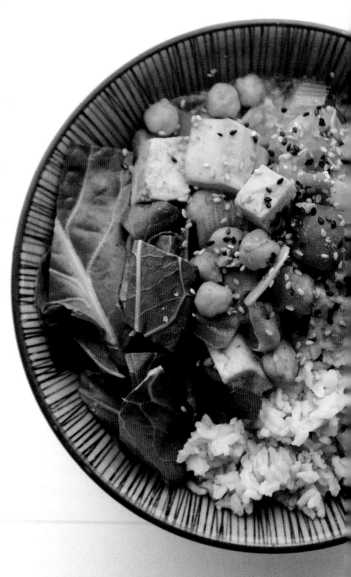

Spanish Pisto with Potatoes

Serves 4

Pisto, a Spanish dish reminiscent of ratatouille, is a great summer meal because it can be served either hot or cold. The potatoes fill out this dish so that it satisfies all by itself, but you can also spoon it over pasta or steamed grains for a heartier meal, or serve it alongside toasted crostini as a zesty appetizer. **Recipe by Darshana Thacker**

1 small onion, cut into ½-inch pieces

¼ cup low-sodium vegetable broth

1 large russet potato, cut into 1-inch cubes

1 red bell pepper, cut into ½-inch pieces

3 garlic cloves, minced

2 teaspoons dried oregano

1 eggplant, peeled and cut into ½-inch cubes

1 small zucchini or summer squash, cut into 1-inch cubes

4 tomatoes, peeled and cut into ½-inch pieces

1 tablespoon paprika

1 tablespoon fresh lemon juice

½ teaspoon sea salt

¼ teaspoon freshly ground black pepper

1 tablespoon chopped fresh parsley

Heat a large deep skillet over medium heat. When hot, add the onion and cook, stirring often, until it begins to stick to the pan and lightly brown, about 4 minutes. Add the broth and stir to deglaze the pan. Add the potatoes, bell pepper, garlic, and oregano and cook, stirring occasionally, until the onion and pepper are tender, about 10 minutes.

Stir in the eggplant, zucchini, tomatoes, paprika, and ½ cup water and cook until the potatoes are tender, 15 to 20 minutes.

Season with the lemon juice, salt, and black pepper. Garnish with the parsley and serve.

Note: To peel fresh tomatoes, bring a medium pot of water to a boil. Set up a large bowl of ice water. Cut an X in the bottom of the tomato skins, then drop the tomatoes into the boiling water. Cook until the tomato skins begin to loosen at the X, about 30 seconds. Use a slotted spoon to transfer the tomatoes to the ice water and let them sit until cool, about 2 minutes. Slip off the skins, using a paring knife if necessary to help remove them.

Per serving: 165 calories, 1 g total fat, 0 g saturated fat, 0 mg cholesterol, 320 mg sodium, 37 g total carbohydrate (9 g dietary fiber, 11 g sugar, 0 g added sugars), 6 g protein, 3 mg iron

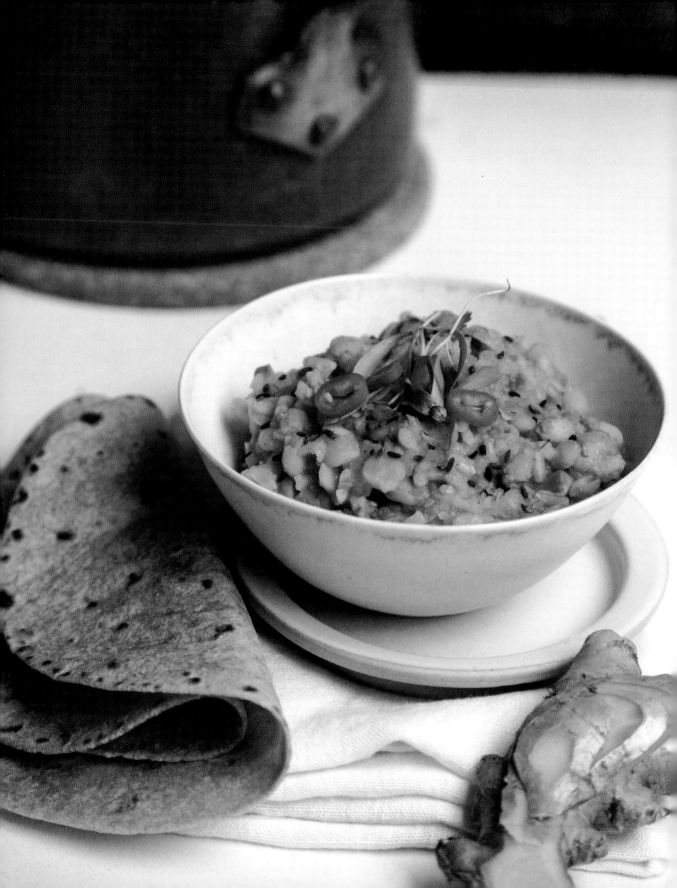

Kitchari with Warm Spices

Serves 4

Kitchari is a term derived from Sanskrit meaning "mixture," and usually refers to a combination of legumes and rice, cooked together. In Ayurvedic practice, this is a traditional healing food. The warming spices and ginger help give your digestive system a much-needed break. You can serve this soothing bowl topped with diced avocado and heaps of fresh cilantro, or try folding in some baby spinach right at the end.

1 cup dried yellow split peas

½ cup chopped sweet white onion

½ cup finely chopped carrot

6 cups low-sodium vegetable broth

½ cup uncooked brown basmati rice, rinsed

1 tablespoon minced fresh ginger

¾ teaspoon sea salt

1 fresh Thai red or serrano chile, halved lengthwise, plus more for garnish, if desired

1 teaspoon ground cumin

1 teaspoon black mustard seeds

1 teaspoon ground coriander

1 teaspoon ground turmeric

Juice of 1 lemon

½ cup chopped fresh cilantro

1 ripe avocado, pitted, peeled, and chopped

Soak the split peas in water to cover overnight. Drain, rinse, and set aside.

Heat a heavy soup pot over medium heat. Add the onion and carrot and dry sauté, stirring now and then, until the vegetables begin to stick to the pan, about 2 to 3 minutes. Add ¼ cup of the broth and stir to deglaze the pan. Stir in the split peas, rice, ginger, salt, and remaining 5¾ cups broth. Add the chile and bring to a simmer. Reduce the heat to medium-low, cover, and simmer gently until the peas begin to fall apart but aren't melting, 30 to 35 minutes.

In a small sauté pan, toast the cumin and mustard seeds over medium-high heat until the seeds are fragrant and begin to pop, 1 to 2 minutes, shaking the pan now and then. Add the coriander and turmeric and toast until fragrant, 15 to 30 seconds, shaking the pan continuously.

Stir the toasted spice mixture into the kitchari. Remove from the heat and stir in the lemon juice and cilantro.

Serve with the avocado and additional sliced fresh chile (if you like it hot).

Per serving: 379 calories, 6 g total fat, 1 g saturated fat, 0 mg cholesterol, 698 mg sodium, 65 g total carbohydrate (17 g dietary fiber, 7 g sugar, 0 g added sugars), 15 g protein, 4 mg iron

Sweet Potato Tagine

Serves 8

The term *tagine* comes from the beautiful North African earthenware pots in which this dish is traditionally slow cooked, allowing its vibrant flavors to infuse the beans and vegetables. If you're feeling inspired, you might try using one—they're easy to find in cookware stores. Serve with couscous and fresh herbs such as mint, cilantro, or parsley.

2 teaspoons coriander seeds

2 teaspoons cumin seeds

½ teaspoon whole black peppercorns

½ teaspoon ground cinnamon

1 cup chopped onion

3 garlic cloves, minced

3 cups low-sodium vegetable broth

3 tablespoons no-added-sodium tomato paste

1 large sweet potato (about 1 pound), peeled and cut into ½-inch pieces

2 cups cooked chickpeas (see page 42) or no-added-sodium canned chickpeas

1 tablespoon grated lemon zest

1 tablespoon fresh lemon juice

½ cup chopped pitted green olives

¼ cup currants or golden raisins

3 tablespoons chopped fresh parsley leaves

3 tablespoons chopped fresh mint leaves

Cooked whole-grain couscous (see page 36; optional)

In a large skillet, toast the coriander, cumin, peppercorns, and cinnamon over medium heat, stirring frequently to prevent scorching, until they are fragrant, 2 to 3 minutes. Remove from the heat and let cool for a few minutes. Transfer to a spice grinder and grind to a powder. Set the spice blend aside.

Return the pan to medium-high heat. When hot, add the onion and dry sauté, stirring often, until it begins to stick to the pan and lightly brown, 3 to 4 minutes. Add the garlic and spice blend and cook for 1 minute. Add ¼ cup of the broth and stir to deglaze the pan. Simmer until the broth has evaporated and the onion begins to stick to the pan again, 2 to 3 minutes more. Stir in the tomato paste until thoroughly combined, then stir in the remaining 2¾ cups broth, the sweet potato, chickpeas, lemon zest, lemon juice, olives, and currants. Bring to a simmer over medium-high heat. Reduce the heat to low, cover, and simmer until the sweet potatoes are fork-tender, about 20 minutes. Stir in the parsley and mint.

Serve with couscous, if desired.

Per serving (without couscous): 171 calories, 2 g total fat, 0 g saturated fat, 0 mg cholesterol, 173 mg sodium, 32 g total carbohydrate (6 g dietary fiber, 8 g sugar, 0 g added sugars), 5 g protein, 2 mg iron

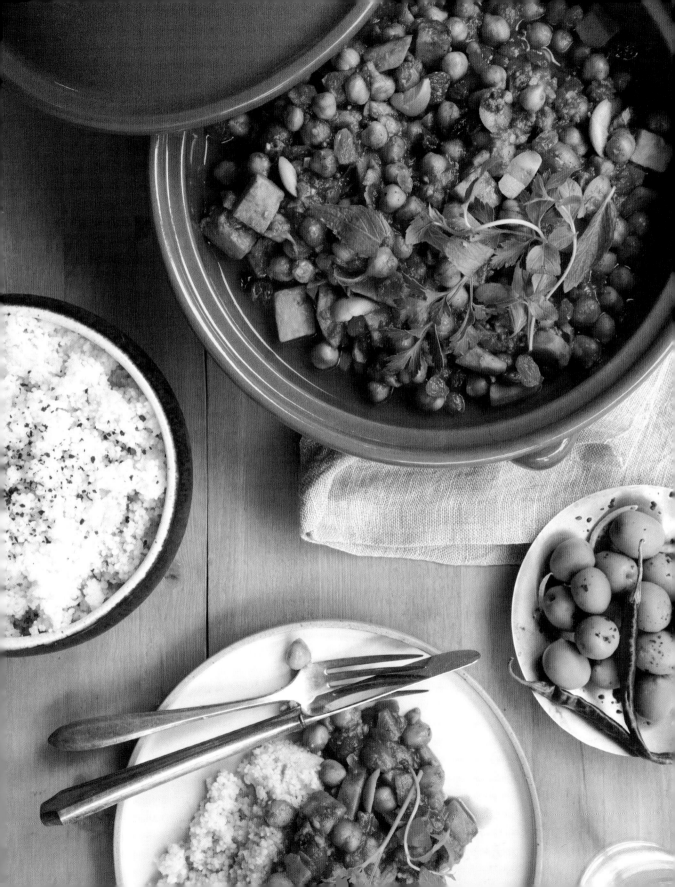

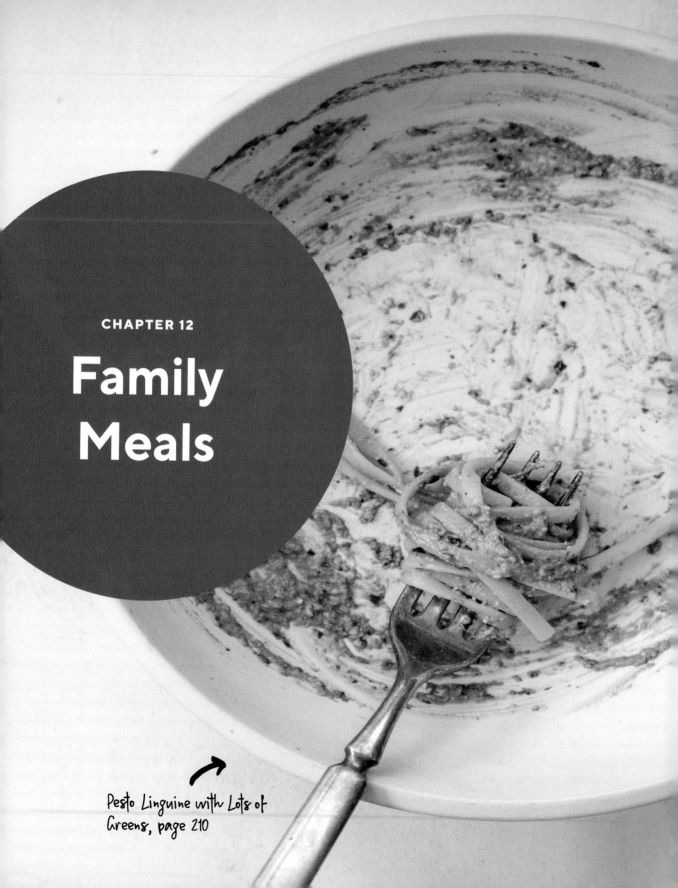

CHAPTER 12

Family Meals

Pesto Linguine with Lots of Greens, page 210

Family dinner: It's a time of warmth, laughter, nourishment, and connection. For many of us, our most cherished memories from childhood revolve around the dinner table, or spending time in the kitchen. Unfortunately, it can also be a time of struggle if the whole household is not into healthy eating, with health-conscious parents trying to coax their children (or spouse) into eating and enjoying foods that will help them grow and thrive.

Here's a great tip for getting kids excited about healthy food: choose whole foods, plant-based variations on simple, time-tested comfort foods; and involve the whole family in the cooking process. Show them how to grow sprouts, or even veggies, if you have a garden. Shop with them and ask them to pick out new types of produce they may be interested in tasting. And invite them into the kitchen—it may be a messy process, but it's sure to pay off in enthusiasm for the finished meal. (See page 23 for more tips on getting the family on board.) In this chapter, we'll help you re-create family favorites: pasta, casseroles, stir-fries, burgers, tacos, and pizza.

Pasta Night

It's hard to beat pasta for a quick, satisfying, and delicious dinner that will please every member of the family. Get the children involved in choosing a colorful sauce (try a new one each week!), picking their favorite pasta shapes, and testing whether they are cooked just right. These days, there are so many whole-grain options, including many gluten-free varieties for those who need them, making pasta a healthy and comforting choice, with little struggle from the small ones.

Choosing the Right Sauce

From simple and comforting tomato sauce to fragrant herb pesto to creamy white sauce and sweet roasted red pepper sauce, your choice of sauce is what brings your pasta dish alive. See pages 208–211 for recipes.

Make it fun by creating a pasta bar! Choose a couple of sauces to highlight at your next buffet dinner, with roasted and steamed vegetable options for guests to mix in (see page 87). Pair with a salad (chapter 9) and the perfect garlic bread (page 71).

Chef's Tip

Sauce is what brings people together; it is the single, essential, most important aspect to any meal. Red sauce, marinara, Nana's gravy—call it what you wish, but know that a good sauce will bring together the meal, and the family.

Choosing a Pasta

To ensure that your pasta retains the nutritious fiber of the original grains, always choose a whole-grain variety rather than the traditional "white" pasta, which is made from refined flour. Whole wheat pasta is readily available, and at many stores you may also find pastas made with ancient wheat varietals like Kamut, farro, or spelt. For those who prefer gluten-free, try brown rice, quinoa, or corn pasta. You might also experiment with legume-based pastas, such as chickpea or lentil. Our favorite variety, which you'll see in a number of the recipes ahead, is brown rice pasta.

Size is everything! Pasta comes in numerous shapes and sizes, which your kids will enjoy. But the designs are not merely decorative. The twists, holes, and grooves are intended to trap the sauce, ensuring that every mouthful is packed with flavor. When choosing pasta, think about the kind of sauce you are making. Is it a thick, creamy sauce that will easily stick to the pasta? In that case, bigger and simpler shapes like rigatoni or penne will work well, as will long noodles with more surface area such as linguine or tagliatelle. Is it a textured sauce like puttanesca, where the small pieces of olive, chile, and tomato would catch in grooves? Choose a straight pasta such as spaghetti or spaghettini. Experiment with different styles and notice the difference.

COOKING PASTA

When cooking pasta, make sure you have a large straight-sided pot, and use plenty of water. Worried about sticking? You don't need to add oil to keep the pasta separated, you just need a big enough pot. Most will season the pasta water with salt, but this step is certainly not needed if you're cutting back on your sodium intake. Bring the water to a rolling boil, add the pasta, and stir while cooking. Timing is key, so read the package and also be sure to test a minute or two before the suggested time is up so that you get the perfect "al dente" consistency. Be sure not to overcook your dried pasta.

When your pasta is cooked, drain it immediately. You might want to save a little of the cooking water to thin your sauce if needed. Pastas containing gluten should not be rinsed, as the starches that have been released in the cooking process will help the sauce to stick. For gluten-free pastas, rinse quickly with hot water before adding the sauce; this will help your gluten-free pasta not be too "gummy."

Building Your Pasta Plate

Don't stop at sauce! Pasta dishes are a great opportunity to get your veggies in. Add plenty of fresh steamed, roasted, or sautéed greens or veggies, toss them up in the sauce, and watch your kids eat them without even noticing. Get sneaky and mince the veggies, or shred them so they "melt" and are hidden in the sauce.

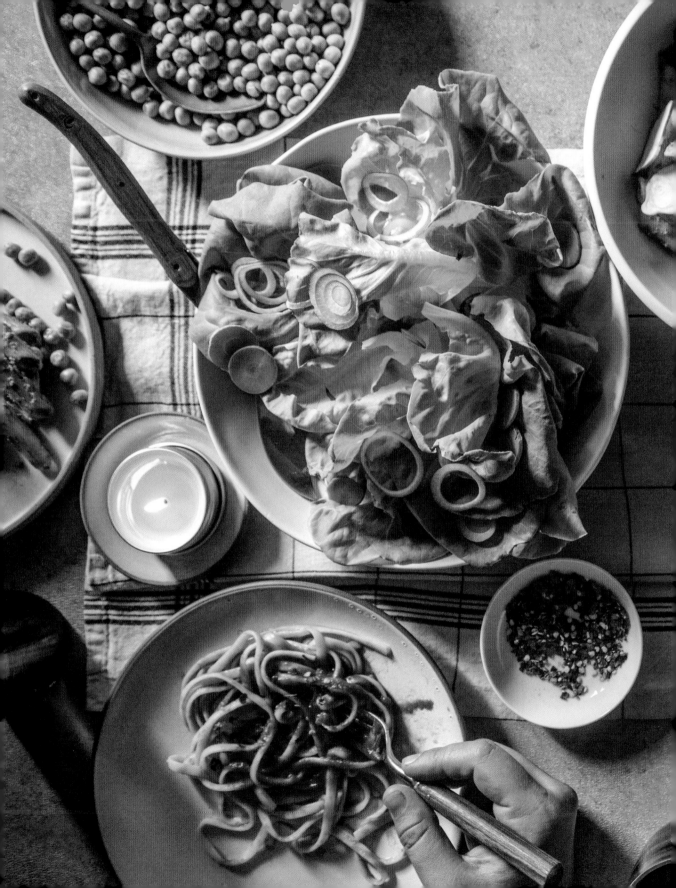

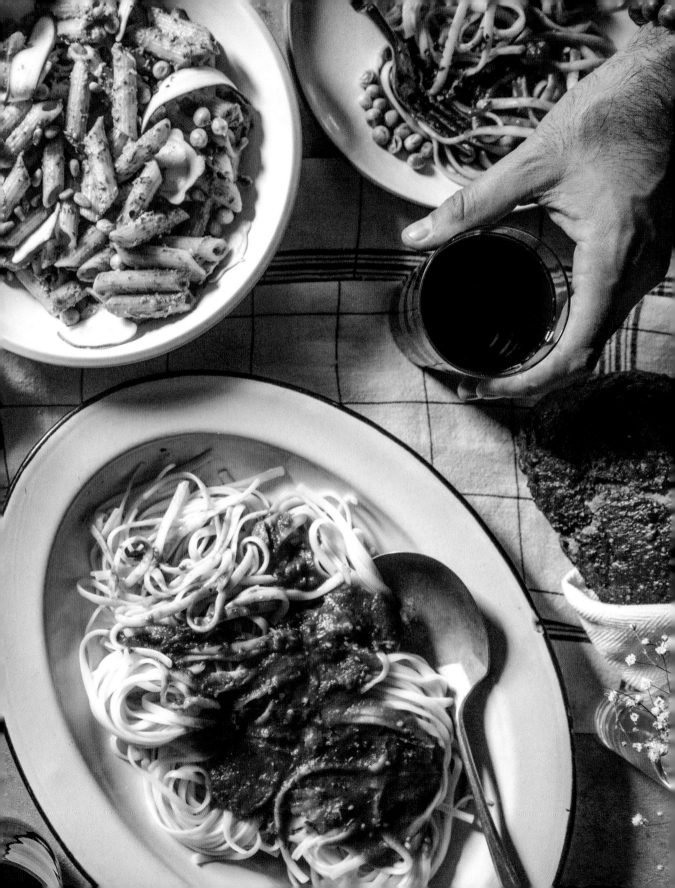

Penne Carbonara with Cauliflower

Serves 4

This nondairy version of the beloved creamy pasta dish is the perfect comfort food. Instead of bacon, we use smoked tofu to capture the signature flavor profile of this traditional recipe. If you can't find smoked tofu, you can use Baked Tofu (page 134). You can also try adding Carrot Lox (page 101). If you like your pasta extra creamy, use 3 cups of cashew cream sauce instead of two. Choose several varieties of cauliflower to serve this with a splash of color.

1 pound whole-grain or legume-based penne pasta

½ cup diced white onion

¼ cup minced cauliflower, plus some florets for garnish

3 garlic cloves, minced

½ cup white wine

2 cups Basic Cashew Cream Sauce (page 165)

⅓ cup low-sodium vegetable broth

½ cup shelled fresh peas or defrosted frozen peas

½ cup ¼-inch-cubed smoked tofu or Baked Tofu (page 134)

Freshly ground black pepper

½ lemon

¼ cup coarsely chopped fresh parsley

¼ teaspoon flaky sea salt, for finishing

Pea tendrils, for garnish

Bring a pot of water to a rolling boil. Add the penne and cook, stirring frequently, until al dente, 6 to 8 minutes.

Heat a large sauté pan over medium-high heat. When hot, add the onion and cauliflower and dry sauté, stirring often, until they begin to stick to the pan and lightly brown, 3 to 4 minutes. Stir in the garlic, then add the wine and stir to deglaze the pan. Cook until most of the liquid has evaporated, about 2 minutes.

Stir in the cashew cream sauce and broth. Reduce the heat to medium-low and stir in the peas, tofu, and pepper.

Finely grate the zest from the lemon half and set aside. Squeeze the juice into the pan (through your hand to catch the seeds) and stir to incorporate into the sauce. Cook until the sauce is bubbling around the edges, about 2 minutes.

Drain the pasta and add it to the pan. Toss to coat with the sauce. Add the parsley and toss to mix.

Divide the pasta among four plates. Sprinkle some of the flaky salt and lemon zest over each serving. Use a mandoline to shave the raw cauliflower florets over each serving, then garnish with pea tendrils.

Per serving: 691 calories, 13 g total fat, 2 g saturated fat, 0 mg cholesterol, 435 mg sodium, 109 g total carbohydrate (7 g dietary fiber, 11 g sugar, 0 g added sugars), 29 g protein, 8 mg iron

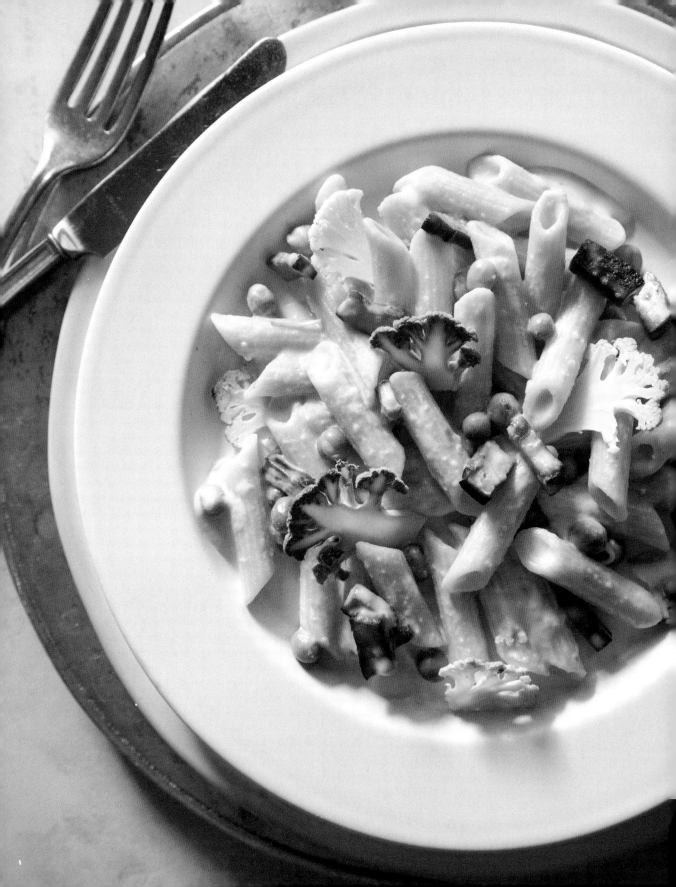

Pesto Linguine with Lots of Greens

Serves 4

Aromatic herbs and leafy greens—this delicious pasta is packed with flavor *and* nutrition. Bump up the red pepper flakes for a bit more of a kick (pictured on page 202).

1 pound whole-grain or legume based linguine

½ cup thinly sliced sweet onion

½ cup low-sodium vegetable broth

1 cup Oil-Free Herb Pesto (page 163)

½ teaspoon red pepper flakes

¼ teaspoon freshly ground black pepper

1 cup lightly packed baby spinach

1 cup thinly sliced kale without tough stems

½ teaspoon sea salt

6 whole walnut halves

Bring a large pot of water to a boil. Add the pasta and cook according to the package directions until al dente.

Meanwhile, heat a large, deep sauté pan or wok over medium-high heat. When hot, add the onion and dry sauté, stirring often, until it begins to stick to the pan, 3 to 4 minutes, stirring often. Add the broth and stir to deglaze the pan. Stir in the pesto, red pepper flakes, and black pepper and bring to a simmer. If the sauce gets too thick, add a splash of the pasta cooking water or more broth.

When the pasta is cooked, stir the spinach and kale into the pesto mixture, then drain the pasta and add it to the sauce. Toss to coat.

Remove from the heat and divide among four bowls. Sprinkle with the salt and use a truffle shaver or Microplane to finely shave the walnuts over each plate.

Per serving: 518 calories, 16 g total fat, 1 g saturated fat, 0 mg cholesterol, 559 mg sodium, 87 g total carbohydrate (3 g dietary fiber, 6 g sugar, 0 g added sugars), 23 g protein, 6 mg iron

Farfalle with Roasted Tomatoes, Leeks, & Lemon Sauce

Serves 6

You can prepare the tomatoes and leeks for this decadent and colorful pasta up to a day ahead and refrigerate them. Simply add them to the pot and cook the pasta in broth—since this is a one-pot meal and no draining of the pasta is required. We're so confident you'll be delighted with the result that we encourage you to cook enough for leftovers, too! **Recipe by Whole Foods Market**

TOMATOES AND LEEKS

1 recipe Roasted Cherry Tomatoes & Garlic (page 88)

2 leeks, white and pale green parts only, cleaned (see Note on cleaning leeks, page 37) and thinly sliced

¼ teaspoon sea salt

¼ teaspoon freshly ground black pepper

¾ cup white wine

LEMON SAUCE AND PASTA

Zest and juice of 1 large lemon

2 tablespoons drained capers

¼ cup Basic Cashew Cream Sauce (page 165) or plain nondairy cream cheese

½ teaspoon sea salt

5 cups low-sodium vegetable broth

1 pound whole grain or legume based farfalle pasta

¼ teaspoon freshly ground black pepper

½ teaspoon red pepper flakes (optional)

Grilled shrimp or chicken (optional)

½ cup shredded fresh basil leaves

For the tomatoes and leeks, prepare the Roasted Cherry Tomatoes & Garlic.

Meanwhile, heat a nonstick skillet over medium-low heat. Add the leeks and season with the salt and pepper. Cook until the leeks begin to stick to the pan, about 5 minutes. Add ¼ cup of the wine and stir to deglaze the pan and loosen the leeks. Repeat this process, cooking the leeks until they stick to the pan, then deglazing with ¼ cup of the wine, until all the wine has been used and the leeks are very soft, almost melted. Stir the melted leeks into the roasted tomatoes. Set aside.

For the lemon sauce, whisk together the lemon zest, lemon juice, capers, cashew cream sauce, and salt. Set aside.

Pour the broth into a large pot. Add the pasta, black pepper, and red pepper flakes (if using) and bring to a boil over medium-high heat. Reduce the heat to low, cover, and simmer, stirring occasionally to prevent sticking, until the pasta is tender but still chewy in the center and only a little liquid is left in the pan, 12 to 14 minutes.

Stir in the tomato and leek mixture, shrimp or chicken (if using), lemon sauce, and basil and cook gently over low heat, stirring well, until slightly thickened and creamy, 2 to 3 minutes.

Serve hot, in shallow bowls.

Note: Try adding chopped mushrooms, chopped asparagus, and/or carrot ribbons to the pot as you're cooking the pasta.

Per serving (without chicken or shrimp): 366 calories, 3 g total fat, 0 g saturated fat, 0 mg cholesterol, 494 mg sodium, 72 g total carbohydrate (2 g dietary fiber, 7 g sugar, 0 g added sugars), 13 g protein, 4 mg iron

Building Casseroles and Layering Dishes

The French term *casserole* is derived from the large, deep ceramic pan used to make these delicious, oven-baked meals. By definition, anything you choose to put in that dish is a casserole, so let your creativity get to work! Casseroles are a great opportunity to experiment with texture and flavor combinations. They are often made in layers (like lasagna), which allows you to play with contrasts—a piquant or spicy layer beneath a rich creamy layer, for example. The slow cooking method gives the flavors plenty of time to develop and marry in the oven. Casseroles make great one-dish family dinners for busy people, because once you put them in the oven, you don't need to worry about them until they are done. They are also a quick heat-and-serve leftover and often taste even better the next day.

Roasted Eggplant with Cashew Cheese

Serves 6

This whole foods, plant-based twist on an Italian classic is easy to make and sure to delight the whole family. You can make the red sauce and cashew cream cheese in advance for quick assembly.

Recipe by Shoshana Pulde

4 large eggplants

1 tablespoon sea salt

1 recipe No-Oil Red Sauce (page 164)

1 recipe Cashew Cream Cheese (page 264) or Kite Hill nondairy ricotta cheese

Peel the eggplant and slice it lengthwise into ¼-inch-thick planks. Place them in a 13 by 9-inch baking dish or a bowl, sprinkle with the salt, and toss gently to coat all over. Let stand for about 1 hour.

Preheat the oven to 350°F.

Rinse the eggplant slices and squeeze out excess moisture. Dry on paper towels.

Rinse and dry the baking dish, then pour a thin layer of the red sauce over the bottom of the dish. Add a single layer of eggplant slices, overlapping the slices slightly if necessary. Spread on one-third of the cheese, then drizzle with another layer of red sauce. Repeat with the eggplant slices, cheese, and red sauce to create two more layers, ending with the sauce.

Bake, uncovered, until the eggplant is very tender when tested with a toothpick, 45 to 50 minutes.

Remove from the oven and let cool until warm. Slice and serve as a side dish.

Per serving: 413 calories, 13 g total fat, 2 g saturated fat, 0 mg cholesterol, 585 mg sodium, 64 g total carbohydrate (20 g dietary fiber, 27 g sugar, 0 g added sugars), 13 g protein, 4 mg iron

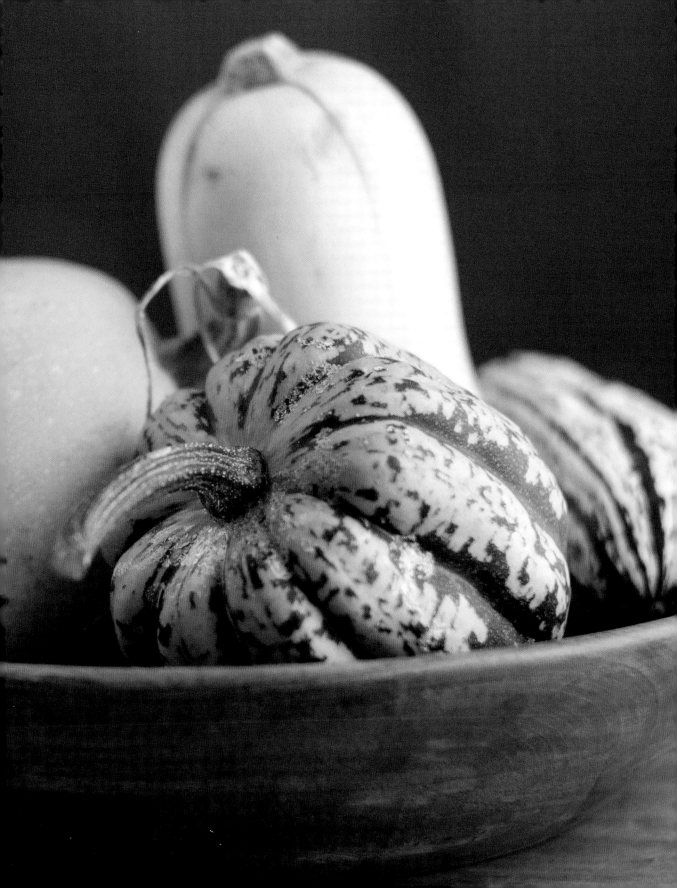

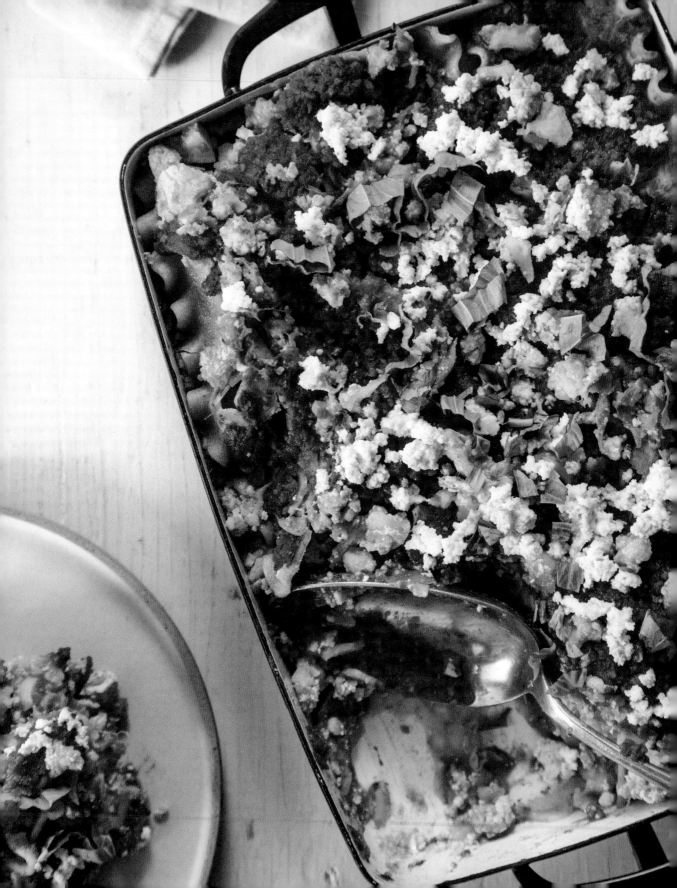

Plant-Powered Lasagna

Serves 8

Everyone loves lasagna, but we don't always love the way we feel after eating a couple of servings. This plant-packed variation on the family favorite will satisfy your appetite and also leave you feeling light and energized, thanks to its vibrant mix of vegetables.

3 cups chopped peeled sweet potatoes

1 head cauliflower, cut into large florets

¼ cup garlic cloves

1 (14-ounce) block extra-firm tofu, drained

½ cup chopped fresh parsley

¼ cup nutritional yeast

1 tablespoon white miso paste

1 teaspoon chopped fresh oregano

½ teaspoon coarse sea salt

1 teaspoon freshly ground black pepper

1 recipe No-Oil Red Sauce (page 164)

1½ cups thinly sliced onions

16 whole-grain lasagna sheets (1 pound)

1 cup nondairy ricotta, such as Kite Hill

Put the sweet potato in a medium saucepan, add water to cover, and bring to a boil over high heat. Boil until the sweet potato is tender, 10 to 12 minutes. Drain and set aside to cool.

Place the cauliflower and garlic in the same saucepan, add fresh water to cover, and bring to a boil over high heat. Reduce the heat to medium-low and cook until the cauliflower is very tender, 10 to 12 minutes. Drain and set aside to cool.

Place the tofu in a large bowl and crumble it with your hands. Add the cooled sweet potato, cauliflower and garlic mixture, parsley, nutritional yeast, miso, oregano, salt, and pepper. With clean hands, mix the ingredients well, breaking them up until the mixture has the consistency of coarse ricotta cheese. Set aside.

Preheat the oven to 350°F. Spread 1 cup of the red sauce evenly over the bottom of a 13 by 9-inch baking dish. Arrange the onion slices in a layer over the sauce. Arrange a single layer of lasagna sheets to cover the entire bottom of the pan. Spread a thick (about ¾-inch) layer of the sweet potato mixture over the lasagna, then spread about 1½ cups of the red sauce over the sweet potato mixture. Repeat this layering two more times, for a total of four layers of lasagna noodles and three layers of filling. Top with a final layer of red sauce and sprinkle about ½ cup of the sweet potato mixture over the top.

Cover with parchment paper and aluminum foil and bake for 35 minutes. Uncover and bake for 10 minutes more to crisp the top. Remove from the oven and let cool for 20 minutes before slicing.

Scatter the ricotta over the top and serve with any remaining sauce on the side.

Per serving: 479 calories, 5 g total fat, 1 g saturated fat, 0 mg cholesterol, 737 mg sodium, 89 g total carbohydrate (12 g dietary fiber, 18 g sugar, 0 g added sugars), 22 g protein, 6 mg iron

Building the Perfect Stir-Fry

Stir-frying is one of the most popular high-heat cooking methods, and a great way to highlight seasonal, or even leftover, veggies! "Stir-fry" is another broad term that leaves plenty of room for culinary creativity. Use high heat with the proper pan, aromatics (ginger, onion, lemongrass, garlic, chiles, etc.), plenty of veggies, and a flavorful and punchy sauce. Choose to add some tofu or tempeh for extra protein if you like. You don't need oil—use the Dry Sauté Method (see page 78) to start your dish. Just keep a closer eye on the pan since it is on high heat. Make sure those onions don't burn!

The traditional and most effective pan to use with high heat is a wok. The sloped sides of the wok enable all the surfaces of the pan to be used in the cooking process. If you have an electric stove, you'll find a flat-bottomed wok to be more effective. As the vegetables cook, use a wooden spatula to push them around so they all touch the pan surface.

Stir-frying is the perfect example of why *mise en place* (see page 27) is critically important for the success of your dishes. With a high-heat cooking method, you can't afford to take time to prep your veggies as you go—you'll overcook the ones already in the pan. Have everything chopped and lined up before you start so all your attention can be at the stove.

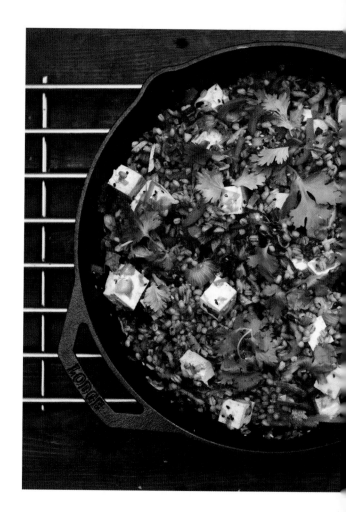

Saag & Tofu Paneer

Serves 4

This Indian-inspired recipe is one of John Mackey's favorites. It is quite simple to make, but it takes a lot of fresh spinach (*saag*) to get the right texture and flavor. Tofu substitutes well for the paneer cheese used in traditional recipes, as it has a similar texture and mild flavor. **Recipe by Dan Marek**

1 (14-ounce) block firm tofu, drained

1 cup unsweetened soy milk or other nondairy milk

½ (15-ounce) can coconut milk

2 tablespoons curry powder

1 teaspoon cayenne pepper

4 tablespoons fresh lemon juice

1 yellow onion, chopped

10 ounces fresh spinach

1 bunch mustard greens, trimmed

4 garlic cloves

1½ tablespoons minced fresh ginger

1 (6-ounce) can no-added-sodium tomato paste

1 teaspoon cumin seed

Wrap the drained tofu in a few layers of paper towels, then sandwich it between two plates and weight down the top plate with a heavy book. Press for at least 10 minutes and up to 1 hour.

Meanwhile, in a medium bowl, stir together the soy milk, coconut milk, curry powder, cayenne, and 2 tablespoons of the lemon juice.

Cut the pressed tofu into roughly ½ by 3-inch strips and place them in the bowl. Cover with the marinade and marinate in the refrigerator for at least 2 hours or up to overnight.

Preheat the oven to 350°F. Line a baking sheet with parchment.

Remove the tofu from the marinade, reserving the marinade. Place the tofu strips on the prepared baking sheet, leaving space between them (if they touch, they will stick together). Bake for 20 minutes, then flip the tofu slices using a spatula and bake until slightly firm to the touch, about 20 minutes more.

Meanwhile, heat a large sauté pan over medium-high heat. When hot, add the onion and dry sauté, stirring to prevent sticking, until translucent, about 4 minutes. Add 2 tablespoons water and stir to deglaze the pan. Remove from the heat and let cool slightly.

Bring a large pot of water to a boil. Submerge the spinach and mustard greens in the boiling water for 30 seconds. Remove with tongs and transfer to a food processor. Add the onion, garlic, ginger, tomato paste, cumin, remaining 2 tablespoons lemon juice, and the reserved marinade. Puree until mostly smooth.

Pour the spinach mixture back into the pan and reheat over low heat. Add the tofu strips and mix gently until coated and warmed through.

Serve hot.

Per serving: 254 calories, 8 g total fat, 1 g saturated fat, 0 mg cholesterol, 210 mg sodium, 25 g total carbohydrate (7 g dietary fiber, 11 g sugar, 0 g added sugars), 21 g protein, 10 mg iron

Stir-Fried Five-Spice Cauliflower

Serves 6

Five-spice powder is one of the essential base seasonings for Chinese cooking. It gives this dish a nice balance of sweet, savory, bitter, and sour flavors. A little goes a long way, so don't overseason. Remember, when stir-frying, all your ingredients should be prepped before you turn on the stove! Serve with rice or Asian noodles.

⅓ cup low-sodium tamari

1 tablespoon white wine or sherry

1 tablespoon date paste (see page 56)

1 teaspoon Chinese five-spice powder

1 head cauliflower, cut into bite-size florets

2 teaspoons white miso paste

6 mini bell peppers, sliced into thin rounds

1 onion, sliced lengthwise into strips

1 garlic clove, minced

¼ cup raw cashews

1 (5-ounce) can no-added-sodium sliced water chestnuts, drained

1 teaspoon cornstarch

2 green onions, chopped

1 teaspoon white and/or black sesame seeds

In a small bowl, stir together the tamari, wine, date paste, and five-spice powder. Place the cauliflower in a large zip-top bag and pour in the tamari mixture. Massage to coat the cauliflower, press out the air, and seal. Marinate in the refrigerator for 4 to 5 hours, tossing occasionally to coat.

In a small bowl or measuring cup, mix the miso with ½ cup hot water until dissolved. Set aside.

When ready to cook, heat a wok or large skillet over medium-high heat. When very hot, add the bell peppers and onion and dry sauté, stirring often, until they begin to stick to the pan and lightly brown, 2 to 3 minutes. Add the garlic and cook, stirring, for 1 minute. Pour in 1 to 2 tablespoons of the miso mixture and stir to deglaze the pan.

Add the cashews, water chestnuts, cauliflower, and half the marinade from the bag to the pan and simmer, stirring often, until the vegetables are tender but still slightly crunchy in the center, 2 to 3 minutes. Discard the remaining marinade. There should only be a little liquid left in the pan when the vegetables are done.

Stir the cornstarch into the remaining miso mixture and pour into the pan. Simmer until the liquid thickens enough to coat the back of a spoon, 3 to 4 minutes. Remove from the heat.

Transfer the mixture to a serving bowl and garnish with the green onions and sesame seeds.

Per serving: 106 calories, 3 g total fat, 1 g saturated fat, 0 mg cholesterol, 402 mg sodium, 17 g total carbohydrate (4 g dietary fiber, 7 g sugar, 0 g added sugars), 6 g protein, 2 mg iron

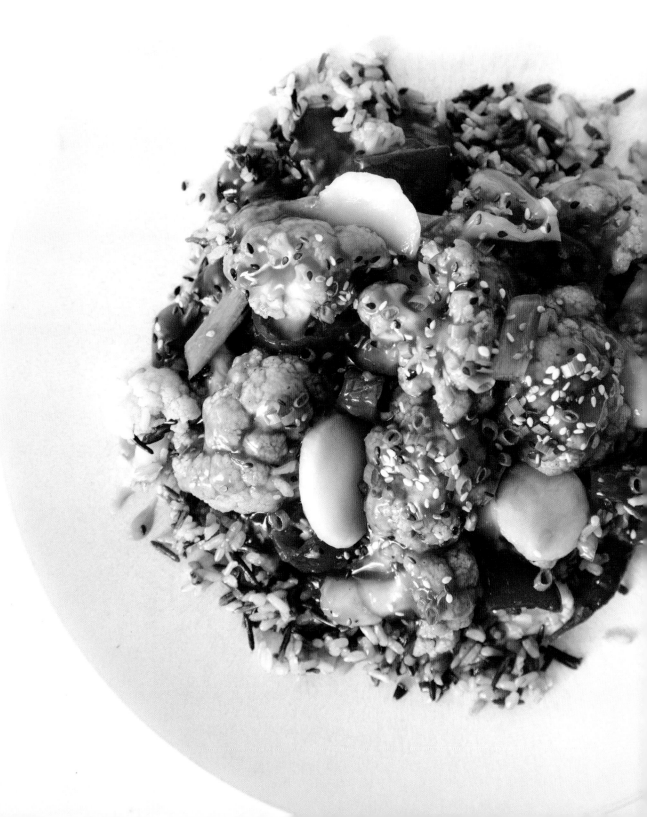

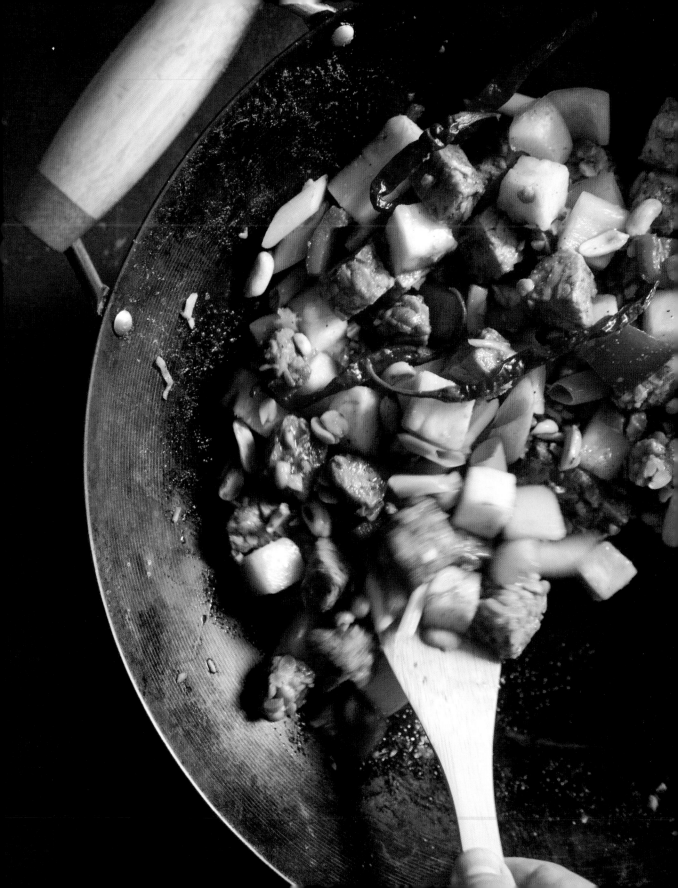

Kung Pao Tempeh with Pineapple

Serves 4

The marriage of sweet and sour flavors is one of the reasons so many of us love Chinese food. Here the sweetness is achieved with pineapple, and the acidity comes from the traditional Shaoxing wine, a form of sherry. The distinctive Chinese five-spice powder adds to the character of this stir-fry, along with fresh ginger, garlic, and chiles. If you want to enhance the spice or sweetness, bump up the chiles or pineapple.

8 ounces firm tempeh, cubed (about 2 cups)

2 teaspoons Chinese five-spice powder

2½ tablespoons cornstarch

1½ teaspoons onion granules

1 teaspoon garlic granules

½ teaspoon freshly ground black pepper

½ cup Shaoxing wine or dry sherry

½ cup low-sodium vegetable broth

1½ tablespoons low-sodium tamari

1 tablespoon minced fresh ginger

4 garlic cloves, minced

3 dried red chiles

3 cups chopped red and yellow bell peppers

1½ cups cubed fresh pineapple

¼ cup dry-roasted unsalted peanuts

¼ cup sliced green onions

Cooked brown rice (see page 36), for serving (optional)

Preheat the oven to 350°F. Line a baking sheet with parchment paper.

Steam cubed tempeh in a covered steamer basket over gently simmering water until just heated through, 4 to 5 minutes.

In a medium bowl, combine the five-spice powder, 1½ tablespoons of the cornstarch, the onion and garlic granules, and the black pepper. Add the tempeh, turning gently until well coated. Arrange the tempeh in a single layer on the prepared baking sheet and bake until crispy, about 20 minutes, turning once halfway through cooking. Remove from the oven.

In a small bowl, whisk together ¼ cup of the wine, the broth, tamari, ginger, garlic, and remaining 1 tablespoon cornstarch. Get the remaining ingredients prepped and ready to go if you haven't already.

Heat a wok or large sauté pan over high heat. When the pan is very hot, add the dried chiles and toast, tossing frequently, until fragrant, about 30 seconds. Add the bell peppers, pineapple, and crispy tempeh and toss. Cook, tossing frequently, until the ingredients start to stick to the pan, about 3 minutes. Add the remaining ¼ cup wine and cook for 2 minutes. Add the broth mixture, peanuts, and green onions and cook, stirring frequently, until the liquid thickens into a sauce, about 3 minutes.

Serve hot, over brown rice (optional).

Per serving: 334 calories, 11 g total fat, 2 g saturated fat, 0 mg cholesterol, 481 mg sodium, 35 g total carbohydrate (3 g dietary fiber, 18 g sugar, 0 g added sugars), 17 g protein, 3 mg iron

Constructing Whole Foodie Veggie Burgers

Burgers are an American favorite, and you don't have to give up that satisfying meal-in-a-bun just because you adopt a whole foods, plant-based diet. Luckily there are plenty of meat-free options available today. However, the veggie burgers you find in the freezer aisle are delicious but don't usually highlight whole foods and are often made from highly processed ingredients. If you have the time to make your own, you can choose all the ingredients going into your better burger, and ensure that they're made with whole ingredients: whole grains, beans, vegetables, and more. Plus, you'll get a nutritional powerhouse to throw on the grill or in the oven. You can also branch out beyond the basic burger and try some creative flavor combinations.

Our simple formula uses equal parts grains, beans, and veggies and a "binder" to hold it all together. Simply combine all the ingredients in a bowl, add herbs and spices, mix thoroughly, form into rounds, and bake. Top with your favorite condiments, fresh vegetables, and some fermented vegetables to add a tangy kick, and serve on a whole-grain bun. It's all about the fixins!

FIX YOUR OWN FAST FOOD

Fast food doesn't have to mean unhealthy food. Make extra burgers using one of the recipes in this section, and stack them with squares of parchment paper in between before freezing. When you need a meal in a hurry, you can grab one, pop it in the toaster or oven and reheat in minutes!

Mushroom & Barley Burgers

Serves 6

The time-tested combination of mushrooms and barley give these veggie burgers a meaty texture and rich umami flavor. This recipe requires some preparation time, but it's well worth the effort. You can get a jump on things by roasting the garlic a day ahead, or using garlic paste (pages 69 and 70) you've stored in the fridge or freezer.

½ yellow onion, chopped

8 ounces cremini (baby bella) mushrooms, chopped

8 ounces oyster mushrooms, chopped

½ teaspoon minced seeded jalapeño

1 teaspoon ground cumin

½ teaspoon fresh thyme leaves

¼ cup low-sodium vegetable broth

¼ cup walnuts

1 tablespoon onion granules

½ teaspoon sea salt

½ teaspoon freshly ground black pepper

3 tablespoons Roasted Garlic Paste (page 69)

2½ cups cooked barley (see page 36)

½ cup oat flour

¼ cup chopped fresh parsley

2 tablespoons potato starch or cornstarch

Heat a large sauté pan over medium-high heat. When hot, add the onion and dry sauté, stirring often, until it begins to stick to the pan and lightly brown, 3 to 4 minutes. Stir in both kinds of mushrooms, the jalapeño, cumin, and thyme and cook until the mushrooms release their liquid and begin to stick to the pan, 4 to 6 minutes. Add the broth and stir to deglaze the pan. Remove from the heat and set aside.

Put the walnuts, onion granules, salt, and pepper in a food processor and grind to a fine meal, about 1 minute. Transfer to a bowl.

Scrape the sautéed mushroom mixture into the food processor (no need to wash it first), add the roasted garlic paste, and blend to a coarse consistency, 1 to 2 minutes. Scrape the mixture into the bowl with walnut meal. Stir in the barley, oat flour, parsley, and potato starch. Mix well; it will be very thick. Cover and chill the mixture for 1 hour to help it firm up.

Preheat the oven to 375°F. Line a baking sheet with parchment paper.

Use your hands to compress and form the mixture into 6 patties. Place them on the prepared baking sheet and bake for 15 minutes. Flip each burger gently, then bake until the burgers have firmed up slightly, 10 to 15 minutes more.

To crisp them up, lightly coat a nonstick skillet with a little spray oil, set it over medium heat, and sear the burgers until crisp on both sides, 2 to 3 minutes per side.

Notes: You can roll this mixture into meatballs and bake them as described for the burgers.

Once baked, you can stack the burgers between squares of parchment or freezer paper and freeze them in zip-top bags for several months.

Per serving: 192 calories, 5 g total fat, 1 g saturated fat, 0 mg cholesterol, 245 mg sodium, 34 g total carbohydrate (5 g dietary fiber, 2 g sugar, 0 g added sugars), 6 g protein, 2 mg iron

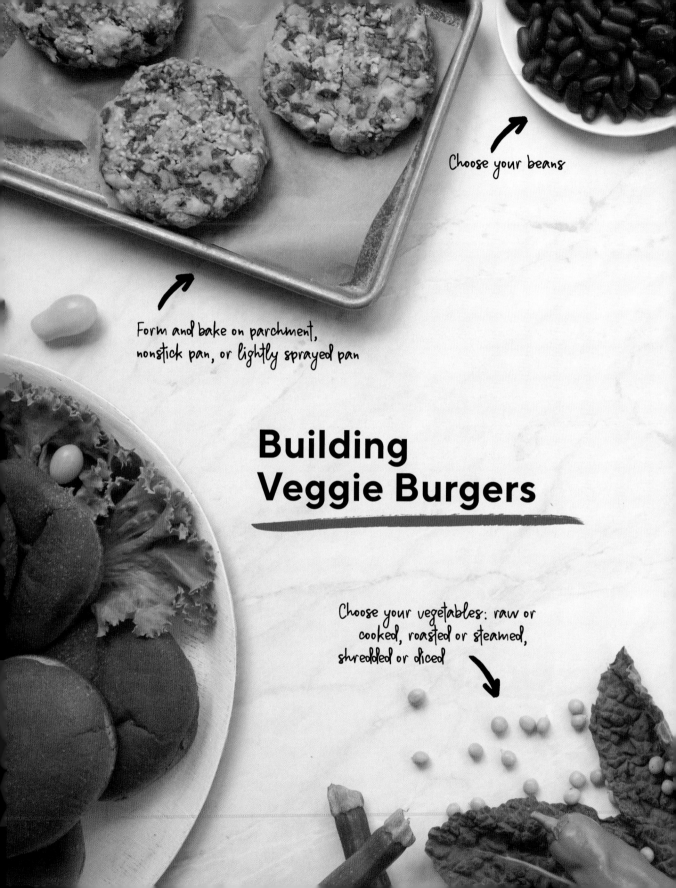

Choose your beans

Form and bake on parchment,
nonstick pan, or lightly sprayed pan

Building
Veggie Burgers

Choose your vegetables: raw or
cooked, roasted or steamed,
shredded or diced

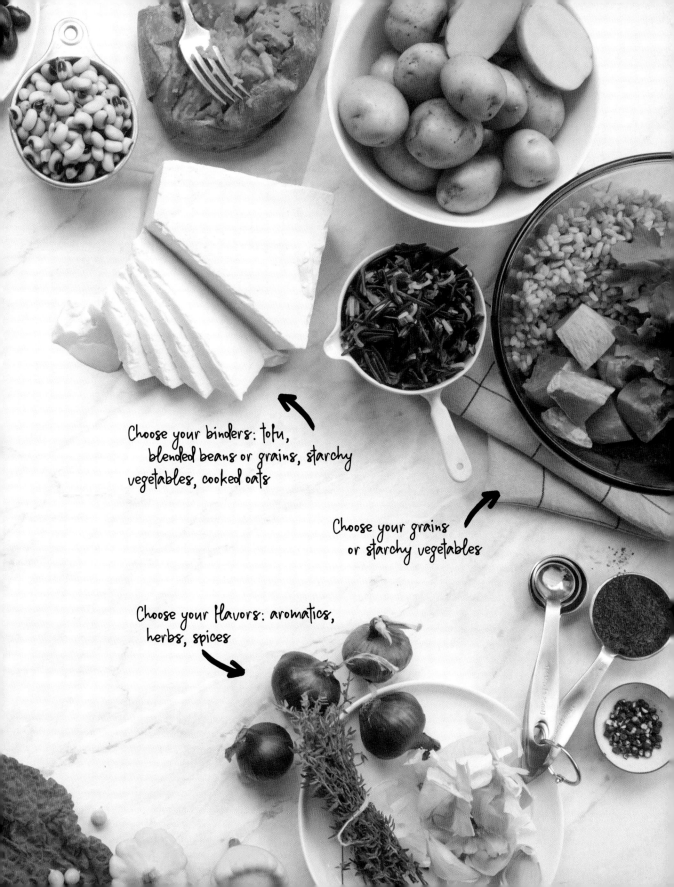

Choose your binders: tofu,
 blended beans or grains, starchy
vegetables, cooked oats

Choose your grains
 or starchy vegetables

Choose your flavors: aromatics,
 herbs, spices

Greek Burgers with Dill Hummus & Cucumber Relish

Serves 6

Plant-based burgers can be delicious and versatile, as this Mediterranean-inspired recipe demonstrates. For more flavor, slice the white onion into discs about ¼ inch thick and grill each disc just until grill marked on both sides, or add your favorite hot sauce or spicy pepper relish. You can make the burgers ahead of time, stack them between squares of parchment paper, and store them in a resealable bag. Refrigerate for up to 3 days or freeze for up to 1 month. Reheat the burgers in a nonstick pan, on the grill, or in a toaster oven.

BURGERS

1 cup cubed peeled russet potatoes

1 cup spinach

¼ cup raw cashews

¾ cup cooked white beans (see page 42) or canned no-added-sodium white beans, drained and rinsed

¼ cup chopped Kalamata olives

⅓ cup chopped roasted red bell peppers

2 tablespoons minced shallot

2 garlic cloves, minced

2 tablespoons minced fresh parsley

1 teaspoon minced fresh oregano

1 teaspoon paprika

½ teaspoon ground cumin

¼ teaspoon freshly ground black pepper

Sea salt, to taste (optional)

TO SERVE

6 soft whole wheat burger buns

1¼ cups Dill Hummus (page 262)

1¼ cups Cucumber Relish (page 228)

Harissa or red pepper relish of your choice (optional)

1 white onion, sliced paper-thin and rinsed

6 leaves butter lettuce

For the burgers, preheat the oven to 400°F. Line a rimmed baking sheet with parchment paper.

Steam the potatoes in a covered steamer basket over gently simmering water until tender, 10 to 12 minutes. Remove and set aside in a large bowl.

Steam the spinach until wilted and bright green, 1 to 2 minutes. Remove and set aside.

Grind the cashews into a fine meal using a food processor (not a high-speed blender, as this will puree the nuts).

Add the beans to the bowl with the potatoes and coarsely mash them together. Add the spinach, cashew meal, olives, roasted peppers, shallot, garlic, parsley, oregano, paprika, cumin, black pepper, and salt to taste and mix until everything is fully incorporated and the mixture holds together.

Using a ring mold, or by hand, form the mixture into burger-size patties and space them evenly on the prepared baking sheet.

Bake until the bottoms are golden brown, about 15 minutes. Flip, using a wide spatula, and bake until the other side is golden brown, 8 to 10 minutes more. Remove from the oven.

To serve, spread both sides of each bun with a generous amount of dill hummus. Place a burger on the bottom bun and top with cucumber relish, harissa (if using), onion, and lettuce.

Per serving: 387 calories, 13 g total fat, 2 g saturated fat, 0 mg cholesterol, 598 mg sodium, 54 g total carbohydrate (8 g dietary fiber, 6 g sugar, 0 g added sugars), 16 g protein, 4 mg iron

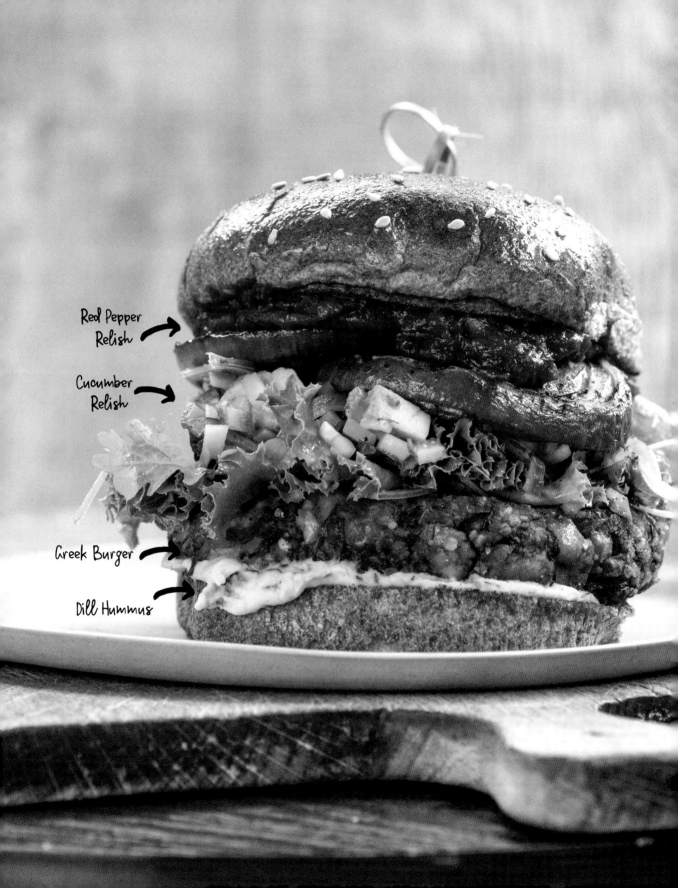

Red Pepper
Relish

Cucumber
Relish

Greek Burger

Dill Hummus

CUCUMBER RELISH

Light, zesty, and fragrant, this relish can be served on crackers and makes a great addition to the Greek Burgers on page 226. **Makes 1¼ cups**

1 cup finely chopped peeled cucumber

¼ avocado, finely chopped

2¼ teaspoons apple cider vinegar

1 tablespoon minced fresh shallot

1 tablespoon sliced fresh mint (leaves stacked and cut into thin strips)

¾ teaspoon grated lemon zest

¼ teaspoon sea salt

¼ teaspoon freshly ground black pepper

Combine all the ingredients in a small bowl, stirring gently to make sure the avocado stays intact. Serve as a condiment or enjoy with crackers or crostini.

Per serving (2 tablespoons): 9 calories, 0.6 g total fat, 0 g saturated fat, 0 mg cholesterol, 59 mg sodium, 1 g total carbohydrate (0 g dietary fiber, 0 g sugar, 0 g added sugars), 0 g protein, 0 mg iron

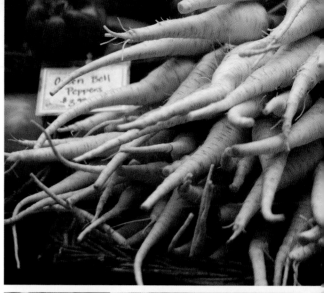

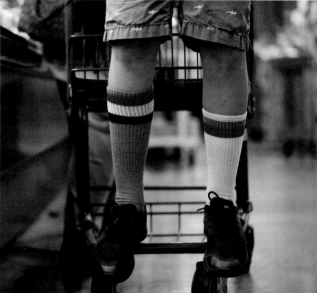

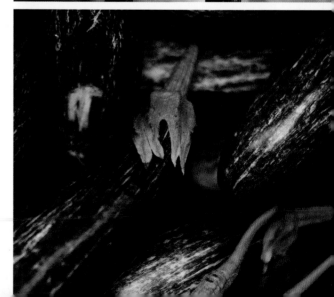

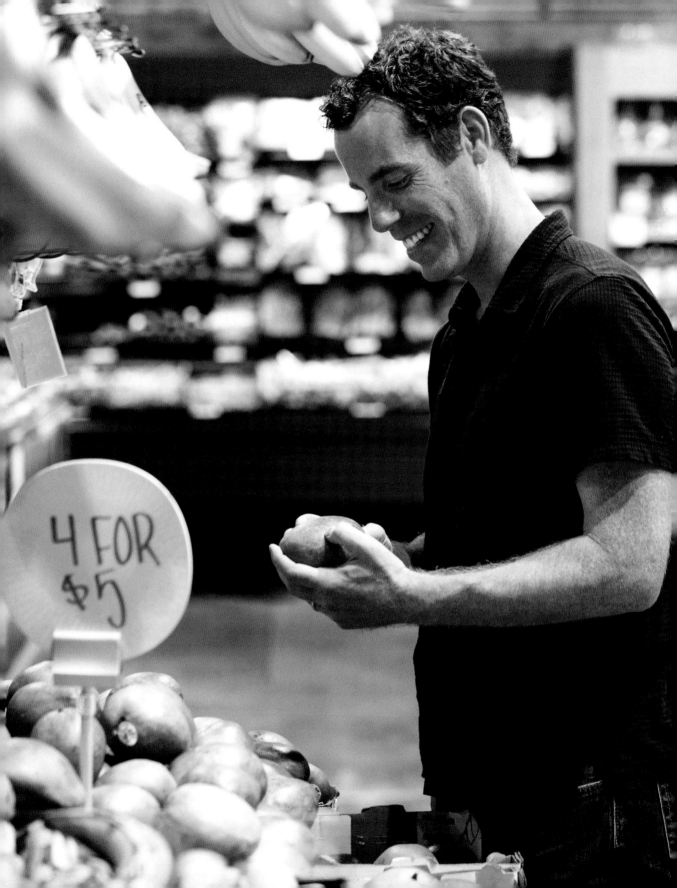

4 FOR
$5

Beet & Bean Burgers

Makes 4 sandwiches

There are so many ways to flavor these burgers. Add your favorite seasonings and vary the beans and veggies when you are familiar with the technique. After the burgers are baked, they can be frozen, so consider doubling the recipe to have a quick meal on hand any night of the week.

¾ cup chopped peeled sweet potato

1 large beet, peeled and shredded (about 2 cups)

1 (15-ounce) can no-added-sodium cannellini beans, drained and rinsed

½ cup old-fashioned rolled oats

2 teaspoons Bragg Liquid Aminos

Spray oil

½ teaspoon freshly ground black pepper

4 whole-grain burger buns, toasted

4 romaine lettuce leaves

4 thick tomato slices

4 thin red onion slices

Preheat the oven to 400°F. Line a baking sheet with parchment.

Steam the sweet potato in a covered steamer basket over gently simmering water until tender, 8 to 10 minutes.

In a medium bowl, stir together the shredded beet, beans, and steamed sweet potatoes. Roughly mash until the beets and sweet potato are evenly incorporated, leaving some chunks of beans in the mixture. Stir in the oats, liquid aminos, and pepper until thoroughly combined.

Form the mixture into four roughly ¾-inch-thick patties. Place the patties on the prepared baking sheet and bake until firm, 45 to 60 minutes.

Heat a large heavy skillet over medium heat. Coat it lightly with spray oil and add the baked burgers. Cook until crispy on both sides, 4 to 5 minutes per side.

Serve the burgers on the buns, with lettuce, tomato, and onion.

Notes: The sky's the limit with condiments: add grainy mustard, unsweetened ketchup, fermented pickles, sauerkraut, chopped avocado, sautéed mushrooms, or whatever you like best. The cooled burgers can be frozen in zip-top freezer bags (stack with squares of parchment paper in between) for up to 1 month. Thaw and cook in the pan as directed.

Per serving: 365 calories, 3 g total fat, 0 g saturated fat, 0 mg cholesterol, 429 mg sodium, 72 g total carbohydrate (15 g dietary fiber, 9 g sugar, 0 g added sugars), 18 g protein, 5 mg iron

Portobello Sliders with Date Mustard & Grilled Endive

Makes 4 sliders

Every now and then, it's nice to a have a veggie burger that's an actual vegetable instead of some form of processed soy. A charcoal grill is the perfect tool for getting smoky flavor on big, meaty mushroom caps marinated in soy sauce and garlic. Portobellos bring the savory, Belgian endive brings the bitter, mustard adds the sharp, and date tames this flavor-packed sandwich with a little sweetness.

¼ cup low-sodium tamari

2 tablespoons balsamic vinegar

2 garlic cloves, minced

4 small (3- to 4-inch diameter) portobello mushrooms caps

3 tablespoons Dijon mustard

½ teaspoon grated fresh horseradish or prepared horseradish

2½ tablespoons date paste (see page 56)

1½ teaspoons minced fresh chives

¼ teaspoon sea salt

¼ teaspoon freshly ground black pepper

Spray oil (for grill)

1 sweet onion, sliced into ¼-inch-thick rounds

2 Belgian endives, halved lengthwise

4 (3- to 4-inch diameter) whole-grain slider buns

¾ cup thinly sliced baby cucumbers

1 avocado, pitted, peeled, and sliced

8 cilantro sprigs

In a shallow bowl or zip-top bag, stir together the tamari, vinegar, and garlic. Add the mushrooms, coat with the marinade, cover or seal the bag, and let marinate at room temperature for at least 1 hour or up to overnight.

Meanwhile, in a small bowl, stir together the mustard, horseradish, date paste, chives, ⅛ teaspoon of the salt, and ⅛ teaspoon of the pepper. Set aside.

Heat a grill to medium-high. Lightly coat the grill grates with spray oil.

Season the onion and endive with the remaining ⅛ teaspoon salt and ⅛ teaspoon pepper. Remove the mushrooms from the marinade and discard the marinade. Grill the mushrooms, onion slices, and endive until nicely grill marked, 3 to 4 minutes per side. During the last minute, toast the buns cut-side down on the grill until golden. Set the buns aside. Transfer the vegetables to a cutting board and chop the endive.

To assemble each sandwich, spread some date mustard on a bun, then layer with a mushroom, an onion slice, some grilled endive, and some cucumbers. Spoon on a little more date mustard, then add the avocado and a couple sprigs of cilantro, and finally the bun top.

Per serving: 243 calories, 7 g total fat, 1 g saturated fat, 0 mg cholesterol, 658 mg sodium, 40 g total carbohydrate (7 g dietary fiber, 14 g sugar, 0 g added sugars), 7 g protein, 2 mg iron

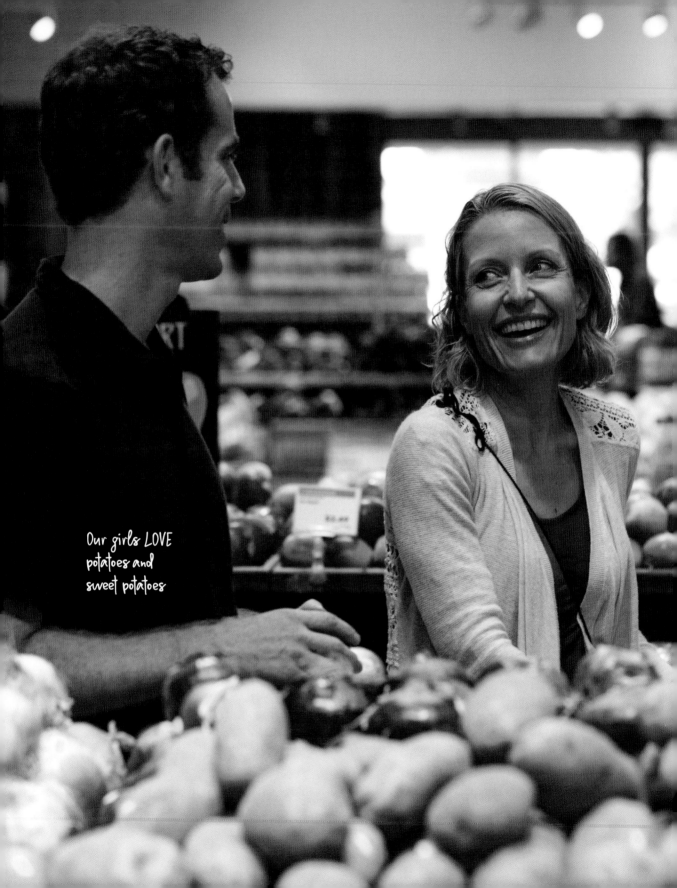

Our girls LOVE
potatoes and
sweet potatoes

Chili Cheeze Fries

Serves 6

Being plant-strong doesn't mean giving up satisfying comfort foods. If you like fries with your burgers, look no further. You won't believe this decadent recipe is 100% plant-strong goodness. Use sweet potatoes instead of russet potatoes, if you like. Serve with a heaping side of greens or a loaded salad! For a richer "cheese" sauce, see page 165. **Recipe by Rip Esselstyn & Ami Mackey of Engine 2**

RIP'S CHEEZE SAUCE

2 russet potatoes, scrubbed

2 large carrots, peeled and cut into a few pieces each

⅔ cup nutritional yeast

⅓ to ⅔ cup unsweetened almond milk or other nondairy milk

Juice of ½ lemon

2 teaspoons Bragg Liquid Aminos

2 teaspoons ground cumin

¼ to ½ teaspoon cayenne pepper

FRIES AND CHILI

6 large russet potatoes, scrubbed and cut into sticks

2 tablespoons salt-free Cajun seasoning

½ cup uncooked brown lentils, rinsed

¼ cup uncooked bulgur wheat

1 (15-ounce) can no-added-sodium black beans, drained and rinsed

½ (15-ounce) can no-added-sodium fire-roasted diced tomatoes, drained

1 tablespoon Bragg Liquid Aminos

1 tablespoon ground cumin

1 tablespoon chili powder

2 teaspoons smoked paprika

For the cheeze sauce, preheat the oven to 400°F.

Pierce potatoes a few times with a fork, then bake them directly on the oven rack until tender, 50 to 60 minutes. Let cool, then peel and discard the skins.

Meanwhile, steam the carrots in a covered steamer basket over gently simmering water until tender, 8 to 10 minutes. Transfer to a food processor or (preferably high-speed) blender. Add the cooked potatoes, nutritional yeast, ⅓ cup almond milk, the lemon juice, liquid aminos, cumin, and cayenne. Blend until smooth, adding a little more almond milk if the sauce is too thick. Use immediately or refrigerate for up to 3 days. Reheat before using.

For the fries and chili, preheat the oven to 425°F. Line two baking sheets with foil.

Coat the potato sticks all over with salt-free Cajun seasoning and arrange them in a single layer on the prepared baking sheets (use more baking sheets if needed to keep the potatoes in a single layer). Bake until brown and crispy, 25 to 35 minutes.

Meanwhile, combine the lentils, bulgur, and 2 cups water in a medium saucepan. Bring to a boil over high heat. Reduce the heat to low and simmer, uncovered, until the lentils are tender, 20 to 25 minutes. Drain any water remaining in the pot. Stir in the beans, tomatoes, liquid aminos, cumin, chili powder, and paprika. Simmer over low heat for 15 minutes.

Arrange the fries on a serving platter or large plate. Pour on the chili and cheese sauce and serve.

Per serving: 525 calories, 3 g total fat, 0 g saturated fat, 0 mg cholesterol, 359 mg sodium, 109 g total carbohydrate (18 g dietary fiber, 8 g sugar, 0 g added sugars), 21 g protein, 7 mg iron

Pizza Party

Who doesn't love pizza? The crispy crust topped with tangy tomato sauce makes a perfect platform to pack on the veggies! In the pages that follow, you can transform this guilty pleasure into a nutritious family feast. Use a whole-grain pizza dough (see recipe below; substitute a non-gluten whole-grain flour if gluten-free). If you don't have time to make your own dough, you can use store-bought frozen whole-grain pizza crusts, pita breads, tortillas, English muffins, whole-grain flatbread, or even a whole-grain baguette (see our mom's delicious recipe for a baguette pizza on page 237).

Whole Wheat Pizza Dough

Makes one big 16 × 8-inch crust

This simple whole wheat dough is used in the Very Veggie Pizza (page 240) and the Sweet Potato BBQ Pizza (page 238). Because the yeast needs a granulated sugar to activate, this recipe uses a small amount of date sugar, made of dried and ground dates, which you can find in the baking section of most natural foods markets. **Recipe by Jess Kolko**

1 (¼-ounce) package active dry yeast

1 tablespoon fine date sugar (see headnote)

3 cups white whole wheat flour, plus more for dusting

1 teaspoon sea salt

Spray oil

In a measuring cup or small bowl, combine 1 cup warm water, the yeast, and the sugar. Let sit until the yeast blooms and the mixture is foamy, about 10 minutes.

Combine the flour and salt in the bowl of a stand mixer. Attach the dough hook, add the yeast mixture, and mix on low speed until the mixture comes together into a dough and forms a ball around the hook, 3 to 4 minutes. If necessary, add more water 1 tablespoon at a time (up to 4 tablespoons) so the dough forms a ball.

Turn the dough out onto a work surface and knead by hand until it springs back lightly when pressed, 3 to 4 minutes. Lightly coat the mixer bowl with spray oil, return the dough to the bowl, and cover with a kitchen towel or plastic wrap. Let stand at room temperature until the dough doubles in size, 1 to 2 hours.

Use right away, store in the fridge in a zip-top bag for up to 5 days, or freeze for a couple of months.

Per serving: 192 calories, 1 g total fat, 0 g saturated fat, 0 mg cholesterol, 291 mg sodium, 41 g total carbohydrate (2 g dietary fiber, 2 g sugar, 2 g added sugars), 5 g protein, 3 mg iron

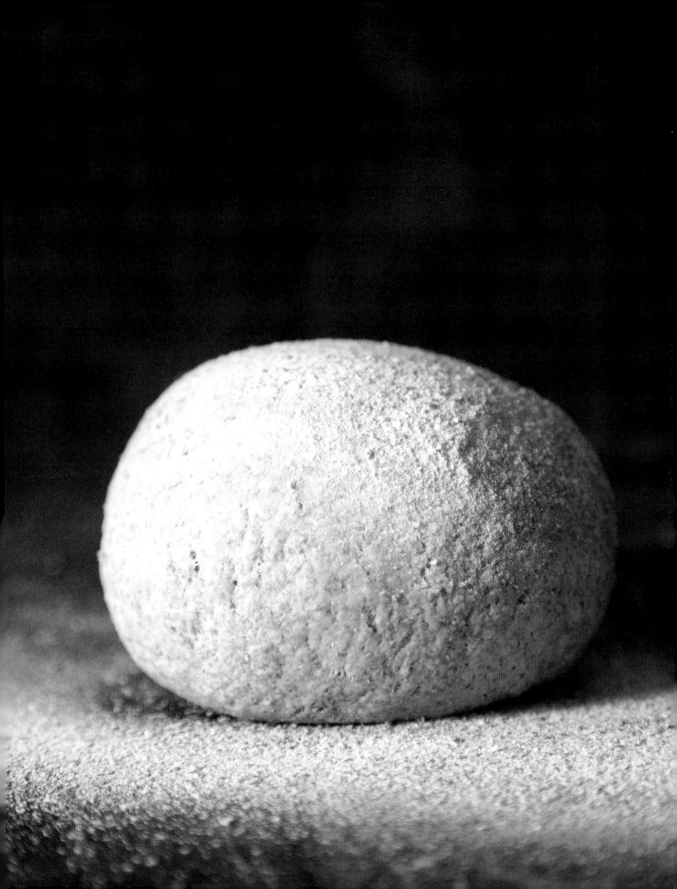

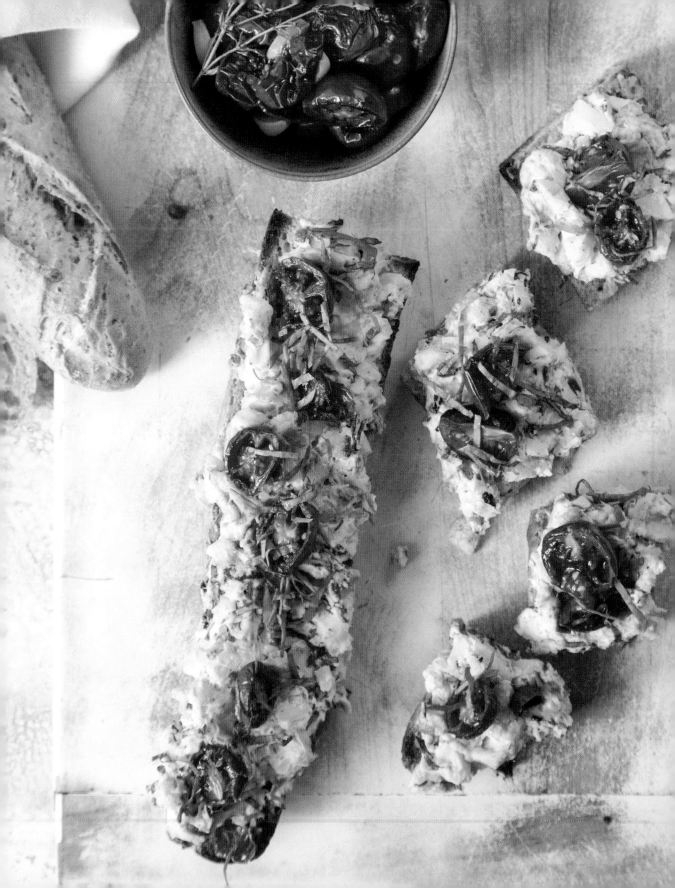

Baguette Pizza with Artichokes, Hearts of Palm, & Roasted Tomatoes

Serves 6 as an appetizer

This creamy topping of artichokes, hearts of palm, and spices is reminiscent of a classic seafood mix. For even more flavor, top with a few drained capers or shredded fresh basil. **Recipe by Beverly Burl, supermom extraordinaire**

1 recipe Roasted Cherry Tomatoes & Garlic (page 88)

1 (16-ounce) can no-added-sodium artichoke hearts, drained

1 (16-ounce) can no-added-sodium hearts of palm, drained

¼ cup Cashew Cream Cheese (page 264) or plain cream cheese

1 small red onion, chopped

¼ cup nutritional yeast

1 teaspoon kelp granules

½ teaspoon Old Bay seasoning

1 cup shredded spinach

1 whole-grain baguette, halved lengthwise

Make the Roasted Cherry Tomatoes & Garlic and have them ready to go. Keep the oven heated to 375°F.

Put the artichoke hearts and hearts of palm in a food processor and pulse a few times, just until chunky. Transfer to a medium bowl and mix in the cashew cream cheese, onion, nutritional yeast, kelp, and Old Bay. (This mixture can also be used as a dip or a sandwich spread.)

Fold in the shredded spinach and spread the artichoke mixture evenly over the cut side of each baguette half. Top with the roasted tomatoes and garlic.

Bake until heated through and the baguette is a bit browned in spots, 8 to 10 minutes.

Let cool slightly, then use a serrated knife to cut into 1-inch-wide slices. Serve.

Per serving (2 slices): 196 calories, 2 g total fat, 0 g saturated fat, 0 mg cholesterol, 328 mg sodium, 37 g total carbohydrate (6 g dietary fiber, 3 g sugar, 0 g added sugars), 9 g protein, 3 mg iron

Sweet Potato BBQ Pizza

Serves 8

This nontraditional pizza, with its sweet, earthy, and tangy flavors, is sure to surprise and delight! If you have a small pizza stone, you can divide the pizza dough in half and make two smaller round pizzas instead of one large rectangular one. It also helps to have all your sauces, dressings, and other ingredients prepped and ready to go before you start pressing out the pizza dough.

1 to 1½ cups Sweet BBQ Sauce (page 161)

1 recipe Whole Wheat Pizza Dough (page 234)

¾ cup shaved red onion

1 sweet potato, peeled and sliced into roughly ¼-inch-thick rounds

Whole grain flour, for dusting

Pinch of sea salt

¼ teaspoon freshly ground black pepper

½ cup thinly shaved red or green cabbage

¼ cup chopped fresh cilantro

1¼ cups Cashew Ranch Dressing (page 156; optional)

Make the BBQ sauce, cooking the sauce until it reduces to the consistency of thick ketchup.

Prepare the pizza dough or have it thawed and ready to go if it was frozen.

Position an oven rack 4 to 6 inches below the broiler and place a pizza stone on the rack. (If you don't have a pizza stone, you can use an upside-down baking sheet, but you'll need to increase the cooking time.) Preheat the oven to its highest temperature (usually 500 to 550°F) for 45 to 60 minutes.

Place the onion in a small bowl of ice water. Let stand at room temperature until you're ready to make pizza.

Steam the sweet potato coins in a covered steamer basket over gently simmering water until tender but not falling apart, 6 to 8 minutes. Remove from the heat and set aside.

Lightly flour a work surface and a wooden pizza peel or cutting board. Stretch the dough on the work surface into an oval or rectangle about 16 inches long and 8 inches wide. Transfer the dough to the pizza peel, reshaping it as necessary.

Drain the onion and pat it dry with paper towels.

Spread 1 cup of the BBQ sauce over the dough, then layer on the sweet potatoes and onion, and season with the salt and pepper.

Shake and slide the pizza onto the hot stone (or baking sheet) and bake for 2 minutes. Rotate the pizza and bake for 2 minutes more. (If using a baking sheet, double these baking times.) Switch on the broiler and broil the pizza until you see some char on the crust, 1 to 2 minutes.

Remove and top with the cabbage and cilantro. Slice and serve with ranch for dipping and additional BBQ sauce, if desired.

Per serving: 161 calories, 1 g total fat, 0 g saturated fat, 0 mg cholesterol, 425 mg sodium, 36 g total carbohydrate (5 g dietary fiber, 7 g sugar, 2 g added sugars), 5 g protein, 2 mg iron

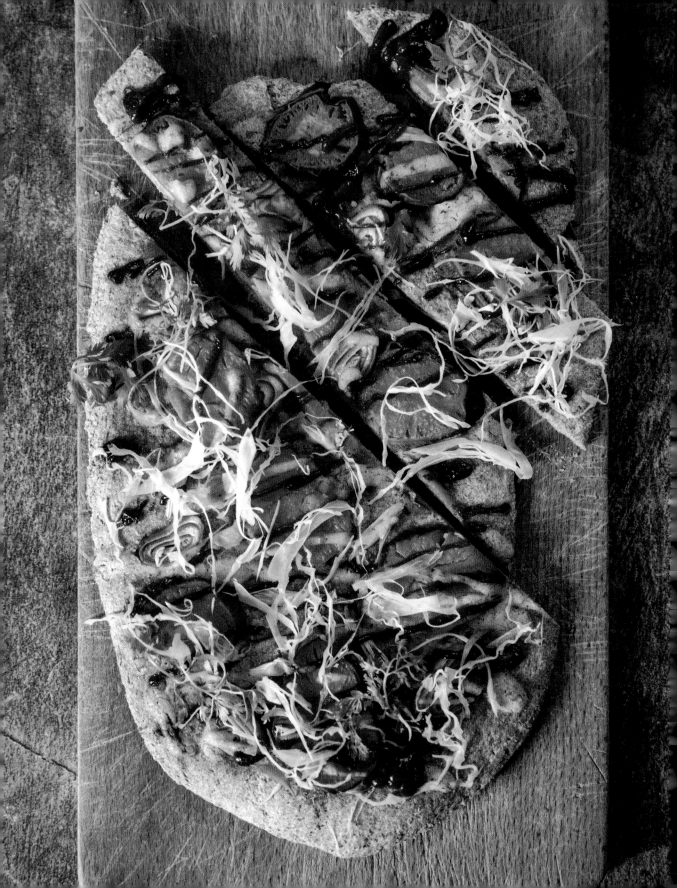

Very Veggie Pizza

Serves 8

How many veggies can you fit on one pizza? This versatile recipe gives you the opportunity to play with your favorites. Get the kids involved in choosing the toppings, too! **Recipe by Jess Kolko**

1 recipe Whole Wheat Pizza Dough (page 234)

1 (14-ounce) block extra-firm tofu, drained

1 cup small broccoli florets

Spray oil (for pan)

8 ounces sliced cremini (baby bella) or other mushrooms

2 cups baby spinach

Whole grain flour (for dusting)

½ to 1 teaspoon red pepper flakes (optional)

⅛ teaspoon sea salt

¾ cup No-Oil Red Sauce (page 164) or Roasted Red Pepper Sauce (page 167)

1 small red bell pepper, seeded and sliced

½ small red onion, sliced

Basic Cashew Cream Sauce (page 165) or Rip's Cheeze Sauce (page 233) (optional)

Prepare the pizza dough or have it thawed and ready to go if it was frozen.

Position an oven rack 4 to 6 inches below the broiler and place a pizza stone on the rack. (If you don't have a pizza stone, you can use an upside-down baking sheet, but you'll need to increase the cooking time.) Preheat the oven to its highest temperature (usually 500 to 550°F) for 45 to 60 minutes.

Meanwhile, wrap the drained tofu in a few layers of paper towels, then sandwich it between two plates and weight down the top plate with a heavy book. Press for at least 10 minutes and up to 1 hour.

Set up a bowl of ice water. Steam the broccoli in a covered steamed basket over gently simmering water until crisp-tender, 2 to 3 minutes. Transfer the broccoli to the ice water to stop the cooking. Let sit for 2 minutes, then drain and set aside.

Cut the pressed tofu into bite-size cubes. Heat a large nonstick skillet over medium heat. When hot, coat lightly with spray oil and add the tofu. Cook, turning often, until browned all over, 10 to 12 minutes. Remove from the pan and set aside.

Return the pan to medium heat and add the mushrooms. Dry sauté, stirring often, until the mushrooms release their liquid and the liquid evaporates, 5 to 6 minutes. Add a splash of water and stir to deglaze the pan, then stir in the spinach and remove from the heat. Stir in the steamed broccoli, red pepper flakes, and salt.

Lightly flour a work surface and a wooden pizza peel or cutting board. Stretch the dough on the work surface into an oval or rectangle about 16 inches long and 8 inches wide.

Transfer the dough to the pizza peel, reshaping it as necessary. Spread the sauce on the dough, then the tofu, then the bell pepper and onion, and finally the broccoli and spinach. If you're using cashew cream sauce or cheeze sauce, drizzle a small amount over the vegetables.

Shake and slide the pizza onto the hot stone (or baking sheet) and bake for 2 to 3 minutes. Rotate the pizza and bake for 2 to 3 minutes more. (If using a baking sheet, double these baking times.) Switch on the broiler and broil the pizza until you see some char on the crust, 1 to 2 minutes.

Remove from the oven, let cool slightly, then slice and serve.

Per serving: 232 calories, 4 g total fat, 1 g saturated fat, 0 mg cholesterol, 371 mg sodium, 40 g total carbohydrate (6 g dietary fiber, 3 g sugar, 2 g added sugars), 12 g protein, 3 mg iron

Get Your Kids Involved with a Pizza Bar

Children are much more likely to eat food they've had a hand in making. Pizza night is a great opportunity to get the little ones in the kitchen. Here's how you can set up your pizza bar:

- Divide your Whole Wheat Pizza Dough (page 234) into individual-size pizzas, or choose a ready-made base like whole grain pita bread, English muffins, or halved baguettes.

- Prepare one or two sauces (try No-Oil Red Sauce, page 164, or Roasted Red Pepper Sauce, page 167).

- Slice up lots of veggies – peppers, tomatoes, onions, zucchini, mushrooms, and more

- Crumble some tofu or choose a nondairy cheese, such as Kite Hill ricotta or Miyoko's mozzarella

- Challenge your kids to make the most colorful pizza! Bake and enjoy.

Taco Tuesday

Interactive, fun, and healthy, Taco Tuesday is one of our favorite nights of the week. Tacos are a great family food—kids will have fun adding toppings and getting their hands messy, all while nourishing themselves with wholesome veggies, grains, beans, and more. And while we love the traditional rice, beans, and salsa, we also enjoy mixing it up and filling our tortillas with flavors from around the world. We hope the recipes in this section will spark your imagination and make you think fresh about what can go in this handheld favorite.

Sweet Potato Enchiladas with Jalapeño Cashew Sour Cream

Serves 6

Soft tacos, filled with flavorful sweet potatoes, corn, and zucchini, smothered in delicious spicy ranchero sauce and baked to perfection—what could be better? You can make the ranchero sauce and cashew sour cream ahead of time and refrigerate them for a few days, and if you find that you have extra, serve them with tortilla chips as a snack!

ENCHILADA FILLING

2 to 3 small zucchini, cut into ¼-inch-thick half-moons (2 cups)

2 cups cubed peeled sweet potatoes

1 cup fresh or frozen corn kernels

1 onion, finely chopped

¼ cup sliced black olives

½ cup chopped fresh flat-leaf parsley

1 tablespoon ground cumin

1 teaspoon freshly ground black pepper

¾ teaspoon granulated garlic

¾ teaspoon granulated onion

½ teaspoon sea salt

½ cup low-sodium vegetable broth

RANCHERO SAUCE

1 (28-ounce) can no-salt-added tomatoes, buzzed in blender until smooth

1 (4-ounce) can green Hatch chiles

¼ cup no-added-sodium tomato paste

1 onion, finely chopped

1 green bell pepper, chopped

1 jalapeño, seeded and chopped

1 tablespoon ground cumin

1 tablespoon minced garlic

½ cup chopped fresh cilantro

½ teaspoon freshly ground black pepper

½ teaspoon sea salt

TO ASSEMBLE

12 corn or whole-grain flour tortillas

Jalapeño Cashew Sour Cream (page 160)

Chopped seeded jalapeño

Chopped fresh cilantro

1 lime, cut into wedges

For the enchilada filling, preheat the oven to 375°F. Line a baking sheet with parchment.

Toss all the filling ingredients together in a large bowl until well coated. Spread the mixture over the prepared baking sheet and roast until browned and soft enough to cut with a fork, 35 to 45 minutes, stirring several times during the cooking time. Remove from the oven and cover to keep warm.

For the ranchero sauce, combine all the sauce ingredients in a medium saucepan and cook over medium-low heat, stirring frequently, for 30 to 35 minutes. Remove from the heat and set aside.

To assemble, warm the tortillas directly over a gas flame on the stovetop or in a hot skillet. Spread about ½ cup of the filling in the center of a tortilla, then fold the sides of the tortilla over the filling. Place two enchiladas on a plate, seam-side down, and smother with ranchero sauce and Jalapeño Cashew Sour Cream. Garnish with jalapeño and cilantro.

Serve with lime wedges for squeezing.

Note: To fill out the meal, serve with stewed black beans and cooked brown rice. For the beans, sauté an onion in a medium saucepan over medium heat, then add 2 (14-ounce) cans black beans (drained and rinsed), a big pinch of granulated garlic, a small pinch of smoked paprika, and about ½ cup vegetable broth. Bring to a boil, then simmer over low heat for 15 minutes. Serve the beans and about 6 cups cooked brown rice alongside the enchiladas.

Per serving: 389 calories, 11 g total fat, 1 g saturated fat, 0 mg cholesterol, 772 mg sodium, 58 g total carbohydrate (8 g dietary fiber, 13 g sugar, 0 g added sugars), 12 g protein, 5 mg iron

It's All About the Salsa!

Zesty, delicious salsa brings tacos alive. You can buy it ready made (choose a brand with no added oil or sugar) but it's so much better made fresh. If you have time, make your salsa a couple of hours ahead of the meal and chill so that the flavors can marry.

Start with a simple, traditional "salsa pico" with fresh, ripe chopped tomatoes, finely chopped red onion, chopped fresh cilantro, lime juice, and sea salt. Add seeded chopped jalapeño if you like it hot. Throw in some cubed avocado to vary the texture.

Or, try our Avocado Salsa (page 246) or Grilled Peach Salsa (page 256).

Get creative and invent your own! Try other fruits like mango or papaya, experiment with different peppers and herbs, add a dash of citrus. The key to a great salsa is to combine sweet, sour, and heat.

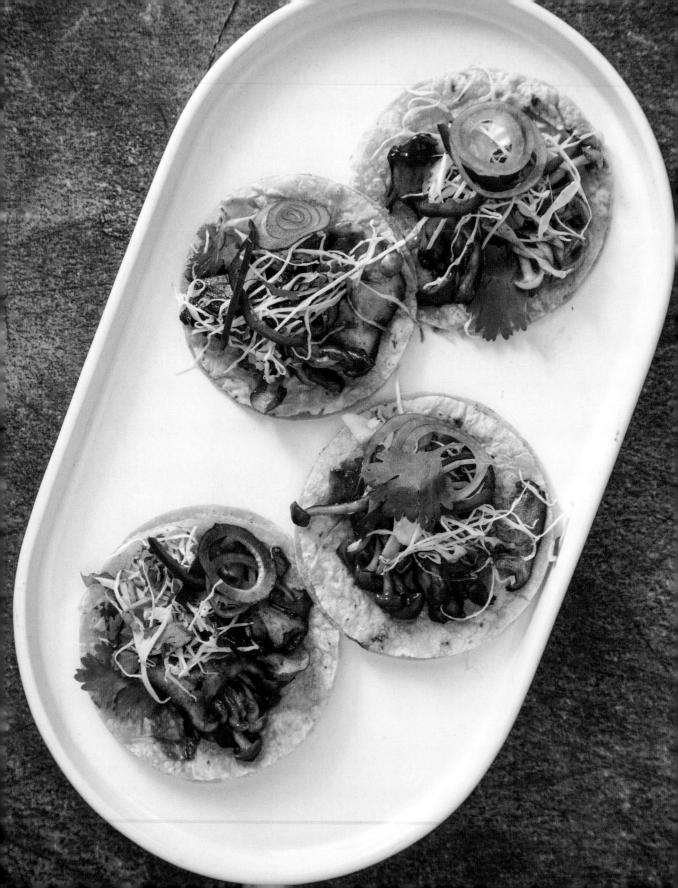

Roasted Mushroom Tacos with Asian BBQ Sauce & Wine-Pickled Onions

Serves 4

Tacos don't have to be limited to traditional Mexican fillings! This recipe gives an Asian twist to the family favorite. Wild mushrooms come in many shapes and sizes—you can use smaller varieties whole, tear the "clustered" varieties like oyster or maitake, and slice larger varieties. You'll want to prepare the pickled onions in advance, since they need to soak for at least four hours.

WINE-PICKLED ONIONS

3 red onions, sliced paper-thin on a mandoline

½ cup red wine vinegar or merlot vinegar

1½ tablespoons apricot paste (see page 56)

¼ teaspoon coarse sea salt

MUSHROOM TACOS

1½ pounds mixed wild mushrooms

1 large onion, cut into matchsticks

1½ cups Asian BBQ Sauce (page 161)

½ large head green cabbage, cut into long, thin strips

Juice of 1 lime

¼ teaspoon sea salt

1 cup fresh cilantro leaves

8 corn tortillas

For the onions, combine all the ingredients in a medium bowl and rub together gently. Set aside to pickle at room temperature for at least 4 hours and up to overnight. Use immediately or refrigerate in a sealed container for up to 1 week.

For the mushrooms, preheat the oven to 375°F. Line a baking sheet with parchment paper.

In a large bowl, combine mushrooms and onion with ¾ cup of the BBQ sauce and mix until coated. Spread the mixture over the prepared baking sheet and roast for 30 minutes, stirring a few times for even cooking. Transfer to a serving bowl.

In a separate bowl, toss together the cabbage, lime juice, salt, and ½ cup of the cilantro.

To assemble, warm the tortillas directly over a gas flame on the stove or in a hot skillet. Add a good-size pinch of the cabbage mixture, then a good-size portion of the BBQ mushrooms, an extra drizzle of BBQ sauce, some onions, and more cilantro leaves. Serve.

Note: Here are some more taco garnishes to try: lime wedges for squeezing, chopped cucumber tossed with chopped fresh mint, paper-thin jalapeño slices, diced avocado tossed with lime juice, Jalapeño Cashew Sour Cream (page 160).

Per serving: 336 calories, 3 g total fat, 0 g saturated fat, 0 mg cholesterol, 602 mg sodium, 72 g total carbohydrate (12 g dietary fiber, 23 g sugar, 0 g added sugars), 11 g protein, 3 mg iron

Rye Tacos with Slow-Roasted Beets & Avocado Salsa

Serves 3

The sweet, smoky beets in this recipe pair beautifully with the soft, earthy rye taco, and the salsa brings a light, fresh finish to the dish. While the beets are roasting, you can prepare everything else. **Recipe by Hiram Camillo**

ROASTED BEETS

5 large beets or 12 baby beets (2-inch diameter), scrubbed, tops removed

TORTILLAS

1 cup filtered water

⅓ cup plus ¼ cup rye flour

1 green onion, thinly sliced

3 large garlic cloves, minced

⅛ teaspoon sea salt

Spray oil (for pan)

AVOCADO SALSA

½ red onion, coarsely chopped

½ large avocado, pitted, peeled, and coarsely chopped

8 cilantro sprigs

3 large garlic cloves, chopped

2 to 3 large jalapeños, seeded and coarsely chopped

2 teaspoons distilled white vinegar

¼ teaspoon sea salt

TOPPINGS

¼ cup thinly sliced red onion

2 baby beets, such as golden or Chioggia, scrubbed, tops removed

1 lime, cut into 6 wedges

For the roasted beets, preheat the oven to 400°F. Line a baking sheet with parchment. Place the scrubbed beets on the pan and roast for 3 hours (1½ hours for baby beets), turning the beets halfway through cooking, until fork-tender, shriveled, and slightly crispy and charred on the exterior. Remove from the oven and let cool. When cool enough to handle, slice into bite-size pieces.

Meanwhile, for the tortillas, in a medium bowl, whisk together the water, flour, green onion, garlic, and salt. The mixture should have the consistency of thick pancake batter.

Heat a low-sided medium sauté pan or tortilla pan over medium heat. When hot, lightly coat the pan with spray oil. Use a rounded ladle or spoon to ladle ¼ cup of the batter into the pan, then quickly spread the batter with the ladle or spoon until it is 4 to 5 inches in diameter. Cook until the edges begin to dry, 1 to 2 minutes per side. The tortilla should have black or dark brown spots throughout. Transfer the tortilla to a plate covered with a clean kitchen towel and wrap to keep warm, or use a tortilla holder. Repeat with the remaining batter. Let the tortillas steam in the towel or holder for 10 minutes so they become pliable.

For the salsa, in a food processor, combine the onion, avocado, cilantro, garlic, jalapeños, vinegar, and salt and pulse until finely chopped but not completely pureed, 30 to 60 seconds total, stopping to scrape down the bowl once or twice.

To assemble the tacos, divide the roasted beets, sliced onion, and salsa among the tortillas. Use a mandoline to shave the golden or Chioggia beets into paper-thin slices over each taco for more crunch and color. Add a squeeze of lime, fold in the sides, and roll up to enclose.

Per serving: 418 calories, 12 g total fat, 1 g saturated fat, 0 mg cholesterol, 621 mg sodium, 73 g total carbohydrate (18 g dietary fiber, 27 g sugar, 0 g added sugars), 12 g protein, 6 mg iron

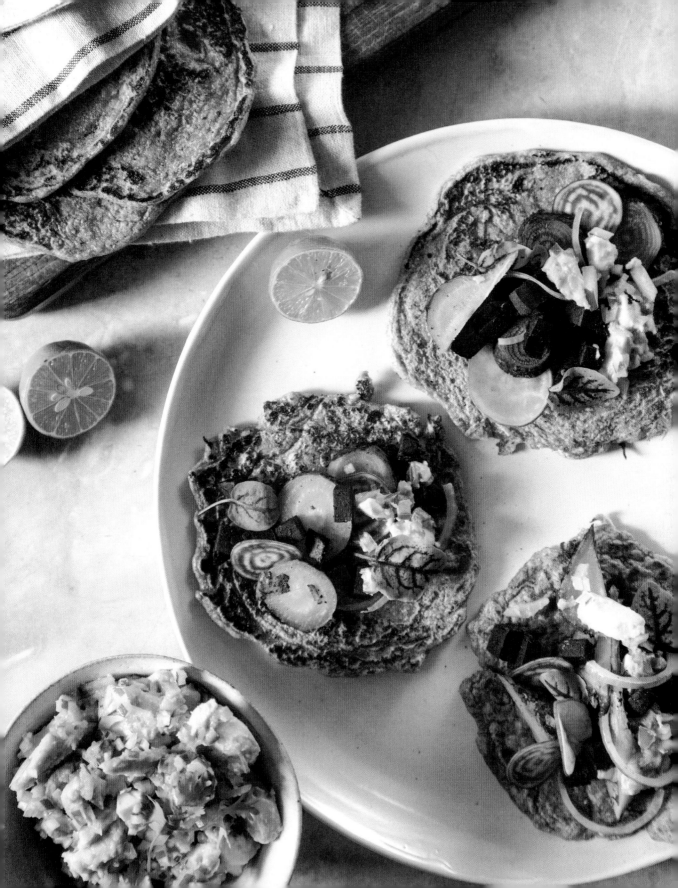

CHAPTER 13

Entertaining with Whole Foods

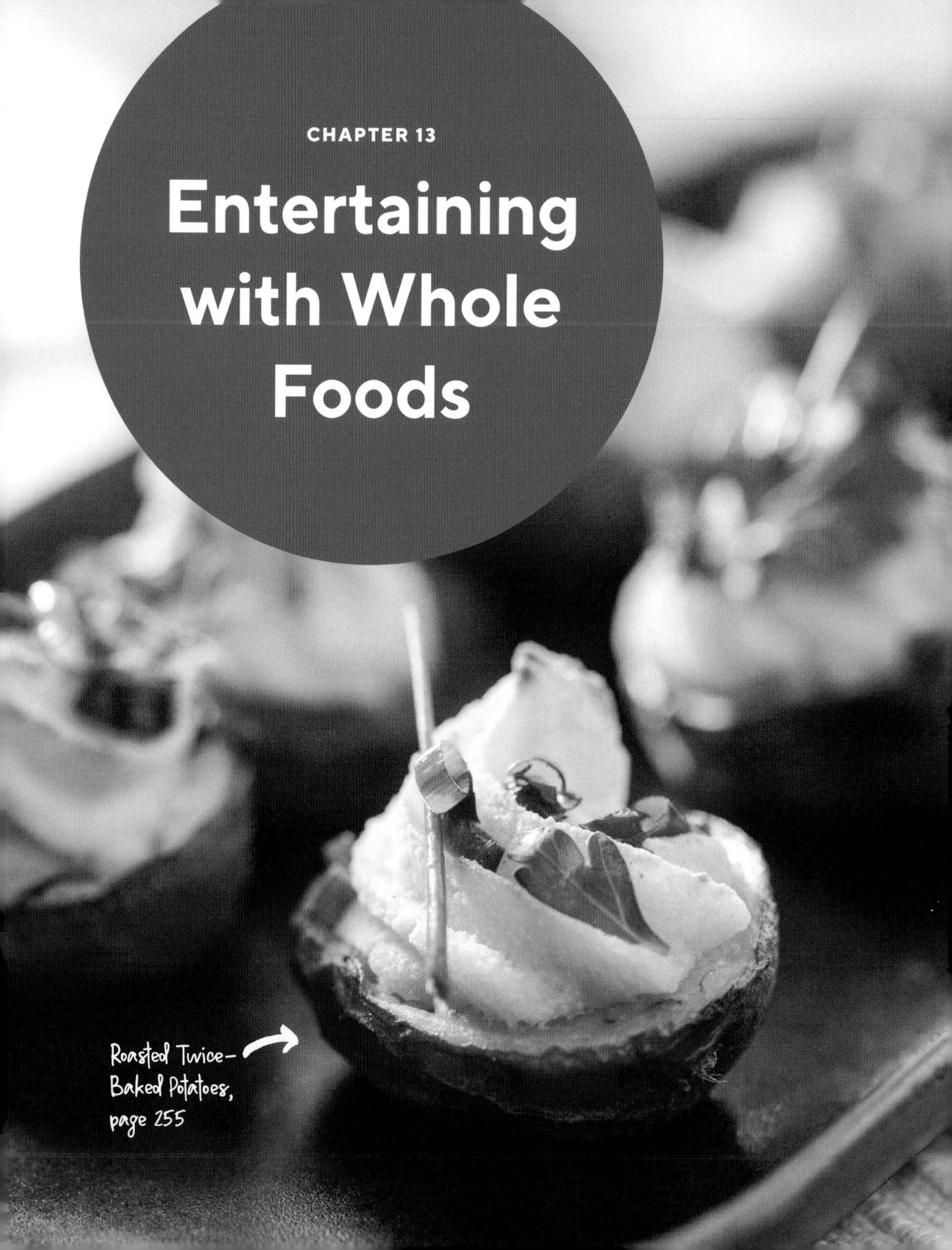

Roasted Twice-
Baked Potatoes,
page 255

Want to amaze your friends? Invite them to a dinner, garden party, or reception where every dish is made from whole, plant foods, and all are delicious *and* nutritious! From small bites to multicourse feasts, you can combine the recipes in this book to create your perfect party menu. At the end of this chapter, you'll find some suggested themed menus that will make every dinner party and event special.

Small Bites

If you're having a cocktail party or a casual reception, small bites can make a big impression. What better way to kick off a dinner party than with some delicious snacks, canapés, or appetizers to welcome your guests? The following recipes are sure to nourish and entertain without requiring anyone to sit down.

Easy Roasted Vegetable Bites

Roasted veggies cut in bite-size pieces and cubed marinated tofu or tempeh make great party foods, especially when jazzed up with a spice blend. See page 87 for instructions and roasting times and try Mum's Spice Blend (page 67) for a flavor-packed coating.

Try a variety of mushrooms, broccoli or cauliflower florets, cubed sweet potato, or baby sweet peppers. Serve on skewers or with cocktail sticks for handheld eating, and add a dipping sauce such as Asian BBQ Sauce (page 161) or Almond-Chile Sauce (page 158)

Tofu Bites

Serves 8

Reminiscent of a tater tot, these crispy tofu cubes make a great snack, appetizer, or party bite. Serve with your favorite dipping sauce. After breading each cube, you could skewer a few for easy party serving. You can also add these to your favorite salad or stir-fry, so be sure to make extra!

½ cup nutritional yeast

1½ tablespoons cornstarch

1 tablespoon ground cumin

1 tablespoon chili powder

1 tablespoon onion powder

1 tablespoon garlic powder

1 teaspoon poultry seasoning

1 teaspoon smoked paprika

1 teaspoon freshly ground black pepper

½ teaspoon sea salt

2 (14-ounce) blocks extra-firm tofu, drained and cut into 1-inch cubes

½ cup lightly packed fresh cilantro leaves

1 small red chile, thinly sliced (optional)

1 cup Rip's Cheeze Sauce (page 233) or your favorite BBQ sauce

Preheat the oven to 350°F. Line a rimmed baking sheet with parchment paper.

In a food processor, combine the nutritional yeast, cornstarch, cumin, chili powder, onion powder, garlic powder, poultry seasoning, smoked paprika, black pepper, and salt and pulse until blended, 20 to 30 seconds. Transfer to a large bowl.

Add the tofu cubes to the bowl and gently roll in the seasoning mixture until evenly coated. Transfer to the prepared baking sheet in a single layer, leaving a little space between each cube.

Bake until lightly browned on the bottom, about 15 minutes. Flip the cubes over with tongs and bake until the second side is lightly browned and crisp, 10 to 15 minutes more. Transfer to a bowl and toss with cilantro and chiles (if using).

Serve with Rip's Cheeze Sauce alongside for dipping.

Per serving: 169 calories, 8 g total fat, 1 g saturated fat, 0 mg cholesterol, 202 mg sodium, 9 g total carbohydrate (2 g dietary fiber, 1 g sugar, 0 g added sugars), 15 g protein, 3 mg iron

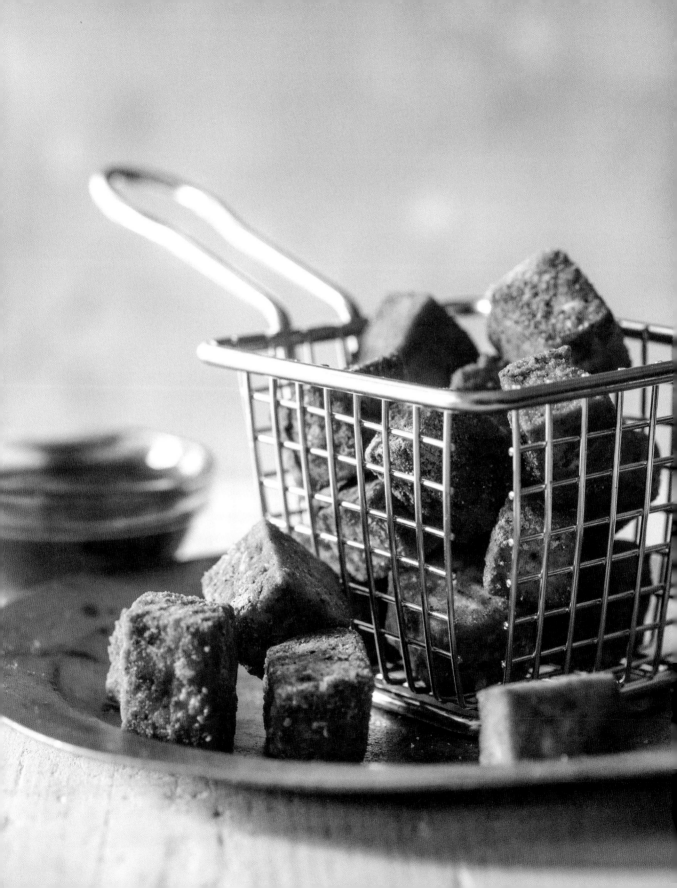

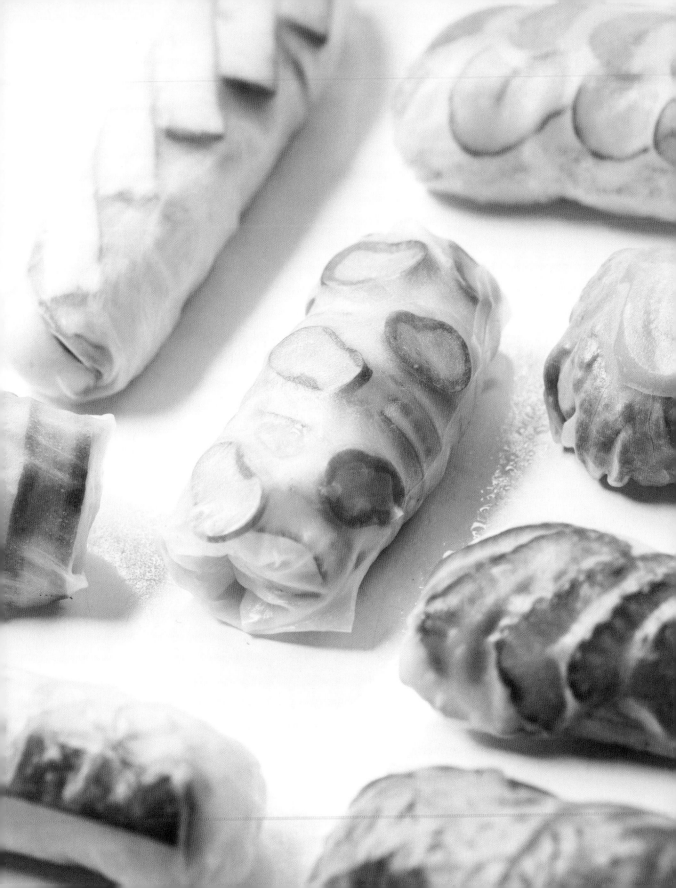

Summer Rolls for All Seasons

A great handheld starter, offering endless opportunities to highlight seasonal fruit and vegetables. Get creative with your own combinations of the ingredients listed below.

Rice paper wrappers

Rice noodles, spiralized zucchini, cucumber, daikon, coconut, or other vegetable noodles

Marinated or raw sliced vegetables, fruits, tofu, or tempeh

Fresh herbs (mint, cilantro, Thai basil, etc.), chiles, toasted nuts or seeds

Condiments such as hot sauce, miso, or Fruit Paste (page 56)

Dipping sauces such as Almond-Chile Sauce (page 158), Citrus-Miso Dressing (page 156), or Spicy BBQ Tahini Sauce (page 158)

Combination Suggestions

- Baked tofu, sprouts, and chiles
- Sliced beets, orange, and greens
- Purple cabbage, toasted sesame, miso paste
- Cucumber, daikon, and chiles
- Shiitake, shallot, and greens
- Avocado, radish, and cilantro
- Carrot Lox (page 101), olives, arugula
- Kiwi, mint, and cucumber
- Sliced strawberries and basil

Fill a medium sauté pan or pie pan with warm water. For each summer roll, dip a rice paper wrapper into the water, coating it completely. Transfer the wrapper to a work surface and let soften for 1 minute (don't leave in water or it will become unusable).

On the bottom third of the paper, stack up layers of noodles, sliced raw vegetables or fruits, herbs and nuts or seeds, and condiments.

Wet your fingers to prevent sticking. Fold the bottom of the paper up and over the filling. Fold in the sides, then roll away from you to enclose the filling. Place the roll seam-side down on a platter and repeat with the remaining ingredients, leaving a little space between each roll on the platter.

Serve with your favorite dipping sauce.

Herbed Apricot & Water Chestnut Lettuce Wraps

Serves 4

These lettuce wraps are simple to put together but make a big impression—perfect for a summer party when stone fruits are in season. Ripe apricots have a lovely warm sweetness with a touch of citrus. You can try using peaches, plums, or nectarines as well.

8 ripe yet firm apricots, pitted and cubed

½ cup chopped water chestnuts

3 tablespoons minced green onion

3 tablespoons chopped fresh cilantro

1 tablespoon chopped fresh mint

½ teaspoon minced red chile

Juice of ½ lime

1 head butter lettuce, leaves separated

¼ cup Citrus-Miso Dressing (page 156)

¼ cup chopped unsalted dry-roasted peanuts or almonds

In a medium bowl, toss the apricots, water chestnuts, green onion, cilantro, mint, chile, and lime juice until combined.

In each lettuce leaf, place a few tablespoons of the apricot mixture. Drizzle with the dressing and garnish with the nuts. Roll up and enjoy.

Notes: For more flavor, halve the apricots, remove the pits, and grill the halves before cubing them.

You can replace the citrus-miso dressing with Almond-Chile Sauce (page 158).

Per serving: 127 calories, 5 g total fat, 1 g saturated fat, 0 mg cholesterol, 164 mg sodium, 19 g total carbohydrate (3 g dietary fiber, 11 g sugar, 0 g added sugars), 4 g protein, 2 mg iron

Roasted Twice-Baked Potatoes

Serves 4 as an appetizer

These addictive little bite-size snacks make perfect party food. Be sure to make enough, because you and your guests won't be able to keep your hands off them! You can also try substituting tiny Yukon Gold or small purple potatoes for the red potatoes. (Pictured on page 248.)

Spray oil (for pan)

6 small red potatoes, halved lengthwise

½ teaspoon freshly ground black pepper

2 teaspoons prepared spicy mustard

¼ cup Basic Cashew Cream Sauce (page 165)

¼ teaspoon sea salt

1 teaspoon chopped fresh chives

¼ cup finely chopped red bell pepper

Smoked paprika, for garnish

Fresh parsley sprigs, for garnish

Flaky sea salt (optional)

Preheat the oven to 400°F. Line a baking sheet with parchment paper and coat the paper lightly with spray oil.

Arrange the potatoes cut-side down on the prepared baking sheet and sprinkle the tops with ¼ teaspoon of the black pepper. Roast until a knife easily pierces a potato, about 30 minutes, without turning. Remove from the oven and let cool completely on the pan.

When cool, use a melon baller to scoop out some of the potato flesh, leaving a ¼-inch-thick layer on the skins; set the skins cut-side up on the baking sheet and set aside. Place the flesh in a medium bowl and add the mustard, cashew cream sauce, salt, and remaining ¼ teaspoon black pepper. Use a potato masher or fork to mash until smooth; the consistency should be smooth but not too wet. Stir in the chives and bell pepper.

Spoon the potato mixture into a zip-top bag and press it into one corner. Snip off the corner of the bag and squeeze the mixture into the potato skins, dividing it evenly.

Return the potatoes to the oven and roast until the filling is golden brown on top, 10 to 12 minutes. Remove from the oven.

Garnish with smoked paprika, parsley, and flaky salt, if desired, and serve.

Per serving: 195 calories, 1 g total fat, 0 g saturated fat, 0 mg cholesterol, 257 mg sodium, 42 g total carbohydrate (5 g dietary fiber, 4 g sugar, 0 g added sugars), 5 g protein, 2 mg iron

Dips and Spreads

Easy and crowd-pleasing, a selection of dips and spreads makes a great party opener. Serve your favorites with raw veggies or chips or spread them on whole-grain and seed crackers.

Grilled Peach Salsa

Makes about 1½ cups

This salsa is a nice mix of sweet and spicy, with the caramelized grilled peaches giving character to this simple condiment. If you like more spice, leave the seeds in the jalapeño! Enjoy as a dip for chips or as an accompaniment to veggie burgers. For those who eat fish, this salsa would also make a nice topping for grilled fish. You can also try this recipe with other fruits instead of the peach, for example, watermelon, mango, or pears. **Recipe by Whole Foods Market**

Spray oil (for grill)

3 ripe yet firm peaches, halved and pitted

½ cup chopped cucumber

1 tablespoon finely chopped seeded jalapeño

½ small red onion, finely chopped

1 tablespoon fresh lime juice

¼ cup chopped fresh cilantro

¼ teaspoon sea salt

Freshly ground black pepper

Heat a grill to medium-high or heat a grill pan over medium-high heat. When hot, coat the grill grates or pan lightly with spray oil. Place the peaches cut-side down on the grill and sear until nicely grill marked, about 4 minutes. Transfer the peaches to a cutting board and let cool slightly. When cool, finely chop and transfer to a medium bowl.

Add the remaining ingredients to the bowl and stir to combine.

Per serving (2 tablespoons): 19 calories, 0 g total fat, 0 g saturated fat, 0 mg cholesterol, 49 mg sodium, 5 g total carbohydrate (1 g dietary fiber, 4 g sugar, 0 g added sugars), 0 g protein, 0 mg iron

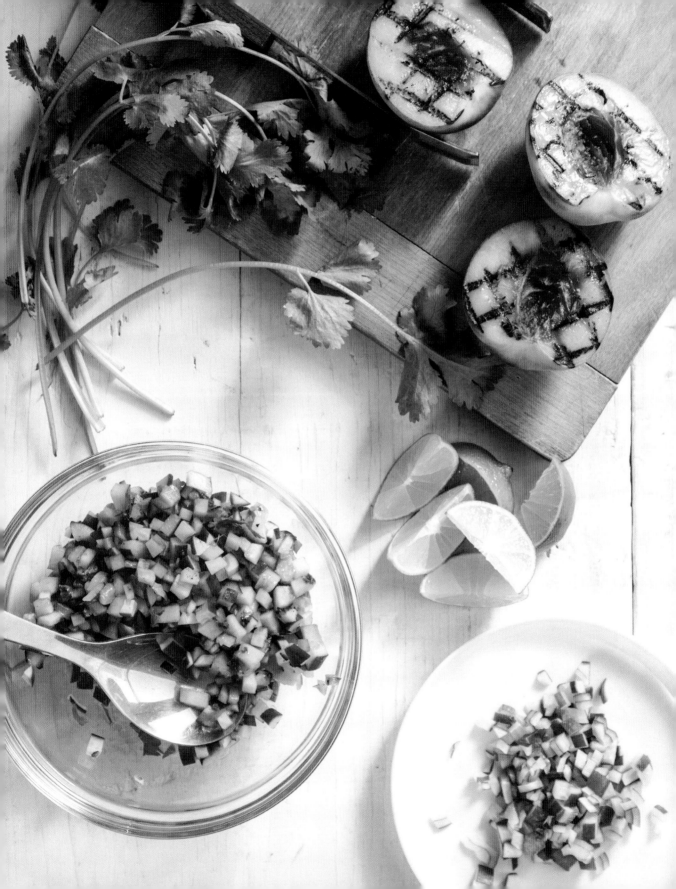

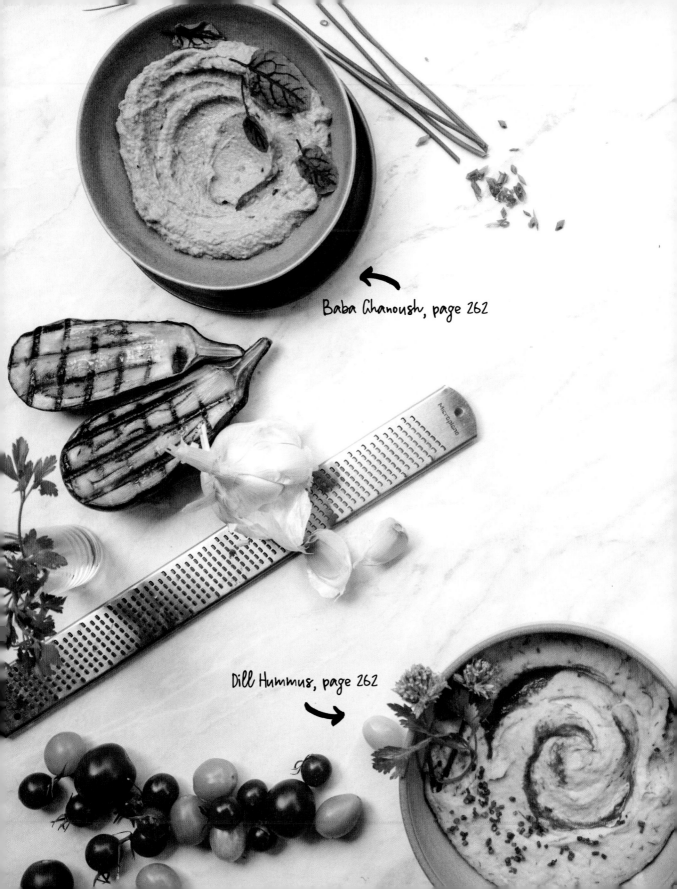

Baba Ghanoush, page 262

Dill Hummus, page 262

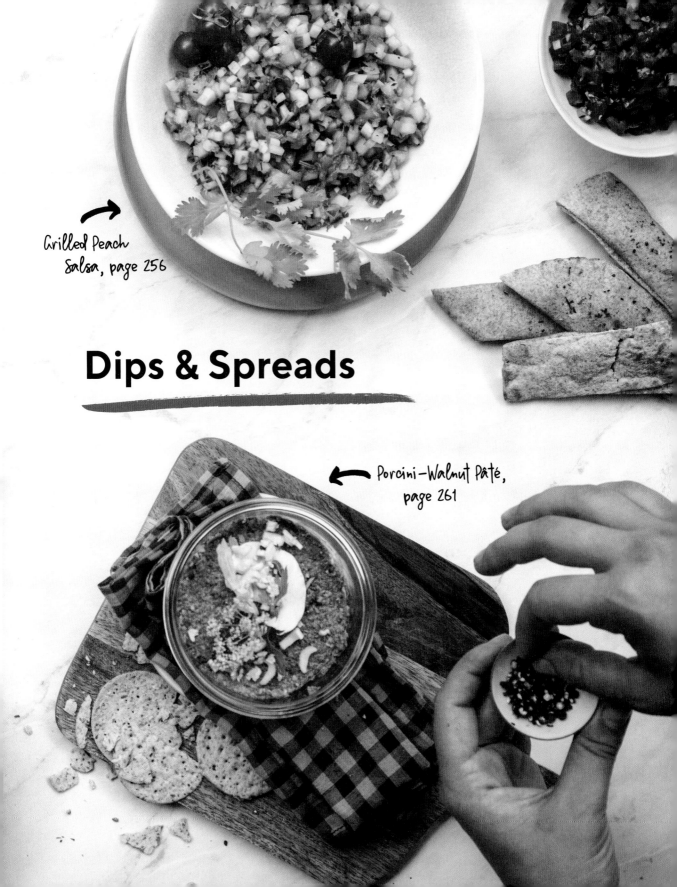

Grilled Peach
Salsa, page 256

Dips & Spreads

Porcini–Walnut Pâté,
page 261

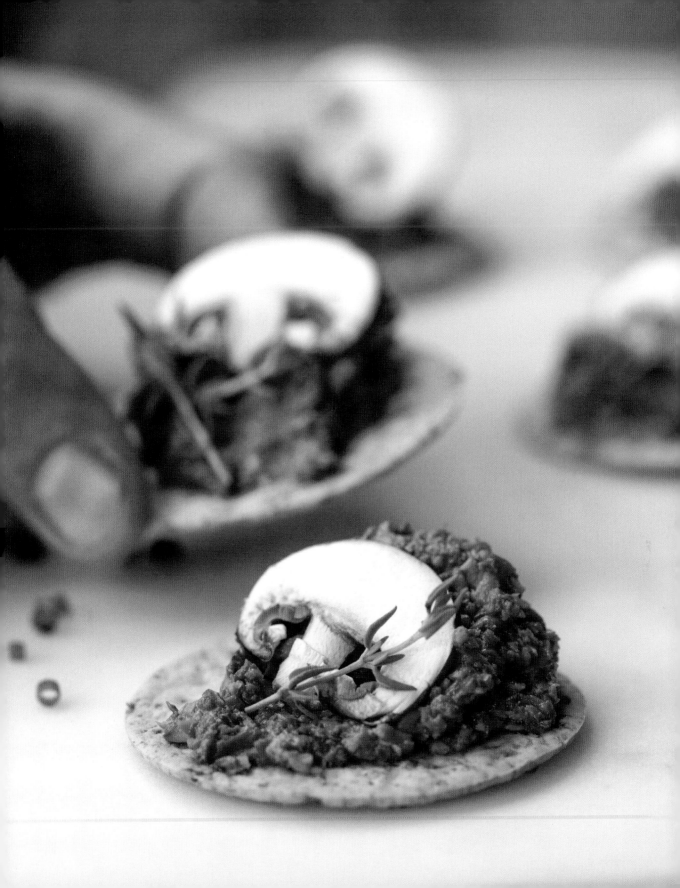

Porcini-Walnut Pâté

Makes about 4 cups

A simple but sophisticated pâté that highlights the earthiness of fresh and dried mushrooms, complemented by the delicate flavors of thyme and parsley. Serve with vegetables or crackers, or in a sandwich wrap with whole-grain flatbread.

½ cup walnuts

¼ cup pine nuts

2 ounces dried porcini mushrooms

4 sun-dried tomato halves

1 onion, diced

¼ cup low-sodium vegetable broth

1 pound cremini (baby bella) mushrooms, chopped

1 teaspoon minced fresh thyme

2 tablespoons dry sherry

¼ cup chopped fresh parsley, plus more for garnish

¼ cup nutritional yeast

1 teaspoon sea salt

½ teaspoon freshly ground black pepper

Place the walnuts and pine nuts in a small bowl and add water to cover. Let soak for at least 8 hours or up to overnight. Drain and rinse, then transfer to a food processor.

Put the dried porcini mushrooms and sun-dried tomato halves in a heatproof bowl and add 1 cup very hot water. Let soak until soft, about 30 minutes. Pluck the porcinis and tomato halves from the water and transfer them to the food processor with the nuts; reserve the soaking liquid.

Process the nuts, mushrooms, and sun-dried tomatoes until finely chopped but not pureed.

Heat a large skillet over medium-high heat. When hot, add the onion and dry sauté, stirring often, until it begins to stick to the pan and lightly brown, 3 to 4 minutes. Add the broth and stir to deglaze the pan.

Stir in creminis and thyme and cook until the mushrooms release their liquid and the liquid evaporates, about 5 minutes. Add the sherry and stir to deglaze the pan. Remove from the heat.

Add the onion mixture to the food processor and process until finely chopped. Scrape down the sides of the processor then, with the machine running, add just enough of the reserved mushroom-tomato soaking liquid to break the mixture down into a thick paste, ¼ to ½ cup total.

Pulse in the parsley, nutritional yeast, salt, and pepper just until incorporated. Transfer to an airtight container and refrigerate until ready to serve, at least thirty minutes and up to 3 days.

Serve garnished with a little parsley.

Per serving (¼ cup): 63 calories, 4 g total fat, 0 g saturated fat, 0 mg cholesterol, 173 mg sodium, 4 g total carbohydrate (1 g dietary fiber, 1 g sugar, 0 g added sugars), 3 g protein, 1 mg iron

Baba Ghanoush

Serves 8 as a dip

This traditional Middle Eastern dip gets its distinctive smoky flavor from the grilled eggplant. Serve with crudités or spread on whole-grain pita bread. **Recipe by Dan Marek**

2 large globe eggplants

Spray oil (for grill)

¼ cup tahini

2 tablespoons low-sodium tamari

5 garlic cloves, or 2 tablespoons garlic paste (pages 69 and 70)

Juice of 2 lemons

Heat a grill to medium-high.

Prick the eggplants all over with a fork. Lightly coat the grill grates with spray oil. Place the eggplants on the grill grates, directly over the heat, cover the grill, and cook until the skin is blistered and blackened all over and the eggplants are tender, 15 to 20 minutes, turning a few times. Remove and let cool.

When cool enough to handle, cut the eggplants in half lengthwise and scoop the flesh into a food processor; discard the skin. Add the remaining ingredients and process until smooth, 2 to 3 minutes.

Serve warm, or refrigerate in an airtight container for up to 3 days. Bring to room temperature before serving.

Per serving: 94 calories, 4 g total fat, 1 g saturated fat, 0 mg cholesterol, 181 mg sodium, 13 g total carbohydrate (5 g dietary fiber, 5 g sugar, 0 g added sugars), 3 g protein, 1 mg iron

Dill Hummus

Makes 1¼ cups

This aromatic fresh bean spread can be served on crackers or as a dip and makes a great addition to the Greek Burgers (page 226).

1 cup cooked white beans (see page 42) or canned no-added-sodium white beans, drained and rinsed

¼ cup tahini

1 tablespoon fresh lemon juice

1 garlic clove

⅛ teaspoon red pepper flakes

½ teaspoon sea salt

1½ tablespoons minced fresh dill

1 tablespoon minced fresh chives

Hot sauce of your choice (optional)

In a food processor, combine the white beans, tahini, lemon juice, garlic, red pepper flakes, and salt. Process to a smooth, thick puree. Add a little water, if needed, to get the mixture moving.

Pulse in the dill and chives just until incorporated.

Use as a spread, or serve as a dip, topped with a drizzle of your favorite hot sauce, if desired.

Per serving (2 tablespoons): 63 calories, 3 g total fat, 0 g saturated fat, 0 mg cholesterol, 119 mg sodium, 6 g total carbohydrate (2 g dietary fiber, 0 g sugar, 0 g added sugars), 3 g protein, 1 mg iron

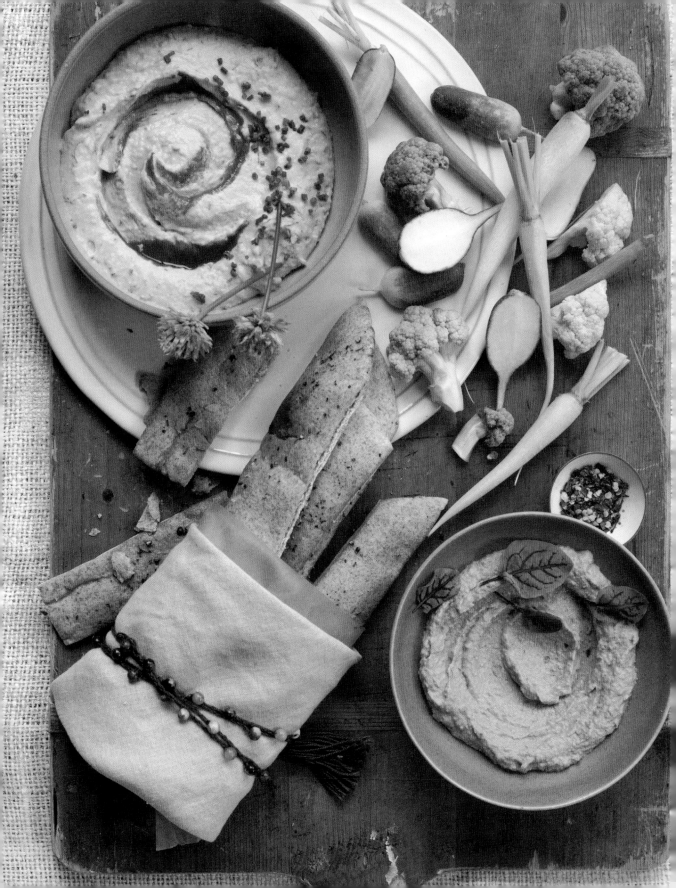

Cashew Cream Cheese

Makes about 1¾ cups

This simple nut cheese has become a staple in many of our recipes over the years. Spread it on whole-grain crackers with a drizzle of White Balsamic Syrup (page 72) or date paste (see page 56) for a simple hors d'oeuvre or after-dinner bite. You can also spread it on bread or whole-grain bagels, and you'll find it layered in the Roasted Eggplant with Cashew Cheese on page 212 and spread on a delicious tartine on page 130. Jazz it up by adding chives or other fresh herbs, tapenade, chopped sun-dried tomatoes, or chopped Carrot Lox (page 101). For best results, use a high-speed blender.

2 cups raw cashews, soaked for a few hours or up to overnight

Juice of 1 lemon

2 tablespoons small-flake nutritional yeast

1 tablespoon onion powder

½ teaspoon fine sea salt

Drain and rinse the cashews and transfer them to a high-speed blender.

Add the lemon juice, nutritional yeast, onion powder, and sea salt. Blend until smooth, adding water as needed, a tablespoon at a time, to get the mixture moving. It should be thick like cream cheese.

Use the cashew cream cheese immediately, or scrape it into an airtight container and refrigerate for up to 4 days.

Note: To flavor the cream cheese, blend in some roasted peppers or stir in chopped chives or other herbs.

Per serving (2 tablespoons): 96 calories, 7 g total fat, 1 g saturated fat, 0 mg cholesterol, 87 mg sodium, 6 g total carbohydrate (1 g dietary fiber, 1 g sugar, 0 g added sugars), 3 g protein, 1 mg iron

The Whole Foodie Dinner Party

Gathering friends and family over a meal that you have put thought and effort into is one of the greatest gifts to share with others. Your dinner party menu doesn't need to be overly complex or ambitious—the secret to wowing your guests is choosing the right combination of dishes so that the ingredients, flavor profiles, and theme of your evening have a chance to shine. Keep it simple, but serve it beautifully.

For more casual events, lay out a sumptuous buffet so guests can sample a variety of dishes. Or create a build-your-own bar for tacos, salads, bowls, or burgers. Most people love to be interactive with food, so make lots of small bowls of prepped vegetables, sauces, grains, beans, and other toppers and let your guests take charge of their plates.

To create a sense of occasion for more formal dinners, separate your menu into several courses, or have a common thread running among all the dishes. Here are some tips for stress-free entertaining.

Setting the Scene: Tips for a Memorable Dinner Party

Welcome your guests. Break the ice and welcome your guests with small bites and a drink, with refills close by. The best way to kick off a special evening, especially for those who are not familiar with a whole foods, plant-based diet, is to let them taste several one-bite appetizers. First impressions go a long way.

Create a unique menu. What's in season? Do you have a new favorite dish? Can your evening be themed to give your guests a particular cultural experience? These are questions to ask when shaping your menu. Consider creating several courses: this allows each dish to be savored and appreciated on its own terms while still working with all the dishes to follow. Rather than serving your main dish with a side and a salad, turn those into three courses. Add a soup course and a dessert, and you've got a grand five-course dinner. Pair with your favorite wines to add flair to the culinary experience.

Talk about the food. Don't be afraid to ask your guests to pause their conversation when a new course is served so you can take a couple of minutes to tell them what they'll be eating and why you love that particular dish. You'll spark conversation about the menu, ingredients, techniques, or flavors used.

Simple is okay. Every course does not have to be elaborate. Simple courses are nice complements to the more complex items on your menu. Have a big salad available for guests who want seconds of greens. Buy some local fresh produce that's in season and highlight those veggies as fillers on the table between courses.

Create a dining experience. Offer dishes that are interactive, such as building rolls or small bites, adding a sauce to the plate at the table, adding toppings to dishes at the table, and so on. Think about temperatures of your dishes—serve warm courses on warm plates/bowls and cold courses on cold plates/bowls.

Gather in the kitchen. Guests will go where the action is, so assume everyone will end up in the kitchen before the sit-down meal. It's futile to resist, so use this as an opportunity to shine, have some snacks ready, and, most important, have your space clean before guests arrive. An organized cook is a successful cook!

Don't stress, and welcome support. Creating a multicourse meal for several people can sometimes be stressful. Take a deep breath—you don't want there to be an atmosphere of stress when your guests walk in. If guests arrive early and offer to help, put them to work assembling small bites or pouring drinks.

Set the scene and the tone for the evening. Have some welcoming music on when guests arrive. Set the table with place cards or a small decoration on each plate, such as a freshly picked sprig of herbs or a small flower. Centerpieces can be more than just flowers as well: get creative with a vegetable and greens bouquet in the middle of the table. It's the little things that add up to a memorable experience.

Be present. This requires being well organized leading up to the dinner party. Guests are there to eat, but also to *be* with you. Every time you get up to prepare something, you leave your guests. *Mise en place* (see page 27) will make putting courses together quick and easy.

Have fun, and celebrate the moment. The point of having a party is to gather with friends and family you love and to have fun. This is the most important thing to remember, from the planning to the final course. If there was a detail that was not perfect or a dish that did not come out the way you intended, your guests will never know. Relax. Enjoy the last bites with your guests and take a breather! You did amazing.

Whole Foodie Menu Suggestions

Whether you're looking for a holiday theme, a special dinner party, or a fun family meal, these suggested menus will be sure to come in handy.

THE PERFECT BRUNCH

Liquid Sunshine Smoothie (page 110)

Whole Foodie Pancakes (page 122)

Tofu Scramble with Spinach, Peppers, & Basil (page 120)

Carrot Lox Tartine with Cashew Cream Cheese, Capers, & Shallot (page 130)

Dark Chocolate Pudding Parfaits with Berries & Cacao Nibs (page 270)

Ma's Wicked Good Zucchini Bread (page 133)

GETTING THE KIDDOS INVOLVED

Tofu Bites (page 250)

Mixed lettuces with Cashew Ranch Dressing (page 156)

Baguette Pizza with Artichokes, Hearts of Palm, & Roasted Tomatoes (page 237)

Very Veggie Pizza (page 240)

Whole Foodie Ice Pops (page 274)

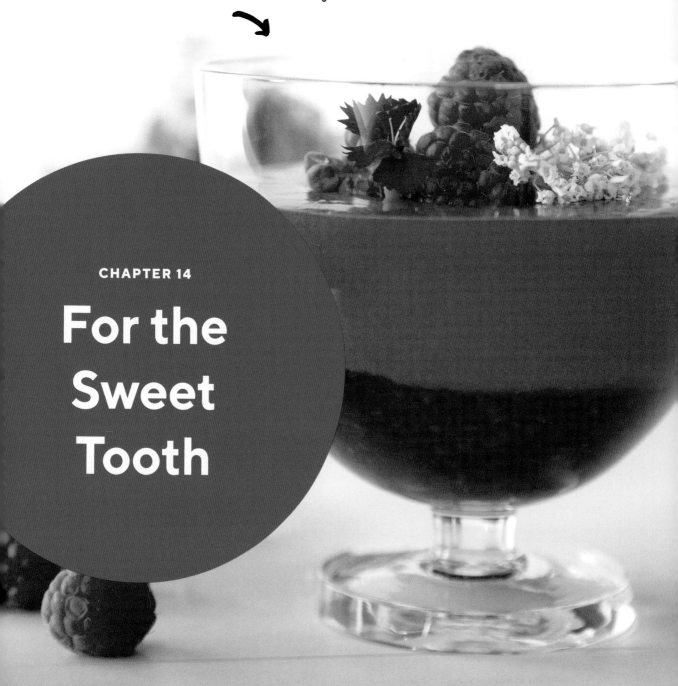

Dark Chocolate Pudding Parfaits with
Berries and Cacao Nibs, page 270

CHAPTER 14

For the Sweet Tooth

A whole foods, plant-based diet doesn't include sugar or other refined sweeteners, but that doesn't mean you have to deprive your sweet tooth! Nature's sweetest gifts—whole fruits—can be used in so many creative ways. Dried fruit pastes can take the place of refined sugars in baking and other desserts, while fresh and frozen fruits add a natural sweetness, flavor, and color to dishes. Nuts, avocado, or tofu can bring creamy and rich textures to complement the acidity of many fruits.

Quick Desserts

Sometimes you need a sweet in a hurry! The recipes in this section will satisfy your cravings without taking up too much of your valuable time. Note that many of the recipes call for fruit pastes; find instructions for making these on page 56.

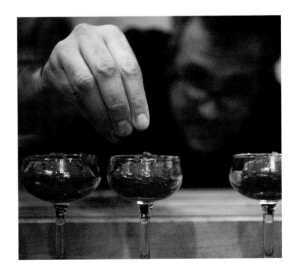

Dark Chocolate Pudding Parfaits with Berries & Cacao Nibs

Serves 4

Silken tofu has a smooth, creamy texture and a neutral taste that make it ideal for desserts. You can usually find it in shelf-stable aseptic packages in the international foods aisle of the grocery store—buy some extra packs to have on hand any time you want to whip up a quick and satisfying dessert. To create a richer pudding for a special occasion, try swapping out the tofu for two ripe avocados. You'll be amazed at the results, and your guests will never guess the secret ingredient. Try these at brunch!

1 (12-ounce) package firm silken tofu, drained

2 very ripe bananas, peeled

¾ cup date paste (see page 56)

½ teaspoon pure vanilla extract

Pinch of sea salt

¾ cup raw unsweetened cacao powder

¼ cup cacao nibs or shaved dark chocolate, plus more for garnish

8 fresh strawberries

½ pint fresh raspberries

In a food processor, combine the tofu, bananas, date paste, vanilla, and salt. Process until very smooth, 2 to 3 minutes. Scrape down the sides as needed. Add the cacao powder and process until smooth. Pulse in the cacao nibs just until evenly distributed. Spoon the pudding into a pastry bag fitted with a star tip, if you like. (You can also just spoon the pudding into serving glasses later.)

Hull the strawberries and finely chop them. Mix the chopped strawberries with the whole raspberries, reserving some raspberries for garnish.

Pipe or spoon ¼ cup of the pudding into each of four ½-pint canning jars, martini glasses, or parfait glasses. Divide the mixed berries among the jars or glasses. Spoon the remaining pudding over fruit, and top each serving with a reserved raspberry. Cover with plastic wrap and chill for at least 1 hour and up to overnight.

Garnish with more cacao nibs or shaved chocolate.

Note: Use your favorite berry compote or fresh fruits of choice instead of the fresh berries. In the photo (page 268), huckleberries poached with orange and date paste are shown.

Per serving: 344 calories, 10 g total fat, 5 g saturated fat, 0 mg cholesterol, 99 mg sodium, 63 g total carbohydrate (16 g dietary fiber, 40 g sugar, 0 g added sugars), 10 g protein, 5 mg iron

Easy Parfaits

In French, *parfait* means "perfect," and these sweet delights really are perfect at any time of the day—for breakfast, as a snack, or as an after-dinner treat. Plus, they're perfectly easy to make. Simply layer a little fruit in the bottom of a bowl, glass tumbler, or stemmed glass, add a layer of cream, then another layer of fruit, then another layer of cream, and top with something crunchy. Easy and delicious!

Fruit	Cream	Crunch
Fresh fruit—berries, tropical fruits, stone fruits, orchard fruits, banana, etc.	Vanilla Coconut Cream (below), or Plain Cashew Cream flavored with vanilla, lemon, cinnamon, fresh mint, etc.	Plantastic Granola (page 117)
Poached fruit (see page 276)	Tofu cream	Toasted nuts or seeds
Roasted fruits	Chocolate cream	Toasted rolled oats or puffed grains
Stewed, marinated, or macerated fruits		

Vanilla Coconut Cream

Makes about 2½ cups

This rich and creamy dessert sauce is a great pairing to many recipes, such as Baked Strawberry & Apple Thyme Crumble (page 280), and Whole Foodie Pancakes (page 122). It's also great for dipping fresh seasonal fruits and layering in a parfait (see above).

⅓ cup cashews, soaked for at least 3 hours or up to overnight

1 (14-ounce) can coconut milk

¼ cup pitted dates, or 3 tablespoons date paste (see page 56)

¾ cup unsweetened soy milk or other nondairy milk

1 vanilla bean, split lengthwise and seeds scraped, or 1 to 2 teaspoons pure vanilla extract

½ teaspoon sea salt

Drain and rinse the cashews and transfer them to a (preferably high-speed) blender.

Add the remaining ingredients to the blender and blend until smooth. Use immediately or refrigerate in an airtight container for up to 2 days.

Per serving (¼ cup): 122 calories, 10 g total fat, 8 g saturated fat, 0 mg cholesterol, 130 mg sodium, 7 g total carbohydrate (1 g dietary fiber, 3 g sugar, 0 g added sugars), 2 g protein, 2 mg iron

"Supercede" Bars

Makes 16 bars

Protein-packed, chewy, and satisfying, these bars are convenient and tasty on-the-go nutrition. You can replace the cardamom with cinnamon or other warming spices, if you like. **Recipe by Chef Pete Cervoni**

1½ cups raw sunflower seeds

2 teaspoons vanilla bean paste

1½ teaspoons ground cardamom

⅛ teaspoon fine pink Himalayan salt

1½ cups large-flake coconut chips

1 cup pitted unsulfured Deglet Noor or Medjool dates

1½ cups raisins

½ cup unsulfured dried apricots

¾ cup whole hemp protein powder (ground whole hemp seeds)

½ cup hulled hemp seeds

Combine the sunflower seeds, vanilla bean paste, cardamom, and salt in a food processor. Pulse until the mixture forms a coarse meal.

Add the coconut chips, dates, raisins, apricots, and protein powder and process until the mixture is fully blended, 1 to 1½ minutes, stopping to scrape down the sides once or twice. Transfer the mixture to a medium bowl.

Fold in the hemp seeds until fully incorporated. The mixture should be thick and sticky enough to hold together in a mass when pinched between your fingers.

Line a quarter sheet pan or shallow 13 by 9-inch baking dish with plastic wrap, leaving excess plastic overhanging all sides.

Press the mixture firmly into the pan using the excess plastic (this keeps your hands from sticking to the mixture). Smooth the top evenly. The mixture will be about ½ inch thick.

Open the plastic and cover the pan with a large cutting board. Invert the pan and cutting board together, then remove the pan and peel off the plastic. Cut the slab into 16 rectangular bars, each about 1 by 5 inches. (To do that, make one lengthwise cut down the middle of the slab, then make seven crosswise cuts.)

Layer the bars in an airtight container, separating them slightly and separating the layers with sheets of parchment or waxed paper. Refrigerate for up to 1 week or freeze for up to 1 month. Enjoy cold or at room temperature.

Notes: You'll need a large food processor to make this mixture in one batch. If you have a small food processor, make it in two batches and then combine the batches at the end.

These are also great just rolled up into balls and stored in the refrigerator in an airtight container between sheets of parchment or waxed paper. Just pop one in your mouth for a pre- or post-workout snack.

Per serving: 263 calories, 13 g total fat, 4 g saturated fat, 0 mg cholesterol, 17 mg sodium, 29 g total carbohydrate (4 g dietary fiber, 20 g sugar, 0 g added sugars), 10 g protein, 4 mg iron

Apricot-Ginger Bites

Serves 4

These tasty little bites make a perfect pocket-size snack for carrying along on family adventures or packing in the kids' lunch boxes. **Recipe by Brian Stafford**

2 cups dried apricots

1 teaspoon grated fresh ginger

2 tablespoons finely chopped blanched hazelnuts

½ cup unsweetened finely shredded coconut

1 bunch Thai mint or Thai basil, minced

Tear off a foot-long sheet of plastic wrap and lay it out on a work surface.

Combine the apricots and ginger in a food processor and process until as smooth as possible, 30 to 60 seconds, stopping to scrape down the bowl as necessary. There should be no chunks of apricot.

Spoon the apricot mixture onto the plastic wrap and use a rubber spatula to press it into a rectangle about 8 by 4 inches and ½ inch thick.

Sprinkle the hazelnuts evenly over the top.

Starting with one long side of the rectangle, roll up the mixture all the way to the other side to create a log. The mixture will be firm yet sticky, so use the excess plastic to help make a tight roll.

Spread the coconut on a large plate or platter and sprinkle it evenly with the mint. Roll the apricot log over the coconut and mint to coat it completely. Slice the roll crosswise into 1-inch-wide pieces. Store the pieces in an airtight container in the refrigerator for up to 1 week.

Per serving: 274 calories, 9 g total fat, 6 g saturated fat, 0 mg cholesterol, 20 mg sodium, 46 g total carbohydrate (8 g dietary fiber, 23 g sugar, 0 g added sugars), 3 g protein, 3 mg iron

Berry Port Compote

Makes 2 cups

This delicious blend of berries and port wine makes a great adults-only topping for Whole Foodie Pancakes (page 122) or layers perfectly in a parfait with Vanilla Coconut Cream (page 271) and Plantastic Granola (page 117). This recipe uses a maceration process, which involves soaking food in sugar or liquid to soften it and infuse it with flavor.

¼ cup port wine

3 tablespoons date paste (see page 56)

Juice of ½ lime

½ vanilla bean, split lengthwise and seeds scraped, or 1 to 2 teaspoons pure vanilla extract

¼ teaspoon sea salt

2 cups fresh raspberries and/or sliced strawberries

In a medium bowl, whisk together the port, date paste, lime juice, vanilla bean seeds, and sea salt until smooth. Add the berries and toss well. Cover and let macerate at room temperature for at least 1 hour or preferably 3 hours.

Refrigerate until cold, about 1 hour or up to 3 days. Serve chilled.

Per serving (¼ cup): 43 calories, 0 g total fat, 0 g saturated fat, 0 mg cholesterol, 73 mg sodium, 9 g total carbohydrate (3 g dietary fiber, 5 g sugar, 0 g added sugars), 1 g protein, 0 mg iron

Whole Foodie Ice Pops

Makes 6 ice pops

Get the kids involved in creating a healthy summer snack they'll love. These refreshing frozen treats offer endless possibilities for highlighting seasonal fruits and herbs. You'll need some ice-pop molds, some small chunks of fresh fruit, a liquid filling (such as blended fruit, unsweetened iced tea, or coconut water), and herbs or spices.

PINEAPPLE TURMERIC LEMONADE

3 cups chopped pineapple

1 teaspoon grated lemon zest

1 (1-inch) piece fresh turmeric, peeled

¼ cup small-diced fresh pineapple

In a food processor, process the pineapple, lemon zest, and turmeric until mostly smooth, about 1 minute.

Put a couple of teaspoons of the diced pineapple in each ice-pop mold. Pour the puree over the top, insert the handles, and freeze until solid.

Per serving: 77 calories, 0 g total fat, 0 g saturated fat, 0 mg cholesterol, 0 mg sodium, 19 g total carbohydrate (1 g dietary fiber, 17 g sugar, 0 g added sugars), 1 g protein, 1 mg iron

WATERMELON AVOCADO

3 to 4 cups cubed seedless watermelon

Juice of 1 lime

½ avocado, pitted, peeled, and cut into small dice

Pinch of sea salt

In a food processor, process the watermelon and lime juice until mostly smooth, about 1 minute.

Put a couple of teaspoons of the diced avocado in each ice-pop mold and sprinkle with the salt. Pour the puree over the top, insert the handles, and freeze until solid.

Per serving: 45 calories, 2 g total fat, 0 g saturated fat, 0 mg cholesterol, 64 mg sodium, 8 g total carbohydrate (1 g dietary fiber, 5 g sugar, 0 g added sugars), 1 g protein, 0 mg iron

BERRY COCONUT

3 cups fresh berries of choice

2 dates, pitted

About ⅓ cup fresh berries, sliced if large

½ cup fresh, sliced, or unsweetened dried coconut flakes (not sweetened shredded coconut)

In a food processor, process 3 cups of the berries and the dates until mostly smooth, 1 minute.

Put a few teaspoons of the sliced berries and the coconut in each ice-pop mold. Pour the puree over the top, insert the handles, and freeze until solid.

Per serving: 58 calories, 3 g total fat, 2 g saturated fat, 0 mg cholesterol, 2 mg sodium, 9 g total carbohydrate (3 g dietary fiber, 6 g sugar, 0 g added sugars), 1 g protein, 1 mg iron

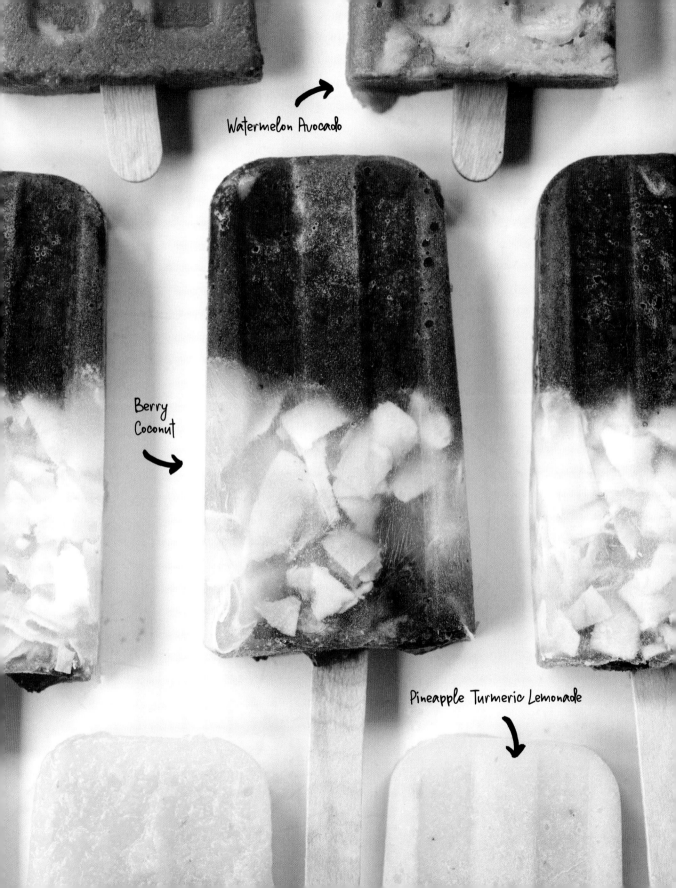

Watermelon Avocado

Berry
Coconut

Pineapple Turmeric Lemonade

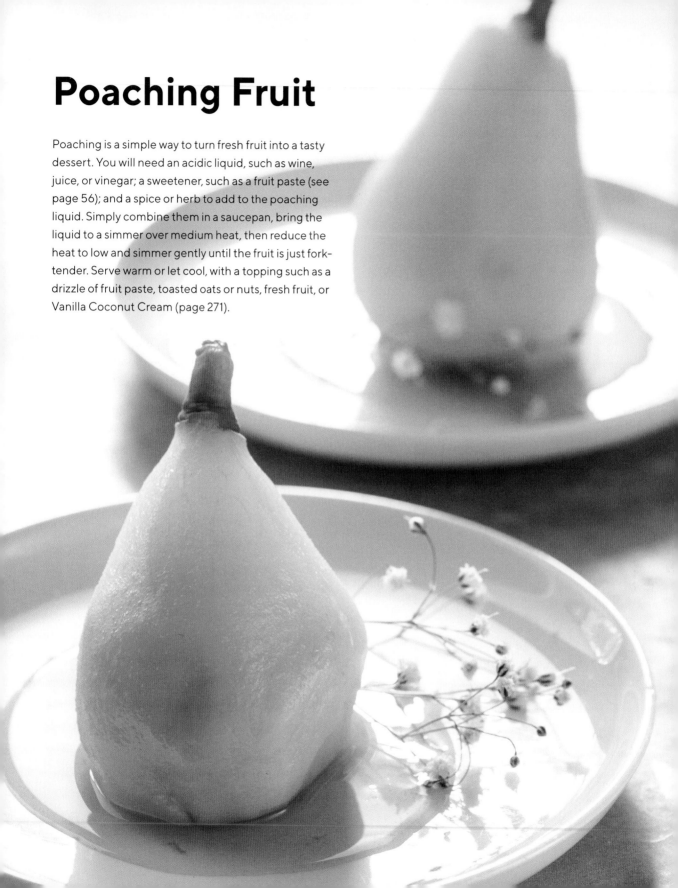

Poaching Fruit

Poaching is a simple way to turn fresh fruit into a tasty dessert. You will need an acidic liquid, such as wine, juice, or vinegar; a sweetener, such as a fruit paste (see page 56); and a spice or herb to add to the poaching liquid. Simply combine them in a saucepan, bring the liquid to a simmer over medium heat, then reduce the heat to low and simmer gently until the fruit is just fork-tender. Serve warm or let cool, with a topping such as a drizzle of fruit paste, toasted oats or nuts, fresh fruit, or Vanilla Coconut Cream (page 271).

Riesling & Orange Poached Pears

Serves 4

This is a simple and sexy way to showcase pears, enhancing their natural flavors. Serve them in the poaching sauce, or make a crowd-pleasing parfait for your next dinner party by layering slices of these pears with Vanilla Coconut Cream (page 271) and Plantastic Granola (page 117).

4 ripe yet firm pears

1½ cups freshly squeezed orange juice

4 cups Riesling or other sweet wine (or fresh fruit juice)

1 tablespoon apricot paste (see page 56)

1 vanilla bean, split lengthwise, or 1 to 2 teaspoons pure vanilla extract

3 star anise pods

Pinch of sea salt

Peel the pears, then use a melon baller or paring knife to remove the core from the bottom only, leaving the pears whole.

Combine the remaining ingredients in a medium saucepan. Bring to a simmer over medium-high heat. Reduce the heat to medium-low so the liquid simmers gently. Add the pears and poach, uncovered, until fork-tender, 15 to 18 minutes (or slightly longer if using Bosc pears), turning the pears during cooking if necessary to cook all sides.

Using a slotted spoon, transfer the pears to a bowl. Bring the poaching liquid to a simmer over high heat and simmer until reduced in volume by about half and thickened slightly, 10 to 12 minutes. Discard the vanilla bean and star anise.

Serve the pears with the warm poaching liquid, or chill the pears in their poaching liquid for up to 2 days and serve cold.

Note: For a thicker sauce, dissolve 1 teaspoon cornstarch in 3 tablespoons water to make a slurry. Stir the slurry into the simmering sauce and cook until thickened, 2 to 3 minutes.

Per serving: 358 calories, 0 g total fat, 0 g saturated fat, 0 mg cholesterol, 96 mg sodium, 49 g total carbohydrate (6 g dietary fiber, 26 g sugar, 0 g added sugars), 2 g protein, 1 mg iron

Suggested Combinations:

CINNAMON APPLES

- **Fruit:** Gala apples, peeled and cored
- **Acid/Liquid:** Orange juice and a touch of white balsamic vinegar
- **Sweet:** Date paste (see page 56)
- **Spice:** Ground cinnamon, freshly grated nutmeg, and vanilla extract

VANILLA PEACHES

- **Fruit:** Peaches, halved and pitted
- **Acid/Liquid:** Apple juice
- **Sweet:** Chopped dried figs
- **Spice:** Vanilla extract

GINGER APRICOTS

- **Fruit:** Apricots, halved and pitted
- **Acid/Liquid:** Orange juice and white wine
- **Sweet:** Apricot paste (see page 56)
- **Spice:** Sliced fresh ginger, cardamom pods, whole star anise, and red pepper flakes

Decadent Desserts

With their sophisticated flavor profiles, these plant-powered treats are the perfect finish to a dinner party. Be sure to tell your guests to leave room—when they discover that these delicious sweets contain no added sugars, they'll be asking for second helpings.

Grilled Pineapple & Sorbet with Coconut & White Balsamic Syrup

Serves 4

This is an impressive dessert to showcase for your next dinner party or share with a loved one. The sweetness of the sorbet and caramelized grilled pineapple pairs perfectly with the sweet acidity of the balsamic syrup.

PINEAPPLE SORBET

¼ cup dried apricots

3 cups cubed pineapple

Juice of ½ lemon

Pinch of sea salt

GRILLED PINEAPPLE

¼ cup white balsamic vinegar

½ teaspoon pure vanilla extract

¼ teaspoon Chinese five-spice powder

4 (¼-inch-thick) pineapple rounds, halved (to make 8 half-moons)

TO SERVE

¼ cup coconut flakes, lightly toasted

3 tablespoons White Balsamic Syrup (page 72)

For the pineapple sorbet, soak the apricots in hot water until softened, about 20 minutes. Drain and transfer to a (preferably high-speed) blender. Add the remaining sorbet ingredients and blend until very smooth.

Transfer the pineapple mixture to a sorbet or ice cream machine and freeze according to the manufacturer's instructions. (If you don't have a sorbet or ice cream machine, pour the mixture into a 2-quart glass baking dish and place it in the freezer. Whisk or stir the mixture every 30 minutes for about 2 hours. The sorbet will have a more rustic texture, similar to granita, because this freezing method creates larger ice crystals.)

For the grilled pineapple, heat a grill to medium-high or heat a grill pan over medium-high heat. In a large shallow dish, whisk together the vinegar, vanilla, and five-spice powder. Add pineapple half-moons and toss gently to coat. Remove the pineapple, reserving the vinegar mixture, and grill it directly over the heat until grill marked on both sides, about 3 minutes per side, drizzling or brushing with the remaining vinegar mixture a couple of times during grilling. Transfer to a plate and set aside.

To assemble, place two slices of grilled pineapple on each plate, followed by a scoop of pineapple sorbet. Sprinkle with toasted coconut flakes and drizzle with balsamic syrup.

Per serving: 202 calories, 3 g total fat, 0 g saturated fat, 0 mg cholesterol, 101 mg sodium, 44 g total carbohydrate (4 g dietary fiber, 36 g sugar, 0 g added sugars), 2 g protein, 1 mg iron

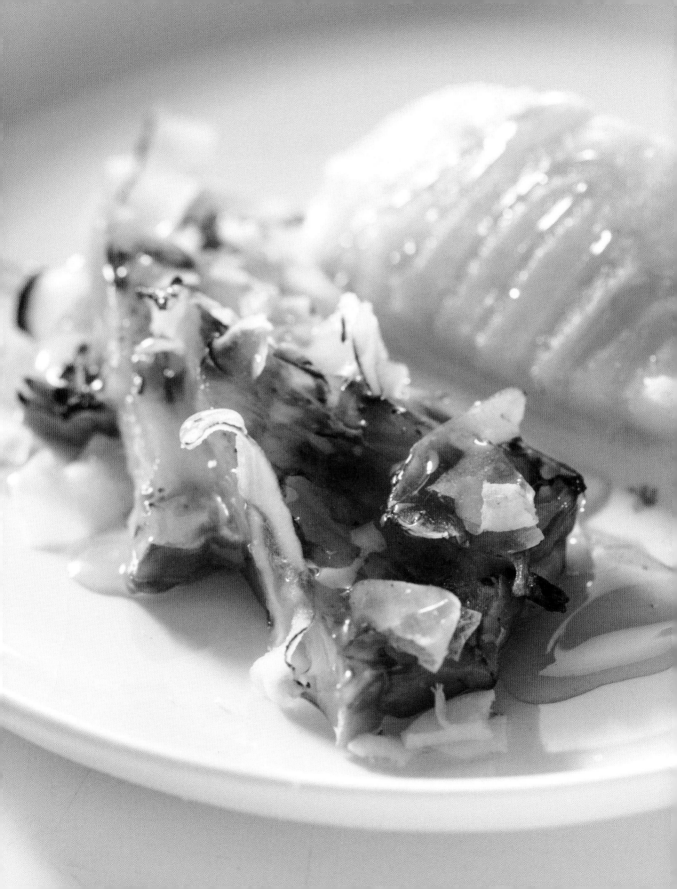

Baked Strawberry & Apple Thyme Crumble

Serves 4

The delicate taste of thyme paired with the berries and apples gives this recipe an unexpected deliciousness. Served warm or cold, it makes a great finish to any meal. For a more decadent dessert, serve with Vanilla Coconut Cream (page 271).

1 (3.5-ounce) bag crispy baked apple chips

¼ cup pitted dates

1 cup old-fashioned rolled oats

1 teaspoon ground cinnamon

4 Pink Lady apples, cored and cut into 1-inch cubes

1 pound fresh strawberries, hulled and sliced

⅓ cup unsweetened applesauce

½ vanilla bean, split lengthwise and seeds scraped, or ½ teaspoon pure vanilla extract

2 tablespoons arrowroot powder

2 tablespoons minced fresh thyme, plus 4 small sprigs for garnish

Vanilla Coconut Cream (page 271; optional)

Preheat the oven to 350°F.

In a food processor, combine the apple chips, dates, oats, and cinnamon. Pulse until the mixture resembles a coarse meal. Pour the mixture into a medium bowl and stir in 1 teaspoon warm water to create a thick and crumbly yet moist topping.

In a medium bowl, combine the apple cubes, strawberries, applesauce, vanilla, arrowroot, and thyme and mix well. Spoon the mixture into four 6-ounce ramekins, dividing it evenly, or a single 8-inch square baking dish. Top with small clusters of the oat topping. Bake until the topping is slightly brown, about 10 minutes.

Serve hot, garnished with thyme sprigs and a drizzle of Vanilla Coconut Cream, if desired.

Per serving: 376 calories, 4 g total fat, 2 g saturated fat, 0 mg cholesterol, 3 mg sodium, 82 g total carbohydrate (13 g dietary fiber, 48 g sugar, 0 g added sugars), 5 g protein, 3 mg iron

Roasted Apples with Chai Streusel & Almond-Date Syrup

Serves 4

Attention, foodies—this recipe turns simple apples into a gourmet dessert. The blend of sweet spices used in chai give this dish a unique finish.

4 Granny Smith apples

1 cup pitted dates, plus 2 chopped pitted dates

½ cup old-fashioned rolled oats

2 tablespoons fine almond flour

½ teaspoon ground cinnamon

¼ teaspoon ground ginger

⅛ teaspoon ground cardamom

Pinch of sea salt

Pinch of freshly ground black pepper

¼ cup almond butter (no added oil, salt, or sugar)

¼ cup unsweetened soy milk or other nondairy milk

1 teaspoon pure almond extract

Preheat the oven to 350°F. Line a small baking dish (just big enough to hold the apples) with parchment paper.

Cut a small slice from the bottoms of the apples so they sit flat, if necessary. Core the apples, hollowing them out to make room for about ¼ cup filling, but leaving the bottoms intact. Place them upright in the prepared baking dish.

Place the whole pitted dates in a medium bowl and cover with very hot water by 1 inch. Let soak for 30 minutes.

Place the chopped dates in a small bowl. Add the oats, almond flour, cinnamon, ginger, cardamom, salt, and pepper. Spoon the almond butter on top and use your fingers to rub it into the oat mixture until it forms pea-size streusel pieces.

Stuff the apples with the streusel. Bake until the apples are tender and the streusel browns, 20 to 25 minutes.

Drain the dates, reserving the soaking water. Place the dates in a (preferably high-speed) blender or a food processor, add the soy milk and almond extract, and blend until very smooth and the consistency of thick maple syrup. Add a little of the reserved soaking water if necessary to reach the desired consistency.

Remove the apples from the oven. Spoon the date syrup over the apples and let cool for 10 minutes before serving.

Per serving: 409 calories, 12 g total fat, 1 g saturated fat, 0 mg cholesterol, 139 mg sodium, 75 g total carbohydrate (12 g dietary fiber, 49 g sugar, 0 g added sugars), 8 g protein, 2 mg iron

Acknowledgments

From the moment of its inception, this book has been a team effort. As authors and chefs, we have enjoyed this opportunity to collaborate with each other, as well as with the many people whose talent, hard work, and dedication have made this book a reality.

Thank you, Ellen Daly, for your tireless dedication to this project and for so eloquently making each of our voices fit into every page.

We are honored to feature recipes by some of our favorite plant-based foodie friends and family in these pages, including Brian Stafford, Jess Kolko, Lisa Rice, Beverly Burl (Wicked Healthy mom), Dan Marek, Rip Esselstyn, Dan Buettner, Darshana Thacker, Peter Cervoni, Hiram Camillo, and Shoshana Pulde. Thank you all for your delectable contributions! Thanks also to Whole Foods Market for providing several recipes.

We are also grateful to the team of enthusiastic home cooks who helped us test, refine, and clarify each of the recipes: Beverly Burl, Jess Kolko, Lisa Rice, Debbie Deisher, Kerry Abdow, Kelly McShane, Char Nolan, Lynne Lamberis, Frederique Pieters, Katie Bozarth, Dianna Carpenter, Greg Zastrow, Kerry Werth, Federica Norreri, Ellen Daly, Kim Smith, Jennifer Alvarado, Lauren Lewis, Stephanie Quilao, Heidi Lekan, John Harsh, Emily Forbes, Chelle Folts Winslow, and Juan Pablo.

David Joachim, our meticulous recipe editor, played an invaluable role in ensuring clarity, consistency, and ease of use, as well as providing nutritional analysis.

Photographs bring a cookbook alive, and we were fortunate to work with the talented Ha Lam, whose camera turns the simplest dish into a work of art. Our thanks to Ha and her team, food stylist Nadine Beauchamp and prop stylist Maya Rossi, for all the food photography. We're also grateful to David Rice, whose portraits and dinner party photographs of the authors captured the spirit of an entertaining and delicious culinary experience.

It was a pleasure to work on this book with the team at Grand Central Life & Style. Thank you to Karen Murgolo, our patient and understanding editor; Morgan Hedden, who kept track of a multitude of details; and Laura Palese, who designed the book's beautiful cover and interior. We are also grateful for the support of our agents, Richard Pine and Eliza Rothstein at Inkwell and Sally Ekus from the Lisa Ekus Group.

Lastly, we are grateful to our families for their unconditional and everlasting support and for inspiring us to work toward a healthier, happier, and better world.

About the Authors

John Mackey, cofounder and CEO of Whole Foods Market, grew the natural and organic grocer, which was acquired by Amazon in 2017, to a $16 billion Fortune 500 company with more than 470 stores and 90,000 team members in three countries. The company has been included on *Fortune* magazine's "100 Best Companies to Work For" list for twenty consecutive years and ranked first in the food and drugstore industry on the magazine's "Most Admired Companies" list in 2016.

While devoting his career to helping shoppers satisfy their lifestyle needs with quality natural and organic foods, Mackey has also focused on building a more conscious way of doing business. He was the visionary for the Whole Planet Foundation, the Local Producer Loan Program, the Global Animal Partnership rating scale for humane farm animal treatment, and the Health Starts Here initiative.

Mackey has been recognized as one of *Fortune*'s "World's 50 Greatest Leaders" and their "Businessperson of the Year," Ernst & Young's "Entrepreneur of the Year Overall Winner for the United States," *Institutional Investor's* "Best CEO in America," *Barron's* "World's Best CEO," MarketWatch's "CEO of the Year," and *Esquire*'s "Most Inspiring CEO."

A strong believer in free market principles, Mackey cofounded the Conscious Capitalism Movement (consciouscapitalism.org) and coauthored the bestseller *Conscious Capitalism: Liberating the Heroic Spirit of Business*. Mackey cut his pay to $1 in 2006, takes no bonus or stock options, and continues to work for Whole Foods Market out of a passion to see the business realize its potential for deeper purpose, for the joy of leading a great company, and to answer the call to service he feels in his heart.

Dr. Alona Pulde is a board-certified practitioner of acupuncture and Eastern medicine and a family medicine physician. **Dr. Matthew Lederman** is a board-certified internal medicine physician. Drs. Pulde and Lederman specialize in reversing disease using nutrition and lifestyle medicine, and created the lifestyle-improvement program used in their medical center and for Whole Foods Market Medical & Wellness Centers. They were featured in the film *Forks Over Knives* and coauthored the *New York Times* bestseller *The Forks Over Knives Plan*, *Forks Over Knives Family*, *Keep It Simple, Keep It Whole*, and, together with John Mackey, *The Whole Foods Diet*. Drs. Pulde and Lederman live in Southern California with their two daughters and work with Whole Foods Market overseeing various health and wellness projects.

Chad Sarno is a cofounder of Wicked Healthy and vice president of culinary at Good Catch Foods. Chad also is an ambassador for Rouxbe, the world's largest online cooking school, where he has launched the Professional Plant-Based Certification course. He spent several years at Whole Foods Market as senior culinary educator, and was media spokesperson for the Global Healthy Eating program. Prior to this, Chad launched a line of boutique restaurants throughout Europe, in Istanbul, Munich, and London.

Derek Sarno is the executive chef and director of plant-based innovations for Tesco, the third-largest food retailer in the world. Derek is a cofounder of Wicked Healthy and of Good Catch Foods. As the former Whole Foods Market senior global executive chef, he catered all of the company's major executive leadership events and oversaw national recipe development. Derek has owned several critically acclaimed restaurants and catering businesses.

Recipe Contributors

Dan Buettner is a *National Geographic* Fellow and *New York Times* bestselling author. His *New York Times Sunday Magazine* article, "The Island Where People Forget to Die," was the second most popular article of 2012. He founded Blue Zones to put the world's best practices in longevity and well-being to work in people's lives.

Beverly Burl is a cooking coach and plant-based recipe developer and is known by many as the Wicked Healthy Mom. Her passion for cooking is also reflected in her sons Chad and Derek, the chefs behind this book.

Peter Cervoni is a classically trained chef who evolved to veganism over twenty years ago. Since that time, he has devoted himself to tasty plant-based and healing foods and has worked all over the world with many luminaries in the health arena.

Rip Esselstyn is the founder of Engine 2 and a healthy eating partner for Whole Foods Market. At Engine 2, Rip develops and implements plant-based programs and products that transform people's health worldwide.

Jess Kolko, RDN, LD: Jess's passion for food started at a young age and led her to begin her career in kitchens across the country. After ten years in the culinary world, she went deep into the science of nutrition and became a registered dietitian. Jess feels strongly that a whole foods, plant-based diet can be healing and nourishing both for the body and for the planet.

Dan Marek is a program manager for the Whole Kids Foundation and runs the Healthy Teachers and Healthy Food Service Programs, which are designed to provide staff with nutrition inspiration and healthy cooking techniques to transform their own well-being and serve as healthy role models for their students. He has been a chef educator in Austin, Texas, for Whole Foods Market and various foundations, is a board member of Slow Food Austin, and runs the catering company Homegrown Vegetarian with his wife, Melissa.

Shoshana Pulde enjoys dabbling in the kitchen, regularly challenging herself to create new, fun, delicious, and nutritious recipes for her family to enjoy!

Lisa Rice is a health coach at the Whole Foods Medical and Wellness Center in Austin, Texas, where she helps patients overcome disease with a whole foods, plant-based diet through one-on-one sessions and group classes. She loves to feed people and is passionate about creating easy, delicious, and healthy recipes for everyone.

Hiram Camillo is a Wicked Healthy advocate and has a thing for plants. As a personal chef, recipe developer, and culinary consultant, Hiram's focus is on clean, inventive cuisine that pushes the limits of flavor and presentation.

Brian Stafford, a chef known for his versatility, is inspired by the beauty and bounty of the Pacific Northwest. Brian gained his knowledge from hands-on experiences working with various cheese artisans, bakeries, small food businesses, retail environments, and restaurants.

Darshana Thacker is chef and culinary project manager for Forks Over Knives. A graduate of the Natural Gourmet Institute, she's known for her hearty and distinctly flavorful creations, which draw inspiration from a wide range of ethnic traditions. Chef Darshana was the recipe author of *Forks Over Knives Family* and a lead recipe contributor for the *New York Times* bestseller *The Forks Over Knives Plan*.

Endnotes

Introduction

1   Michael Pollan, *Cooked: A Natural History of Transformation* (New York: Penguin Press, 2013), 128.

Chapter 1

1   Dan Buettner, *The Blue Zones Solution: Eating and Living Like the World's Healthiest People* (Washington, DC: National Geographic, 2015).

2   John Mackey, Matthew Lederman, MD, and Alona Pulde, MD, *The Whole Foods Diet* (New York: Grand Central Life & Style, 2017).

3   David L. Katz, MD, MPH, "Diets, Doubts, and Doughnuts: Are We TRULY Clueless?" *Huffington Post*, August 13, 2016, http://www.huffingtonpost .com/entry/diets doubts and doughnuts are we truly clueless_us_57af2fe9e4b0ae60ff029f0d.

4   David Katz and Stephanie Meller, "Can We Say What Diet Is Best for Health?" *Annual Review of Public Health* 35 (2014): 83–103.

5   Michael Greger, MD, *How Not to Die: Discover the Foods Scientifically Proven to Prevent and Reverse Disease* (New York: Macmillan, 2015), 264.

Chapter 2

1   Nicola M. McKeown et al., "Whole and Refined Grain Intakes Are Differentially Associated with Abdominal Visceral and Subcutaneous Adiposity in Healthy Adults: The Framingham Heart Study," *American Journal of Clinical Nutrition* 92, no. 5 (2010): 1165–1171.

2   John McDougall, *The Starch Solution* (New York: Rodale Books, 2013), 3.

3   D. Aune et al., "Whole Grain Consumption and Risk of Cardiovascular Disease, Cancer, and All Cause and Cause Specific Mortality: Systematic Review and Dose Response Meta Analysis of Prospective Studies" *BMJ* 353 (i2716) (2016), DOI: 10.1136/bmj.i2716.

4   E. Q. Ye et al., "Greater Whole Grain Intake Is Associated with Lower Risk of Type 2 Diabetes, Cardiovascular Disease, and Weight Gain," *Journal of Nutrition* 142, no. 7 (2012): 1304–1313, DOI: 10.3945/ jn.111.155325.

5   Robert E. Post, MD, MS, Arch G. Mainous III, PhD, Dana E. King, MD, MS, and Kit N. Simpson, DrPH, et al., "Dietary Fiber for the Treatment of Type 2 Diabetes Mellitus: A Meta Analysis," *Journal of the American Board of Family Medicine* 25, no. 1 (2012): 16–23.

6   Y. Papanikolaou and V. L. Fulgoni III, "Bean Consumption Is Associated with Greater Nutrient Intake, Reduced Systolic Blood Pressure, Lower Body Weight, and a Smaller Waist Circumference in Adults: Results from the National Health and Nutrition Examination Survey 1999–2002," *Journal of the American College of Nutrition* 27, no. 5 (2008): 569–576.

7   Vanessa Haetal,"Effect of Dietary Pulse Intake on Established Therapeutic Lipid Targets for Cardiovascular Risk Reduction: A Systematic Review and Meta Analysis of Randomized Controlled Trials," *Canadian Medical Association Journal* 186, no.8 (2014): 252–262, DOI: 10.1503/ cmaj.131727.

8   Dan Buettner, in conversation with the authors, July 2016.

9   I. Darmadi Blackberry et al., "Legumes: The Most Important Dietary Predictor of Survival in Older People of Different Ethnicities," *Asia Pacific Journal of Clinical Nutrition* 3, no. 2 (2004): 217–220.

10 Hong Mei Zhang et al., "Research Progress on the Anticarcinogenic Actions and Mechanisms of Ellagic Acid," *Cancer Biology & Medicine* 11, no. 2 (2014): 92–100.

11   E. E. Devore, J. H. Kang, M. M. B. Breteler, and F. Grodstein, "Dietary Intakes of Berries and Flavonoids in Relation to Cognitive Decline," *Annals of Neurology* 72, no. 1 (2012): 135–143, DOI: 10.1002/ana.23594.

12   Iris Erlund et al., "Favorable Effects of Berry Consumption on Platelet Function, Blood Pressure, and HDL Cholesterol," *American Journal of Clinical Nutrition* 87, no. 2 (2008): 323–331; M. L. McCullough et al., "Flavonoid Intake and Cardiovascular Disease Mortality in a Prospective Cohort of US Adults," *American Journal of Clinical Nutrition* 95, no. 2 (2012): 454–464.

13   Monica H. Carlsen et al., "The Total Antioxidant Content of More than 3100 Foods, Beverages, Spices, Herbs and Supplements Used Worldwide," *Nutrition Journal* 9, no. 3 (2010).

14   Isao Muraki et al., "Fruit Consumption and Risk of Type 2 Diabetes: Results from Three Prospective Longitudinal Cohort Studies," *BMJ* 347 (f5001) (2013).

15   G. Murillo and R. G. Mehta, "Cruciferous Vegetables and Cancer Prevention," *Nutrition and Cancer* 41, no. 1–2 (2001): 17–28.

16   Joel Fuhrman, *Super Immunity: The Essential Nutrition Guide for Boosting Your Body's Defenses to Live Longer, Stronger, and Disease Free* (San Francisco: HarperOne, 2011), 69.

17   Joel Fuhrman, *Eat to Live: The Amazing Nutrient-Rich Program for Fast and Sustained Weight Loss* (New York: Little, Brown and Company, 2011), 72.

18   H. C. Hung et al., "Fruit and Vegetable Intake and Risk of Major Chronic Disease," *Journal of the National Cancer Institute* 96, no. 21 (2004): 1577–1584.

19   P. Carter et al., "Fruit and Vegetable Intake and Incidence of Type 2 Diabetes Mellitus: Systematic Review and Meta Analysis," *BMJ* 341 (c4229) (2010).

20   Latetia Moore, Jordana Turkel, and Joy Dubost, "Adults Meeting Fruit and Vegetable Intake Recommendations—United States, 2013," *Morbidity and Mortality Weekly Report* 64, no. 26 (2015): 709–713.

21   Union of Concerned Scientists, *Extra Daily Serving of Fruits or Vegetables Can Save Lives and Billions in Health Care Costs*, press release, August 7, 2013, http://www.ucsusa.org/news/press_release/produce-saves-lives-money-0398.html#.V2wgrFeHClw.

22   Emilio Ros, "Health Benefits of Nut Consumption," *Nutrients* 2, no. 7 (2010): 652–682; Ying Bao, MD, ScD, et al., "Association of Nut Consumption with Total and Cause Specific Mortality," *New England Journal of Medicine* 369, no. 21 (2013): 2001–2011, DOI: 10.1056/NEJMoa1307352; Emilio Ros and Frank B. Hu, "Consumption of Plant Seeds and Cardiovascular Health," *Circulation* 128, no. 5 (2013): 553–565, originally published July 29, 2013, http://dx.doi.org/10.1161/CIRCULATIONAHA.112.001119.

23   "The Adventist Health Study: Findings for Nuts," Loma Linda University, accessed October 2016, http://publichealth.llu.edu/adventist-health-studies/findings/findings-past-studies/adventist-health-study-findings-nuts.

24   J. Sabaté, "Nut Consumption and Body Weight," supplement, *American Journal of Clinical Nutrition* 78 no. S3 (2003): 647S–650S.

Index